Recent Advances in Gastroenterology-14

Recent Advances in Gastroenterology-14

Her Hsin Tsai MD FRCP
Editor-in-Chief
GastroHep
An International Gastroenterology Journal

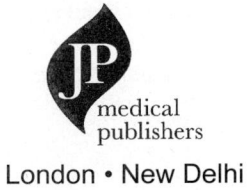

London • New Delhi

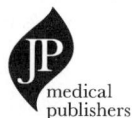

Headquarters
Jaypee Brothers Medical Publishers (P) Ltd
4838/24, Ansari Road, Daryaganj
New Delhi 110 002, India
Phone: +91-11-43574357
Fax: +91-11-43574314
E-mail: jaypee@jaypeebrothers.com

Overseas Office
J P Medical Ltd
83 Victoria Street, London
SW1H 0HW (UK)
Phone: +44 20 3170 8910
Fax: +44 (0)20 3008 6180
E-mail: info@jpmedpub.com

Website: www.jaypeebrothers.com
Website: www.jaypeedigital.com

© 2021, Jaypee Brothers Medical Publishers

The views and opinions expressed in this book are solely those of the original contributor(s)/author(s) and do not necessarily represent those of editor(s) of the book.

All rights reserved. No part of this publication may be reproduced, stored or transmitted in any form or by any means, electronic, mechanical, photocopying, recording or otherwise, without the prior permission in writing of the publishers.

All brand names and product names used in this book are trade names, service marks, trademarks or registered trademarks of their respective owners. The publisher is not associated with any product or vendor mentioned in this book.

Medical knowledge and practice change constantly. This book is designed to provide accurate, authoritative information about the subject matter in question. However, readers are advised to check the most current information available on procedures included and check information from the manufacturer of each product to be administered, to verify the recommended dose, formula, method and duration of administration, adverse effects and contraindications. It is the responsibility of the practitioner to take all appropriate safety precautions. Neither the publisher nor the author(s)/editor(s) assume any liability for any injury and/or damage to persons or property arising from or related to use of material in this book.

This book is sold on the understanding that the publisher is not engaged in providing professional medical services. If such advice or services are required, the services of a competent medical professional should be sought.

Every effort has been made where necessary to contact holders of copyright to obtain permission to reproduce copyright material. If any have been inadvertently overlooked, the publisher will be pleased to make the necessary arrangements at the first opportunity. The **CD/DVD-ROM** (if any) provided in the sealed envelope with this book is complimentary and free of cost. **Not meant for sale.**

Inquiries for bulk sales may be solicited at: jaypee@jaypeebrothers.com

Recent Advances in Gastroenterology-14

First Edition: **2021**

ISBN: 978-1-78779-128-2

Printed at: Sterling Graphics Pvt. Ltd.

Dedicated to
The loving memory of my father

Contributors

Alexandre Loktionov MD PhD
Director
Diag Nodus Ltd
Babraham Research Campus
Babraham, UK

Ali Abdullah MD
Senior Physician
Department of Internal Medicine C
Kaplan Medical Center
Rehovot, Israel

AR Jayakumar PhD
General Medical Research
Neuropathology Section
R&D Service
Bruce W Carter Department of Veterans
Affairs Medical Center
Miami, Florida

Arjun Sugumaran MBBS FRCP FRACP
Consultant Gastroenterologist
Hutt Hospital
Hutt Valley District Health Board
Lower Hutt, New Zealand

Aung Hlaing Bwa
MBBS DipBiomedSc MRCP FRCP Edin
Consultant Physician
Department of Hepatology
Yangon GI and Liver Centre
Yangon, Myanmar

Catriona Scicluna MD MRCP MSc
Higher Specialist Trainee
Department of Gastroenterology
Mater Dei Hospital
Msida, Malta

Christopher Harmston
MBChB FRCS FRACS
Consultant Colorectal Surgeon
Whangarei Hospital
Whangarei, New Zealand

Corinna Hauff MRCP FRCR
Consultant Radiologist
Hull and East Yorkshire University
Hospitals NHS Trust, Hull, UK

Her Hsin Tsai MD FRCP
Editor-in-Chief
GastroHep
An International Gastroenterology
Journal

J Zizzo MD
Medical Research
Neuropathology Section
R&D Service
Bruce W Carter Department of Veterans
Affairs Medical Center
Miami, Florida

Javier P Gisbert MD
Gastroenterology Unit
Hospital Universitario de La Princesa
Madrid, Spain

John Schembri MD MRCP MSc
Resident Specialist
Department of Gastroenterology
Mater Dei Hospital
Msida, Malta

Khin Maung Win
MBBS MMedSc MRCP FRCP Edin
FRCP London FAASLD
Director
Yangon GI and Liver Centre, Myanmar
Honorary Professor
Department of Hepatology
Yangon GI and Liver Center
Yangon, Myanmar

Olga P Nyssen MD
Gastroenterology Unit
Centro de Investigación Biomédica
en Red de Enfermedades Hepáticas y
Digestivas (CIBEREHD)
Instituto de Investigación Sanitaria
Princesa (IIS-IP)
Hospital Universitario de La Princesa
Universidad Autónoma de Madrid
Madrid, Spain

Pierre Ellul MD PhD FRCP MS
Consultant Gastroenterologist
Mater Dei Hospital, Msida, Malta

Pradeep Bhandari
MBBS MD FRCP
Professor
Department of Gastroenterology
Queen Alexandra Hospital
Portsmouth, UK

Si Thu Sein Win MBBS
Senior Medical Officer
Department of Hepatology
Yangon GI and Liver Centre
Yangon, Myanmar

Soe Thiha Maung MBBS MRCP
Senior Medical Officer
Department of Hepatology and
Endoscopy Unit
Clinical Manager
Yangon GI and Liver Centre, Myanmar
Chief Medical Officer
Win Sammering Specialist Clinic and
Medical Check-up Centre
Yangon, Myanmar

Sreedhari Thayalasekaran
MBBS MRCP
Research Fellow
Department of Gastroenterology
Queen Alexandra Hospital
Portsmouth, UK

Stephen Malnick
MA (Oxon) MSc MBBS (Lond) AGAF
Clinical Associate Professor of Medicine
Director
Department of Internal Medicine C
Kaplan Medical Center, Rehovot, Israel

Z Rahaman MD
South Florida Veterans Affairs
Foundation for Research and
Education Inc
Bruce W Carter Department of Veterans
Affairs Medical Center, Miami, Florida

Preface

As clinical and basic research in the specialty of gastroenterology continues to advance at an unrelenting pace, keeping step with these advances can be challenging. Gastroenterology is a wide, diverse specialty and *Recent Advances in Gastroenterology* aims to be a digest where the busy clinician and the budding trainee can delve into and acquire the expanding knowledge base in a single tidy volume. To this end, I have been tasked to put together an anthology of topics in gastroenterology, focusing on areas where there is considerable clinical interest, and anticipating areas where there may be significant important future developments. My task has been greatly facilitated by an eminent international team of experts in their field. We have contributors from no less than seven nationalities across the four continents of Europe, Asia, North America, and Oceania.

The topics chosen reflect the diverse and varied specialty. Selecting the right topics for review was challenging. I have avoided repetition of topics covered in the last iteration and picked areas that have seen rapid advancements and significant changes and focusing on areas where there have been developments in clinical management. Hence, there is a brace of inflammatory bowel disease (IBD) chapters, in medical and surgical aspects of ulcerative colitis management. This is followed by two other luminal gastroenterology chapters on rarer but important gastrointestinal (GI) conditions—the evolving scene of microcytic colitis and eosinophilic enteropathy. Upper GI diseases are represented by a *Helicobacter pylori* eradication master class. There are three chapters of endoscopy/imaging related topics with one on the growing influence of artificial intelligence (AI) in diagnostic imaging. There follows a chapter on improving polyp detection and one on reducing post-endoscopic retrograde cholangiopancreatography (ERCP) pancreatitis. This is intercalated by two chapters on basic science which the clinicians will find stimulating and may provide the basis of future therapy. The first is on the role of eosinophils and the gut and the second is on gut mucin and its role in health and disease by an eminent GI scientist. Then, there are the chapters on hepatology, reflecting the state-of-the-art with hepatitis C therapy with an Asian perspective and the growing importance of nonalcoholic fatty liver disease (NAFLD) and concluding with a chapter on hepatic neurological changes. Finally, we cannot ignore the current global pandemic of COVID-19 and I have included a reflection of its impact on gastroenterology.

I would like to thank my contributors who have delivered their chapters on time in the very tight time constraints imposed on them. They have done a superb job indeed.

Her Hsin Tsai
Beverley, UK

Acknowledgments

I would like to thank all my contributors who have delivered their excellent chapters in a timely fashion. We are especially thankful to Shri Jitendar P Vij (Group Chairman), Mr Ankit Vij (Managing Director), Mr MS Mani (Group President), Ms Chetna Malhotra Vohra (Associate Director—Content Strategy), Ms Pooja Bhandari (Production Head), and Ms Nikita Chauhan (Senior Development Editor) of M/s Jaypee Brothers Medical Publishers (P) Ltd, New Delhi, India.

Contents

1. **Advances in the Treatment of Moderate-to-severe Ulcerative Colitis: Anti-TNFs and Beyond** 1
   Her Hsin Tsai
   - Optimizing Conventional Therapies   *2*
   - Optimizing Anti-TNF Treatments   *5*
   - New Drugs   *7*

2. **Surgical Management of Ulcerative Colitis** 19
   Christopher Harmston
   - The Surgeon as Part of the Multidisciplinary Team   *19*
   - Indications for Surgery   *19*
   - Surgical Technique   *22*

3. **Microscopic Colitis** 29
   Catriona Scicluna, John Schembri, Pierre Ellul
   - Epidemiology   *29*
   - Pathophysiology   *29*
   - Genetic Factors and Microscopic Colitis   *30*
   - Environmental Factors   *31*
   - Clinical Features   *33*
   - Diagnosis   *34*
   - Management   *38*

4. **Eosinophilic Gastroenteritis: Eosinophilic Gastrointestinal Disorders Distal to the Esophagus** 49
   Her Hsin Tsai
   - Epidemiology   *50*
   - Pathogenesis   *50*
   - Clinical Features   *50*
   - Clinical Assessment   *50*
   - Diagnosis   *55*
   - Differential Diagnosis   *55*
   - Natural History and Clinical Course   *58*
   - Management   *58*

5. **Eosinophils and the Gut: Eosinophils in the Human Intestinal Tract in Normal Conditions and Major Colorectal Diseases** 65
   Alexandre Loktionov
   - Structural and Functional Characteristics of Mature Eosinophils 65
   - Migration of Eosinophils to the Gut 67
   - Functions of Eosinophils in the Normal Gut 68
   - Eosinophils in the Major Colorectal Diseases 70

6. **Gut Mucus and its Functional Significance in Health and Disease** 86
   Alexandre Loktionov
   - Mucus Composition and Structure Throughout the Gastrointestinal Tract 86
   - Mucus as a Component of the Intestinal Protective Barrier 88
   - Gut Mucus and Microbiome 90
   - Host Cell Exfoliation and Migration from the Epithelial Surface to Mucus Layers in Normal Physiological Conditions 91
   - Gut Mucus Changes Associated with Inflammatory Bowel Disease 92
   - Gut Mucus Changes Associated with Colorectal Cancer 95

7. **Ten Common Errors in the Treatment of *Helicobacter Pylori* Infection** 106
   Javier P Gisbert, Olga P Nyssen
   Common Errors in the Treatment of *Helicobacter Pylori* Infection 107

8. **Artificial Intelligence in Gastroenterology** 151
   Corinna Hauff, Her Hsin Tsai
   - Application of Artificial Intelligence in Gastrointestinal Radiology 155
   - Artificial Intelligence in Gastrointestinal Endoscopy 159
   - Key Points for Clinical Practice 164

9. **Improving Polyp Detection at Colonoscopy** 167
   Sreedhari Thayalasekaran, Pradeep Bhandari
   - Simple Measures 168
   - Water-assisted Colonoscopy 170
   - Colonoscopy Technology 170
   - Artificial Intelligence 177

10. **Post-endoscopic Retrograde Cholangiopancreatography Pancreatitis** 184
    Arjun Sugumaran
    - Complications Following an ERCP 185
    - Post-ERCP Pancreatitis 185

11. Management of Nonalcoholic Fatty Liver Disease 196
Stephen Malnick, Ali Abdullah

- Dietary Changes   197
- Lifestyle Changes   198
- Bariatric Surgery   199
- Medical Therapy of Nonalcoholic Fatty Liver Disease   199
- Where do we Go from Here?   206

12. Management of Hepatitis C 223
Soe Thiha Maung, Aung Hlaing Bwa, Si Thu Sein Win, Khin Maung Win

- Epidemiology   223
- Pathogenesis   224
- Clinical Presentations and Natural History of Diseases   225
- Diagnosis   227
- Treatment   229

13. Neurological Complications in Liver Diseases 238
J Zizzo, Z Rahaman, AR Jayakumar

- Hepatic Encephalopathy   239
- Hepatitis   241
- Hepatic Myelopathy   249

14. The Impact of COVID-19 on Gastroenterology 261
Her Hsin Tsai

- The Structure of SARS-CoV-2   261
- Epidemiology   262
- The Effect of SARS-CoV-2 on the Gastrointestinal Tract   263
- Effect of COVID-19 on Gastrointestinal Endoscopy   264
- Effect of COVID-19 on Patients with Pre-existing Gastrointestinal Diseases   265
- Effect of COVID-19 on Delivery of Gastrointestinal Services   265

Index 269

CHAPTER

1

Advances in the Treatment of Moderate-to-severe Ulcerative Colitis: Anti-TNFs and Beyond

Her Hsin Tsai

INTRODUCTION

The incidence and prevalence of inflammatory bowel disease (IBD) have been increasing globally, with the highest incidence in Europe and North America. Ulcerative colitis (UC) is the most common form of IBD with the annual incidence of about 5–20 per 100,000 person years and prevalence of up to 500 cases per 100,000 in some parts of the world. UC affects a variable extent of the colon from the rectum extending proximally with primarily mucosal inflammation. Clinically, it presents as bloody diarrhea, urgency, and abdominal pain, and runs a relapsing and remitting course. It is associated with significant morbidity, with an estimated 30–60% of patients experiencing at least one relapse per year, and approximately 20% of patients suffering from severe form of the disease. These symptoms have a major impact on sufferer's quality of life.

Treatment depends on severity and extent of the disease. The aim is to induce symptom-free remission of the disease and maintaining it. For mild-to-moderate disease, 5-aminosalicylate (orally and rectally) remains useful in both induction and maintenance therapy for UC. For moderate-to-severe disease, corticosteroids remain the primary therapy of UC but are limited by serious side effects. Should induction be successful the steroids are withdrawn and replaced by immunosuppressants such as thiopurine analogs, e.g., azathioprine (AZA) and 6-mercaptopurine (6MP).

More targeted therapies have been developed that specifically inhibit the mediators of gut inflammation. Infliximab is the first, an intravenously administered chimeric monoclonal antibody targeting tumor necrosis factor-alpha (TNF-α), a key proinflammatory cytokine involved in gut inflammation. The ACT 1 trial showed that patients with moderate-to-severe UC had a clinical response rate to infliximab of 65.5% at week 8, and almost 50% maintained response at week 30.[1] Adalimumab, a subcutaneously administered humanized anti-TNF antibody, was subsequently developed, with the ULTRA 2 trial demonstrating a clinical response rate of nearly 50% at week 8.[2] These biologic therapies are well established and most physicians caring for these patients are comfortable with their use. They are also demonstrably cost effective, as prices have tumbled with the advent of generic biosimilars.[3]

In this chapter, we shall discuss recent advances in the treatment of moderate-to-severe UC. It is not meant to be a comprehensive discussion on the clinical management of UC. It will focus on evolving clinical concepts in optimizing of treatment and new and emerging drug therapy that will likely impact on the clinical management of UC either already licensed or likely to be in the very near future. The number of treatment choices are growing at a remarkable rate and is by understanding the mode of action of the drugs and trial data that the optimal choices can be made for the specific clinical problem.

OPTIMIZING CONVENTIONAL THERAPIES

It is a common tendency to move onto a new treatment before optimizing current and often cheaper or less toxic treatments. This may be due to pressures put onto the physician either from patient or carer or from pharmaceutical sales pitch. There are several questions the physician should ask before escalation of treatment. This is particularly true of IBDs.

1. Are you treating the right disease?

It might seem an obvious question but there are a number of differential diagnoses that may ensnare the physician. The diagnosis is reached by a combination of clinical, radiological, endoscopic, and histological features. This is why a multidisciplinary approach is desirable, even essential if mistakes are to be not made.

2. Has the severity and extent of ulcerative colitis been properly assessed?

It is a common mistake to equate subjective patient symptom reporting with disease activity. While all reported symptoms need to be addressed with a treatment plan, only mucosal inflammation will respond to immunological modulation. There is understandably often a large functional element in the patient's symptoms. Irritable bowel syndrome (IBS) often coexists with IBD and the physician will need to be cautious in equating symptoms with disease severity. Hence before escalation of treatment, the patient needs to be reassessed. The best tool is colonoscopy. It will demonstrate extent and severity of inflammation. A form of mucosal inflammation scoring should be adopted [e.g., Mayo score or Ulcerative Colitis Endoscopic Index of Severity (UCEIS)] and extent recorded. Biopsies may be helpful. In acute severe disease, it should be done cautiously and once it is clear that the disease is severe (Mayo 3; UCEIS > 7) then the scope may be withdrawn and a plain abdominal X-ray taken. This is not only safer but remarkably helpful in demonstrating extent of disease, presence of mucosal thickening, and serious complication of a dilated colon. CT scans (or MRI) can also be very helpful in the severe cases (**Figs. 1A and B**). In the non-urgent cases, colonoscopy is by far the most useful assessment tool.

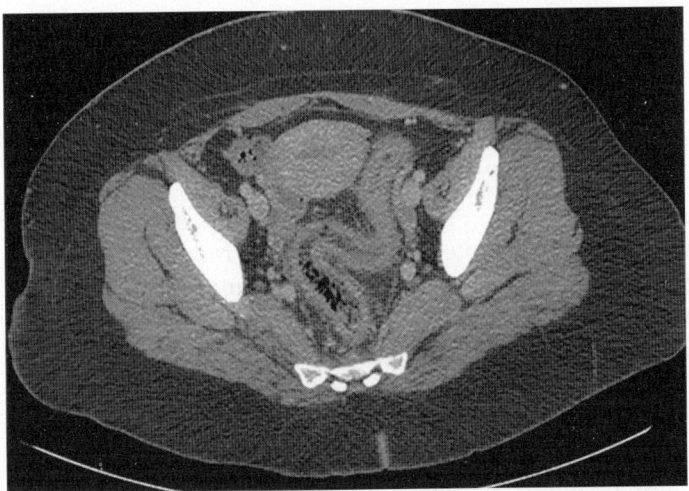

Fig. 1A: Sigmoid inflammation in patient with severe ulcerative colitis.

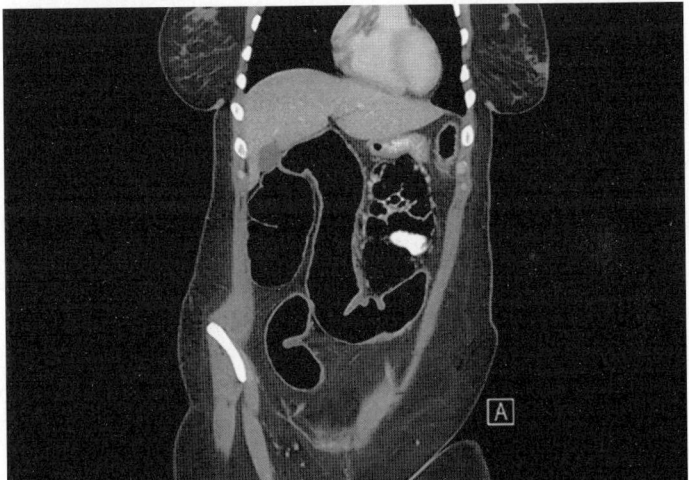

Fig. 1B: Colonic dilatation in acute severe ulcerative colitis.

In recent years, fecal calprotectin has emerged as a useful tool in monitoring disease activity of UC. If done regularly, serial fecal calprotectin may be indicator of disease flare. However, the test in not reliable in predicting severity or extent of disease and should not be used as a justification for treatment escalation but should be used only as supporting evidence of mucosal inflammation.[4]

3. Is the disease acute severe?

Acute severe UC is a potentially life-threatening condition and patients are at risk for progressing to toxic megacolon **(Fig. 1B)** or bowel perforation. Hence recognition of this clinical condition is vital. In the original Truelove and Witts'[5] criteria, it is characterized by:

- Bloody stool frequency ≥6 per day

PLUS at least one of the following evidence of systemic toxicity:
- Fever (temperature ≥ 37.8°C)
- Tachycardia (heart rate ≥ 90 beats/min)
- Anemia (hemoglobin < 105 g/L)
- Elevated inflammatory marker [C-reactive protein (CRP) > 100 g/L, erythrocyte sedimentation rate)

A subgroup with abdominal distension and pain is described as acute fulminant colitis.[5]

Patients with acute severe disease have a high risk of requiring colectomy and need to be recognized and admitted as an acute emergency and treated with fluids and intravenous steroids. They should be assessed frequently and if they do not respond within 3-5 days or if day 3 CRP remains very elevated, then they should be considered for treatment with cyclosporine or infliximab or surgery.[6] Comparative trials have shown no difference between cyclosporine and infliximab.[7,8] Furthermore, there is no evidence that medical therapy results in lower long-term colectomy rates but it is generally accepted that elective surgery carries a lower morbidity.[9,10] The surgical management is discussed in the following chapter.

4. Have you optimized 5-ASA therapies?

5-aminosalicylic acid (5-ASA) treatments are the mainstay in the management of mild-to-moderate UC. This is particularly true of distal disease such as proctitis where the patient may experience a lot of urgency and frequency but may have very limited overall inflammatory load. Formal assessment may classify these patients as having moderate-to-severe disease even though the extent of inflammation may be very limited because of the dependence of scoring systems on bowel frequency counts. In this scenario, immunosuppression may not be the best treatment. Local treatment with 5-ASA products is often the key, with high dose oral and rectal 5-ASA preparations having demonstrable efficacy. This approach is often underused.[11]

5. Have you optimized immunosuppressive therapies?

Immunosuppressive therapy, mainly the use of AZA and 6MP, is the cornerstone of management of moderate-to-severe UC. Patience is required as the drug is slow acting, taking at least 3 months and sometimes up to 6 months to act. It may be used alongside 5-ASA or as monotherapy in patients intolerant of 5-ASA. It should also be used with biologic therapy where it acts synergistically by suppressing antibody formation.

These drugs have many toxic effects and as many as 25% of patients are intolerant of the drug but only 1-2% develop serious toxicity. Liver toxicity and myelosuppression are the principal severe adverse reactions. Thus physicians may adopt a taciturn approach to the drug use for fear of toxicity and is a reason for suboptimal dosing in UC treatment. Enzyme testing and drug metabolite testing is helpful to in optimizing treatment.

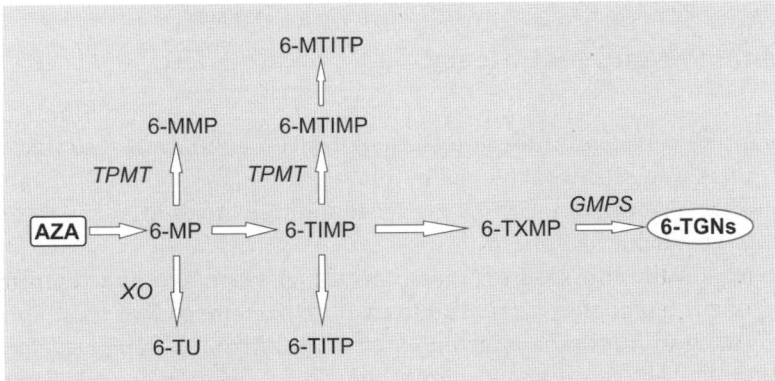

Fig. 2: *Azathioprine metabolism*: Azathioprine is serially converted to 6-TGNs and metabolized in a rate-limiting fashion into 6-MMP by TPMT enzyme.
(AZA: azathioprine; GMPS: guanosine monophosphate synthetase; 6-MP: 6-mercaptopurine; 6-MMP: 6-methylmercaptopurine; TGN: thioguanine nucleotide; TPMT: thiopurine methyltransferase; XO: xanthine oxidase; TIMP: thioinosine monophosphate; TXMP: thioxanthine monophosphate; TITP: thioinosine triphosphate; TU: thiouric acid; GMPS: guanidine monophosphate synthetase; MTIMP: methylthioinosine monophosphate)

Thiopurine methyltransferase (TPMT) is the critical **(Fig. 2)** enzyme in AZA and 6-MP metabolism and determines the levels of active molecule 6-thioguanine (6-TG) and toxic metabolite 6-methylmercaptopurine (6-MMP) levels. Approximately 89% of the population has wild type TPMT, which is associated with normal or "high" TPMT enzyme activity, while 11% are heterozygous and have corresponding low TPMT enzyme activity. A small number (1 in 300) of the population is homozygous for mutations of TPMT and thus have negligible activity, which causes 6-MP to be preferentially metabolized to produce high levels of 6-TG, which then leads to bone marrow suppression. Very high levels of TPMT may result in increased accumulation of 6-MMP increasing risk of liver toxicity. Thus determining the activity of TPMT may help optimize treatment.

Direct measurements of drug metabolite levels are available. Levels of 6-MMP can also be helpful to predict liver toxicity. The active moiety 6-TG can be a good measure of optimal dose of the drug. A recent meta-analysis of studies looking at 6-TG levels also demonstrated that clinical remission was significantly more likely among patients with 6-TG levels over a cut-off value between 230 and 260 (odds ratio 3.2, 95% CI 2.4–4.1).[12]

OPTIMIZING ANTI-TNF TREATMENTS

When it is clear that in the patient who has failed or is intolerant of the conventional treatments for UC, and that the patient has disease of at least moderate severity, then a biologic drug is the next step. It is usual to choose an anti-TNF as it is well established and availability of biosimilars has made it more affordable. There are some recent evolving concepts that may help optimize therapy.

Addition of Immunosuppressives to Anti-TNF Treatment Improves Efficacy

In a clinical trial of infliximab monotherapy versus infliximab plus azathioprine versus azathioprine alone (UC-SUCCESS), corticosteroid-free remission at week 16 was achieved by 39.7% of patients receiving infliximab/azathioprine, compared with 22.1% receiving infliximab alone ($p = 0.017$) and 23.7% receiving azathioprine alone ($p = 0.032$).[13] The effect is likely to be due to improved infliximab serum concentrations due to reduced antibody development in patients on combination therapy. Sub-analyses of a similar Crohn's study (SONIC) showing higher week 30 infliximab trough levels with combination versus infliximab monotherapy, 3.5 µg/mL versus 1.6 µg/mL ($p < 0.001$), and lower incidence of anti-infliximab antibody, 0.9% versus 14.6%. Interestingly, serious adverse events were actually lower with combination versus infliximab monotherapy (15.1% vs. 23.9%, $p = 0.04$).[14]

The dose and length of AZA treatment required remain uncertain but antibody suppression requires only a small dose of AZA, hence it is sensible to keep the patient on AZA for at least 3 months.

Treatment Goals and Targets

It has been noted in many trials involving infliximab that patients who had achieved mucosal healing had a more durable remission than those with symptom resolution without complete mucosal healing.[15] In 2015, the Selecting Therapeutic Targets in Inflammatory Bowel Disease (STRIDE) committee defined the treat-to-target approach for *IBD*, which shifted the goal of UC treatment from short-term symptom resolution to long-term prevention of disease complications (dysplasia/cancer, hospitalizations, and colectomy).[16] The three most promising composite targets for UC were symptom resolution (normalization of bowel habit and absence of rectal bleeding), endoscopic mucosal healing (Mayo or UCIES inflammation score of 0), and fecal calprotectin <100 µg/g. Although this area is still subject to ongoing long-term clinical investigation, early indication is that target achievement with aggressive medical therapy is associated with better outcome, lower colectomy rates, and hospitalizations.[17]

Personalizing Treatment

The ultimate refinement in the management of UC is to accurately personalize treatments for the individual patient. This depends on the ability of the clinician to accurately predict the likely clinical course and prognosis of the disease. This can be difficult to achieve. Currently we depend on clinical features, endoscopic appearance, and response to therapy to help us predict those who are likely to relapse or end up with colectomies. These measures are not adequate. Genetic studies have not been very helpful. Current best practice of personalizing treatment is based on optimizing treatments and selecting the right targets as already discussed above. The future may be the identification of biomarkers that can accurately predict the patients who are likely to have more aggressive disease. One concept is to identify T-cell transcriptional signatures using machine learning and a promising biomarker may soon be available.[18]

Prospective and Scheduled Therapeutic Drug Monitoring

Therapeutic drug monitoring is now widely available both for thiopurines and anti-TNFs. With anti-TNFs both trough drug levels taken just before a scheduled dose and antibody levels are available. Currently, the majority of clinicians perform trough and antibody levels reactively in response to suboptimal treatment response. Prospective scheduled monitoring is regarded as expensive but with costs of therapeutic drug monitoring falling due to the economies of scale, scheduled testing may become increasingly the norm. There is no doubt that it improves patient outcome and gastroenterological associations are recommending its more widespread use.[19] Recent studies suggest that prospective therapeutic drug monitoring may be highly cost effective.[20]

NEW DRUGS

Although anti-TNFs have revolutionized treatment of UC, some 40–60% still fail to respond. If the patient initially responded but then lose response (secondary failure to respond) or if antibody formation is identified as the reason for failure, then switching to a different drug within this class may be appropriate. But when the patient never responded to anti-TNFs (primary failure to respond) or when anti-TNFs have been optimized by scheduled therapeutic drug monitoring and patient still has inadequate response to therapy then a change in class of drug is indicated. Fortunately, there are several such drugs to choose from, some already licensed and others in various stages of development and certification.

Anti-adhesion Agents

One of the key components of the inflammatory response is the ability of the body's immune system to recruit immune modulator cells to the part of the body where they are needed. This is through trafficking of inflammatory cells via the circulatory system. To facilitate this, the vascular endothelium of vessels neighboring the areas where inflammatory cells are required express on its surface the mucosal addressin-cell adhesion molecule (usually abbreviated, MadCAM-1) which binds to integrins expressed on circulatory T-cells **(Fig. 3)**. These integrins are heterodimeric receptors composed of an α and β subunit, that is expressed on the surface of circulating lymphocytes

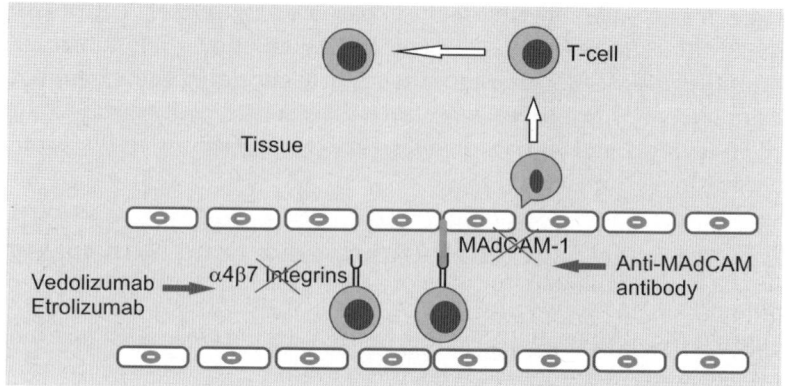

Fig. 3: T-cell trafficking.
(MAdCAM: mucosal addressin-cell adhesion molecule)

when they are activated. This process leads to the binding of circulating lymphocytes onto the endothelium and migration into the lamina propria and tissue, contributing to the inflammatory process in IBD.[21]

These integrins and MAdCAM-1 are thus potential therapeutic targets for IBD therapy. Integrin antagonists are a class of monoclonal antibodies that can block the trafficking of lymphocytes to the intestinal endothelium. The first integrin antagonist to emerge is natalizumab, a humanized IgG4 monoclonal antibody that leads to inhibition of the α4 integrin. Unfortunately, the use of natalizumab was limited by associated increased incidence of progressive multifocal leukoencephalopathy (PML), a fatal demyelinating disease of the central nervous system (CNS) caused by the opportunistic human John Cunningham (JC) virus. Vedolizumab (also known as LDP-02 and MLN02, MLN002), a humanized monoclonal IgG1 antibody, was subsequently developed as a gut selective anti-integrin specifically targeting α4β7 integrins in the gut and importantly not the integrins found in the CNS.[21,22]

The efficacy of vedolizumab was demonstrated in two integrated regulatory trials (GEMINI 1). Response rates at week 6 were found to be 47.1% and 25.5% among patients in the vedolizumab group and placebo group, respectively (95% CI, 11.6–31.7; $p < 0.001$). At week 52, 41.8% of patients who continued to receive vedolizumab every 8 weeks were in clinical remission [Mayo Clinic Score (MCS) ≤2 and no subscore >1], as compared with 15.9% of patients who switched to placebo (95% CI, 14.9–37.2; $p < 0.001$).[23,24]

There may be advantages of using vedolizumab as a second line biologic therapy in UC. Its mode of action is very different from anti-TNF and represents a change in class. In theory, changing of one anti-TNF to another would only be effective if there is drug tolerance due to antibody formation. Primary infliximab failures, that is, those who have never responded to anti-TNF, are not likely to respond to another anti-TNF. The mode of action of vedolizumab also appears more benign compared to anti-TNFs as it does not interfere with critical antibacterial, especially anti-mycobacterial, pathways which make anti-TNFs so hazardous in TB positive individuals. In this respect, there are compelling reasons to suggest that vedolizumab is less harmful than anti-TNFs.[25]

Treatment is given as an IV infusion with an induction of 300 mg at weeks 0, 2, and 6 followed by 8 weekly dosing of 300 mg. There are indications from studies that vedolizumab may take longer than anti-TNFs to achieve therapeutic results. Clinical response may not be apparent until week 10 and hence a little patience from the clinician and forewarning to the patient would be judicious. Some would advocate an additional dose at week 10 if there is a lack of adequate response at week 8.

Using vedolizumab as a first line biologic therapy also can be considered. At present, the cost differential to generic infliximab is too high to make it a cost effective strategy. This is based on equal efficacy of both biologic treatments. However recent data may suggest otherwise. A network meta-analysis has suggested that vedolizumab is superior to adalimumab.[26] This finding is now confirmed by a head-to-head study between adalimumab and vedolizumab. In a randomized trial comparing vedolizumab with adalimumab in over 700 patients with moderately-to-severely active UC, vedolizumab resulted in a significantly higher rate of clinical remission (31% vs. 22%).[27] The rate of serious infections was similar in both groups (<2%). The therapeutic gain may well be sufficiently large to make vedolizumab a cost-effective first line therapy for UC.

Etrolizumab is very similar, being a humanized monoclonal antibody against the β7 subunit of integrins α4β7 and αEβ7. Studies on the induction and maintenance treatment of UC are very promising.[28,29] At the time of writing, the drug has not yet been approved by the FDA.

An antibody to the adhesion MadCAM-1 is also under development.[30]

Anti-interleukin Inhibitors

The proinflammatory cytokines interleukin 12 (IL-12) and interleukin 23 (IL-23) play an important role in the pathophysiology of Crohn's disease (CD) and possibly UC.[31] These cytokines bind to receptors of CD4+ T-cells and lead to their differentiation into activated Th1 and Th17 cells **(Fig. 4)**. There are multiple lines of evidence suggesting that UC is mediated by Th1 and CD by a combination of Th1 and Th17 cells.[32] Furthermore, the IL-23 receptor mutation has been identified as a possible IBD gene.[33] Ustekinumab, a fully human immunoglobulin G1 kappa monoclonal antibody that binds with high affinity to the p40 subunit of human IL-12 and IL-23, has recently been approved for the treatment of moderately to severely active CD in adults. Ustekinumab prevents IL-12 and IL-23 bioactivity by preventing their interaction with their cell surface receptor protein IL-12Rβ1. Through this mechanism of action, ustekinumab effectively neutralizes IL-12 (Th1)- and IL-23 (Th17)-mediated cellular responses.

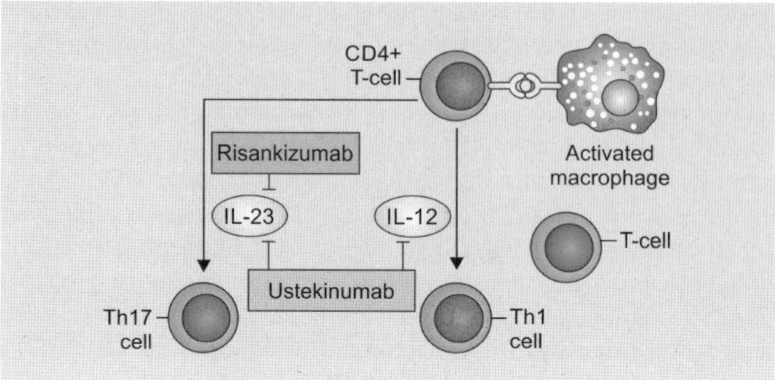

Fig. 4: The role of IL-23 and IL-12.

Evidence for the efficacy of ustekinumab in UC had been investigated and encouraging results published recently.[34] In this study, the percentage of patients who had clinical remission at week 8 among patients who received intravenous ustekinumab at a dose of 130 mg (15.6%) or 6 mg/kg (15.5%) was significantly higher than that among patients who received placebo (5.3%) ($p < 0.001$ for both comparisons). Among patients who had a response to induction therapy with ustekinumab and underwent a second randomization, the percentage of patients who had clinical remission at week 44 was significantly higher among patients assigned to 90 mg of subcutaneous ustekinumab every 12 weeks (38.4%) or every 8 weeks (43.8%) than among those assigned to placebo (24.0%) ($p = 0.002$ and $p < 0.001$, respectively). The incidence of serious adverse events with ustekinumab was similar to that with placebo. However, there were two deaths (one each from acute respiratory distress syndrome and hemorrhage from esophageal varices) and seven cases of cancer (one each of prostate, colon, renal papillary, and rectal cancer and three nonmelanoma skin cancers) among 825 patients who received ustekinumab and no deaths and one case of cancer (testicular cancer) among 319 patients who received placebo. Although these do not constitute a clear hazard signal, some caution must be taken until more data becomes available.

Risankizumab, an IL-23 antibody, is currently being assessed in UC after encouraging results in CD.[35]

JAK/STAT Pathway Inhibitors

Cytokines are released by the immune system in response to a signal principally by gut stellate cells or macrophages in response to a signal. They bind to specific receptors on the T-cell, triggering activation and synthesis of specific proteins that initiate the immune response. Cytokines can take the form of many structurally unrelated proteins that are typed according to their binding to distinct receptor families, which include type I cytokine receptors, type II cytokine receptors, the TNF receptor family, and the IL-1

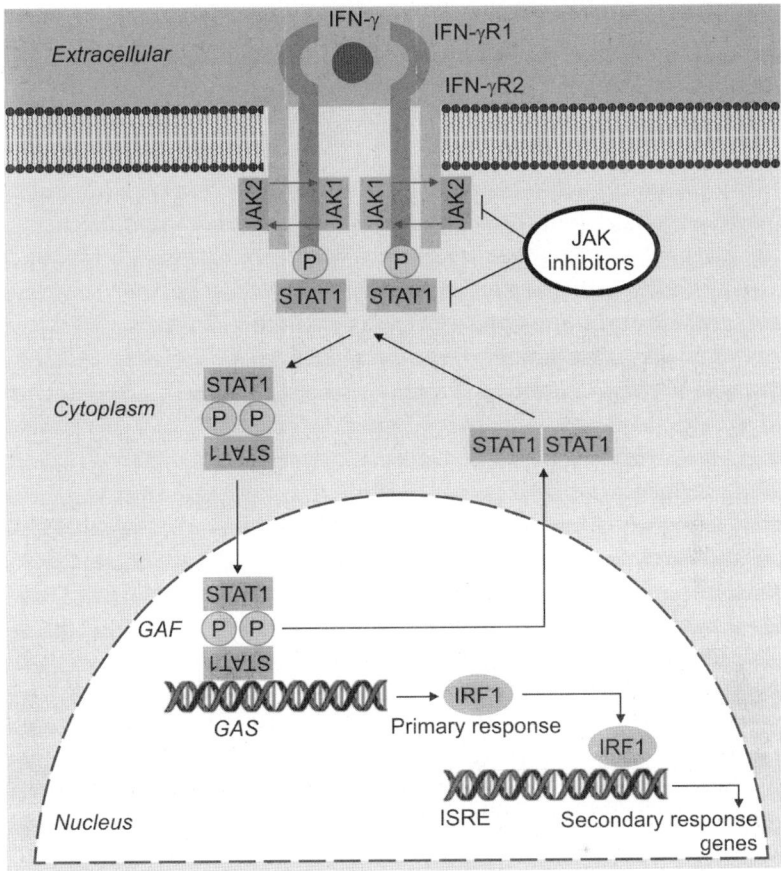

Fig. 5: The JAK-STAT pathway.
(ISRE: interferon-stimulated response element; GAF: gamma activation factor; GAS: gamma activated sequence; IFN: interferon; IRF: interferon regulatory factor)

receptor family receptors. The cytokines bind to the relevant receptor and trigger intracellular changes, resulting in signal transduction and trigger gene expression. The signal transduction is via various protein kinases. The Janus kinase (JAK) is a family of receptor-associated tyrosine kinases that are essential for the cytokine signaling cascade **(Fig. 5)**, downstream of type I and type II cytokine receptors.[36] The JAK-**s**ignal **t**ransducers and **a**ctivators of **t**ranscription (STAT) pathway plays an important role in innate immunity, adaptive immunity, and hematopoiesis, participating in cellular processes such as cell growth, survival, differentiation, and migration. There are four members of the JAK family (JAK1, JAK2, JAK3, and TYK2) and seven signal transducers and transcription activators called signal transducer and activator of transcription, or STAT (STAT 1–4, 5a, 5b, and 6). The unique structure of each JAK clearly distinguishes them from other members of the protein tyrosine kinase family.[37]

Ulcerative colitis and Crohn's disease involve many cytokine signaling which in turn depend on JAK-STAT pathway for immune cell gene transcription. The key cytokines in the pathogenesis of IBD belong to type I and type II cytokines receptors. These are the receptors of certain key cytokines namely IL-6, IL-5, IL-9, IL-10, IL-13, IL-12/23, IL-22, granulocyte-macrophage colony-stimulating factor (GM-CSF), and IFN-γ. All these cytokines signal through the JAK/STAT pathway. In contrast, the cytokines TNF, IL-1, and IL-17, which are the other major drivers of IBD, do not use the JAK-STAT pathway in their signaling pathways but they do however induce the expression of a wide range of downstream proinflammatory cytokines that, in turn, depend on JAK/STAT signaling.[38]

Thus specific inhibitors of these kinases are a logical target as a treatment of inflammatory conditions. Several of these molecules are in development and are small, orally active molecules. Tofacitinib is the first JAK inhibitor to be approved for the treatment of moderate to severely active UC by the FDA (US) and EMA (European) agencies. Several other molecules are undergoing trials and are in advanced stages of development. Tofacitinib (Xeljanz, Pfizer) is a pan-JAK inhibitor that preferentially inhibits JAK1 and JAK3, in a dose-dependent fashion. Oral tofacitinib is well absorbed and is cleared principally by the liver. It has a short half-life of 3 hours.[39]

Tofacitinib was found to be effective for induction of remission for patients with UC. In two randomized trials (OCTAVE Induction 1 and 2 trials of 598 and 541 patients, respectively), patients with moderate-to-severe UC who received tofacitinib 10 mg twice daily experienced remission at 8 weeks more frequently compared with those receiving placebo; for OCTAVE 1, 18% versus 8% (absolute difference 10, 95% CI: 4–16) and for OCTAVE 2, 17% versus 4% (absolute difference 13, 95% CI: 8–18).[40] In the OCTAVE Sustain trial, 593 patients who had a clinical response to induction therapy were randomly assigned to receive maintenance therapy with tofacitinib (either 5 mg or 10 mg twice daily) or placebo for 52 weeks. The primary end point was remission at 52 weeks which occurred in 34.3% of the patients in the 5-mg tofacitinib group and 40.6% in the 10-mg tofacitinib group versus 11.1% in the placebo group ($p < 0.001$ for both comparisons with placebo).[40]

The onset of action of tofacitinib varies greatly with some patients have responding rapidly, while for other patients, response may take up to 8 weeks. Caution should be used when prescribing tofacitinib for patients with a history of thromboembolic disease, cardiovascular disease, or those ≥50 years old with at least one cardiovascular risk factor because of an increased risk of thromboembolic events and mortality in patients who were treated with tofacitinib.

Sphingosine-1-phosphate Receptor Modulators

Sphingosine-1-phosphate (S1P) is a signaling sphingolipid becoming the active moiety by phosphorylation of sphingosine which is catalyzed by sphingosine kinase, an enzyme found in the cytosol and endoplasmic

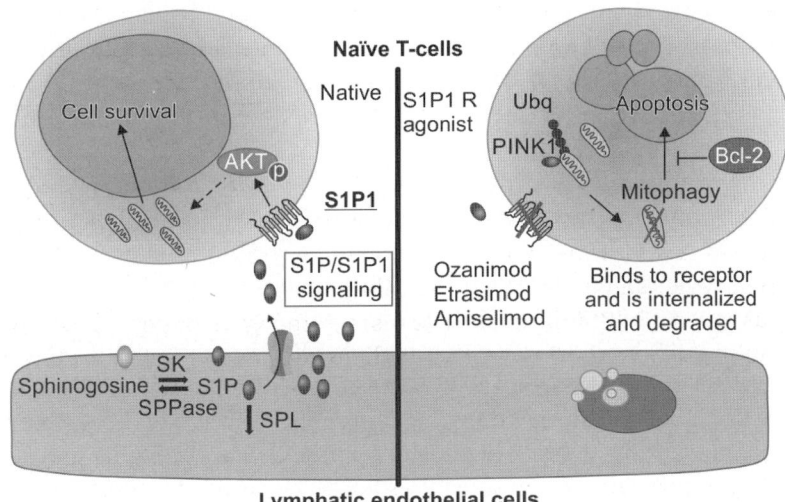

Fig. 6: Sphingosine-1-phosphate (S1P) signaling and receptor modulation.
(SL: sphingosine lyase; SK: sphingosine kinase; PINK1: PTEN-induced kinase 1)

reticulum of various types of cells and S1P can be dephosphorylated to sphingosine by sphingosine phosphatases. S1P produced in endovascular or lymphatic endothelial cells is secreted into the vasculature through the specific transporter SPNS2 **(Fig. 6)**.

Sphingosine-1-phosphate is of importance in the entire human body; it is a major regulator of vascular and immune systems. In the vascular system, S1P regulates angiogenesis, vascular stability, and permeability. In the immune system, it is now recognized as a major regulator of trafficking of T- and B-cells. S1P interacts with its specific receptors S1PR of which there are five subtypes 1–5. S1P1, S1P4, and S1P5 are involved in regulation of the immune system, while S1P2 and S1P3 may be associated with cardiovascular and pulmonary system, and lead to cell proliferation and theoretical cancer-related risks. S1PR1 is of particular importance in immune regulation as it is found on T-cells. It appears to function as an elixir of life to the T-cells ensuring cell survival while a deficiency of S1P results in apoptosis and cell death. There is a concentration gradient between the lymphoid tissue in thymus or nodes and the lymphatic vessels and as the T-cells are attracted to the higher concentration in the vessels, it leads to egress of immune cells from the lymphoid organs (such as thymus and lymph nodes) into the lymphatic vessels.[41]

Sphingosine-1-phosphate is thus a promising target for pharmacologic intervention. When a synthetic agonist targets the S1PR receptor, the receptor–drug complex is internalized and voided and the T-cell loses its ability to respond to the S1P concentration gradient and thus remains the lymphoid tissue rather than egress into the lymphatic vessels and thus into the wider circulation and to the target organ like the gut in IBDs.[42] Several small molecule agonists of S1PR have been developed.[43] Selective targeting S1P receptors for inflammatory conditions is important to avoid unwanted vascular and proliferative effects. Three S1P modulators with differing selectivity for S1P receptors were in clinical development for IBD—ozanimod, etrasimod, and amiselimod.

In the ozanimod study, the primary outcome of remission occurred in 16% of the patients who received 1 mg of ozanimod and in 14% of those who received 0.5 mg of ozanimod, as compared with 6% of those who received placebo ($p = 0.048$ and $p = 0.14$, respectively, for the comparison of the two doses of ozanimod with placebo). Clinical response (decrease in MCS of ≥3 points and ≥30% and decrease in rectal bleeding subscore of ≥1 point or a subscore ≤1) at 8 weeks occurred in 57% of those receiving 1 mg of ozanimod and 54% of those receiving 0.5 mg, as compared with 37% of those receiving placebo. At week 32, the rate of clinical remission was 21% in the group that received 1 mg of ozanimod, 26% in the group that received 0.5 mg of ozanimod, and 6% in the group that received placebo; the rate of clinical response was 51%, 35%, and 20%, respectively. At week 8, absolute lymphocyte counts declined 49% from baseline (BL) in the group that received 1 mg of ozanimod and 32% from BL in the group that received 0.5 mg. There were no safety concerns.[44]

In the OASIS study, etrasimod 2 mg improved change from BL in 3-component MCS versus placebo (difference, 0.99 points; 90% CI, 0.30–1.68; $p = 0.009$). More patients receiving etrasimod 2 mg achieved endoscopic improvement (41.8% vs. 17.8% for PBO; $p = 0.003$). At week 12, there was a significant decrease in circulating lymphocyte counts from BL with etrasimod 1 mg and 2 mg relative to PBO (37.2% and 57.3%, respectively; $p < 0.001$ for both).[45]

Etrasimod demonstrated durable clinical remission in the treatment of moderate to severely active UC in a phase 2 open-label extension study. The 34-week open-label extension study explored the long-term safety, tolerability, and efficacy of etrasimod in 118 patients who completed the 12-week phase 2 OASIS randomized controlled trial. Researchers analyzed the data to determine clinical response, clinical remission, and endoscopic improvement at the end of 46 weeks of treatment. Of the patients who completed 2 mg of etrasimod treatment during the extension study ($n = 84$), 79% achieved clinical response, 39% achieved clinical remission, and 51% had endoscopic improvement by the end of the study. Among patients who also received 2 mg of etrasimod during the OASIS trial ($n = 22$), 82% experienced clinical response, 50% were in clinical remission, and 55% had endoscopic improvement. For patients who achieved clinical response or clinical remission after the OASIS trial, 93% experienced sustained response and 75% experienced sustained remission at both 12 and 46 weeks. Investigators found that adverse events in the extension study were mild-to-moderate and did not discover any new safety concerns.[45]

Choosing a Second (or Third)-line Biologic Therapy

As these newer biologic therapies undergo regulatory trials to achieve certification, the best drug for each clinical scenario is still to be worked out. Until further studies are available, a sensible strategy based on currently available data can be adopted. After optimizing conventional therapies of 5-ASA and immunosuppressives, anti-TNFs in combination with thiopurines can be used a sensible first-line biologic. There may be a case for the use of vedolizumab as a first-line biologic but based on cost and physician familiarity, most experts would regard anti-TNFs to be the logical choice. There may also be a case for using infliximab in preference to adalimumab or golimumab based on network meta-analyses.[46]

In terms of treatment targets, the best single marker is still endoscopic mucosal resolution.[47] Hence an assessment colonoscopic examination at 6 months after commencement of the drug is sensible. If treatment target is not achieved and if trough drug levels are adequate, then a change in class of drug is indicated. Currently, there are three licensed drugs that may be used; vedolizumab, ustekinumab, and tofacitinib. Vedolizumab is probably the best second line drug after anti-TNF failure. If an oral agent is to be preferred, then a case for tofacitinib can be made. Ustekinumab can be held for use as a third line drug.

The pace of change in the landscape of UC therapy continues unabated and it is challenging for the gastroenterologist to keep in step. However, with a sound grounding in scientific basis of the biology of the disease and with a critical eye over trial data, the IBD physician can optimize and personalize treatment of this disabling disease.

REFERENCES

1. Rutgeerts P, Sandborn WJ, Feagan BG, Reinisch W, Olson A, Johanns J, et al. Infliximab for induction and maintenance therapy for ulcerative colitis. N Engl J Med. 2005;353(23):2462-76.
2. Sandborn WJ, van Assche G, Reinisch W, Colombel JF, D'Haens G, Wolf DC, et al. Adalimumab induces and maintains clinical remission in patients with moderate-to-severe ulcerative colitis. Gastroenterology. 2012;142(2):257-65.
3. Tsai HH, Punekar YS, Morris J, Fortun P. A model of the long-term cost-effectiveness of scheduled maintenance treatment with infliximab for moderate-to-severe ulcerative colitis. Aliment Pharmacol Ther. 2008;28(10):1230-9.
4. Reenaers C, Bossuyt P, Hindryckx P, Vanpoucke H, Cremer A, Baert F. Expert opinion for use of faecal calprotectin in diagnosis and monitoring of inflammatory bowel disease in daily clinical practice. United European Gastroenterol J. 2018;6(8):1117-25.
5. Truelove SC, Witts LJ. Cortisone in ulcerative colitis; final report on a therapeutic trial. Br Med J. 1955;2(4947):1041-8.
6. Travis S, Satsangi J, Lémann M. Predicting the need for colectomy in severe ulcerative colitis: a critical appraisal of clinical parameters and currently available biomarkers. Gut. 2011;60(1):3-9.

7. Williams JG, Alam MF, Alrubaiy L, Arnott I, Clement C, Cohen D, et al. Infliximab versus ciclosporin for steroid-resistant acute severe ulcerative colitis (CONSTRUCT): a mixed methods, open-label, pragmatic randomised trial. Lancet Gastroenterol Hepatol. 2016;1(1):15-24.
8. Laharie D, Bourreille A, Branche J, Allez M, Bouhnik Y, Filippi J, et al. Ciclosporin versus infliximab in patients with severe ulcerative colitis refractory to intravenous steroids: a parallel, open-label randomised controlled trial. Lancet. 2012;380(9857):1909-15.
9. Laharie D, Bourreille A, Branche J, Allez M, Bouhnik Y, Filippi J, et al. Long-term outcome of patients with steroid-refractory acute severe UC treated with ciclosporin or infliximab. Gut. 2018;67(2):237-43.
10. Assche GV, Vermeire S, Rutgeerts P. Management of acute severe ulcerative colitis. Gut. 2011;60(1):130-3.
11. Seibold F, Fournier N, Beglinger C, Mottet C, Pittet V, Rogler G, et al. Topical therapy is underused in patients with ulcerative colitis. J Crohns Colitis. 2014;8(1):56-63.
12. Moreau AC, Paul S, Del Tedesco E, Rinaudo-Gaujous M, Boukhadra N, Genin C, et al. Association between 6-thioguanine nucleotides levels and clinical remission in inflammatory disease: a meta-analysis. Inflamm Bowel Dis. 2014;20(3):464.
13. Panaccione R, Ghosh S, Middleton S, Márquez JR, Scott BB, Flint L, et al. Combination therapy with infliximab and azathioprine is superior to monotherapy with either agent in ulcerative colitis. Gastroenterology. 2014;146(2):392-400.
14. Colombel JF, Sandborn WJ, Reinisch W, Mantzaris GJ, Kornbluth A, Rachmilewitz D, et al. Infliximab, azathioprine, or combination therapy for Crohn's disease. N Engl J Med. 2010;362(15):1383-95.
15. Colombel JF, Rutgeerts P, Reinisch W, Esser D, Wang Y, Lang Y, et al. Early mucosal healing with infliximab is associated with improved long-term clinical outcomes in ulcerative colitis. Gastroenterology. 2011;141(4):1194-201.
16. Colombel JF, Narula N, Peyrin-Biroulet L. Management strategies to improve outcomes of patients with inflammatory bowel diseases. Gastroenterology. 2017;152(2):351-61.
17. Ungaro R, Colombel JF, Lissoos T, Peyrin-Biroulet L. A treat-to-target update in ulcerative colitis: a systematic review. Am J Gastroenterol. 2019;114(6):874-83.
18. Biasci D, Lee JC, Noor NM, Pombal DR, Hou M, Lewis N, et al. A blood-based prognostic biomarker in inflammatory bowel disease. Gut. 2019;68(8):1386-95.
19. Feuerstein JD, Nguyen GC, Kupfer SS, Falck-Ytter Y, Singh S; American Gastroenterological Association Institute Clinical Guidelines Committee. American Gastroenterological Association Institute Guideline on Therapeutic Drug Monitoring in Inflammatory Bowel Disease. Gastroenterology. 2017;153(3):827-34.
20. Gettigan NM, Keogh A, McCarthy O, McNally M, Deane C, Slattery E. The effects of proactive therapeutic drug monitoring versus reactive therapeutic drug monitoring in a virtual biologic clinic, a retrospective cohort study. GastroHep. 2019;1(6):274-83.
21. Lau MS, Tsai HH. Review of vedolizumab for the treatment of ulcerative colitis. World J Gastrointest Pharmacol Ther. 2016;7(1):107-11.
22. Tsai HH, Black C. A review of the cost-effectiveness of vedolizumab for treating moderate-to severely active ulcerative colitis. Expert Rev Pharmacoecon Outcomes Res. 2016;16(6):679-83.

23. Feagan BG, Rutgeerts P, Sands BE, Hanauer S, Colombel JF, Sandborn WJ, et al. Vedolizumab as induction and maintenance therapy for ulcerative colitis. N Engl J Med. 2013;369(8):699-710.
24. Sandborn WJ, Feagan BG, Rutgeerts P, Hanauer S, Colombel JF, Sands BE, et al. Vedolizumab as induction and maintenance therapy for Crohn's disease. N Engl J Med. 2013;369(23):2183-96.
25. Bickston SJ, Behm BW, Tsoulis DJ, Cheng J, MacDonald JK, Khanna R, et al. Vedolizumab for induction and maintenance of remission in ulcerative colitis. Cochrane Database Syst Rev. 2014;(8):CD007571.
26. Tsai HH. Editorial: tofacitinib and biologics for moderate-to-severe ulcerative colitis–what is best in class? Aliment Pharmacol Ther. 2018;47(4):539-40.
27. Sands BE, Peyrin-Biroulet L, Loftus EV Jr, Danese S, Colombel JF, Törüner M, et al. Vedolizumab versus adalimumab for moderate-to-severe ulcerative colitis. N Engl J Med. 2019;381(13):1215-26.
28. Vermeire S, O'Byrne S, Keir M, Williams M, Lu TT, Mansfield JC, et al. Etrolizumab as induction therapy for ulcerative colitis: a randomised, controlled, phase 2 trial. Lancet. 2014;384(9940):309-18.
29. Rosenfeld G, Parker CE, MacDonald JK, Bressler B. Etrolizumab for induction of remission in ulcerative colitis. Cochrane Database Syst Rev. 2015;(12):CD011661.
30. Vermeire S, Sandborn WJ, Danese S, Hébuterne X, Salzberg BA, Klopocka M, et al. Anti-MAdCAM antibody (PF-00547659) for ulcerative colitis (TURANDOT): a phase 2, randomised, double-blind, placebo-controlled trial. Lancet. 2017;390(10090):135-44.
31. Uhlig HH, McKenzie BS, Hue S, Thompson C, Joyce-Shaikh B, Stepankova R, et al. Differential activity of IL-12 and IL-23 in mucosal and systemic innate immune pathology. Immunity. 2006;25(2):309-18.
32. Geremia A, Arancibia-Cárcamo CV, Fleming MP, Rust N, Singh B, Mortensen NJ, et al. IL-23-responsive innate lymphoid cells are increased in inflammatory bowel disease. J Exp Med. 2011;208(6):1127-33.
33. Duerr RH, Taylor KD, Brant SR, Rioux JD, Silverberg MS, Daly MJ, et al. A genome-wide association study identifies IL23R as an inflammatory bowel disease gene. Science. 2006;314(5804):1461-3.
34. Sands BE, Sandborn WJ, Panaccione R, O'Brien CD, Zhang H, Johanns J, et al. Ustekinumab as induction and maintenance therapy for ulcerative colitis. N Engl J Med. 2019;381(13):1201-14.
35. Feagan BG, Sandborn WJ, D'Haens G, Panés J, Kaser A, Ferrante M, et al. Induction therapy with the selective interleukin-23 inhibitor risankizumab in patients with moderate-to-severe Crohn's disease: a randomised, double-blind, placebo-controlled phase 2 study. Lancet. 2017;389(10080):1699-709.
36. Schwartz DM, Kanno Y, Villarino A, Ward M, Gadina M, O'Shea JJ. JAK inhibition as a therapeutic strategy for immune and inflammatory diseases. Nat Rev Drug Discov. 2017;16(12):843-62.
37. Banerjee S, Biehl A, Gadina M, Hasni S, Schwartz DM. JAK–STAT signaling as a target for inflammatory and autoimmune diseases: current and future prospects. Drugs. 2017;77(5):521-46.

38. Olivera P, Danese S, Peyrin-Biroulet L. JAK inhibition in inflammatory bowel disease. Expert Rev Clin Immunol. 2017;13(7):693-703.
39. Hemperly A, Sandborn WJ, Vande Casteele N. Clinical pharmacology in adult and pediatric inflammatory bowel disease. Inflamm Bowel Dis. 2018;24(12):2527-42.
40. Sandborn WJ, Su C, Sands BE, D'Haens GR, Vermeire S, Schreiber S, et al. Tofacitinib as induction and maintenance therapy for ulcerative colitis. N Engl J Med. 2017;376(18):1723-36.
41. Pérès M, Montfort A, Andrieu-Abadie N, Colacios C, Ségui B. S1P: the elixir of life for naive T cells. Cell Mol Immunol. 2018;15(7):657-9.
42. Wollny T, Wątek M, Durnaś B, Niemirowicz K, Piktel E, Żendzian-Piotrowska M, et al. Sphingosine-1-phosphate metabolism and its role in the development of inflammatory bowel disease. Int J Mol Sci. 2017;18(4):741.
43. Peyrin-Biroulet L, Christopher R, Behan D, Lassen C. Modulation of sphingosine-1-phosphate in inflammatory bowel disease. Autoimmun Rev. 2017;16(5):495-503.
44. Sandborn WJ, Feagan BG, Wolf DC, D'Haens G, Vermeire S, Hanauer SB, et al. Ozanimod induction and maintenance treatment for ulcerative colitis. N Engl J Med. 2016;374(18):1754-62.
45. Sandborn W, Peyrin-Biroulet L, Trokan L, Zhang J, Kűhbacher T, Chiorean M, et al. A randomized, double-blind, placebo-controlled trial of a selective, oral sphingosine 1-phosphate (S1P) receptor modulator, Etrasimod (A PD334), in moderate to severe ulcerative colitis (UC): Results from the OASIS study. Am J Gastroenterol. 2018;113:S327-8.
46. Bonovas S, Lytras T, Nikolopoulos G, Peyrin-Biroulet L, Danese S. Systematic review with network meta-analysis: comparative assessment of tofacitinib and biological therapies for moderate-to-severe ulcerative colitis. Aliment Pharmacol Ther. 2018;47(4):454-65.
47. Lichtenstein GR, Rutgeerts P. Importance of mucosal healing in ulcerative colitis. Inflamm Bowel Dis. 2010;16(2):338-46.

CHAPTER 2

Surgical Management of Ulcerative Colitis

Christopher Harmston

INTRODUCTION

Medical management forms the mainstay of treatment for patients with ulcerative colitis (UC), but despite advances in medical care, surgery is still often required or chosen for patients in both the emergency and elective setting. Surgery also remains the only curative option for patients with UC. Despite the increasing incidence of UC diagnosis, however, the likelihood of requiring colectomy appears to be decreasing over time from up to 50% in historical studies to around 10% at 10 years in more recent cohorts.[1-3] Around two-thirds of colectomies are performed in an elective setting, and a high proportion of colectomies occurs within 2 years of diagnosis.

This chapter aims to outline the indications for surgery, surgical options, and expected outcomes in patients requiring surgery for UC.

THE SURGEON AS PART OF THE MULTIDISCIPLINARY TEAM

Surgical treatment in patients with UC is best delivered by a multidisciplinary team. Patients who are offered, or considering surgery, should be given information on the available treatment options, risk and benefits of treatment, and potential harmful effects of pursuing nonsurgical options. The patients should also be seen by a person who has knowledge of stomas to give specific information on the siting, care, and management of stoma.[4] Ideally all patients with UC should be managed by a colorectal surgeon with experience of dealing with inflammatory bowel disease. High-volume centers have better outcomes in patients undergoing both emergency and elective operations for UC.[5,6] Referral to a specialist unit, especially in the elective setting, should therefore be considered.

INDICATIONS FOR SURGERY

Acute Indications

Patients with UC may present in the acute setting with a variety of problems, some of which can be life-threatening. It is in the acute surgical setting that patient outcomes are worse, and the risk of mortality is significant if management is not optimal.

Acute Severe Colitis

Acute severe colitis (ASC) occurs in up to 15% of patients with UC and occurs as a first presentation in 10–20% of patients with UC.[7] Emergency colectomy occurs in approximately 20% of patients with acute severe colitis, and around 20–40% of patients who avoid an emergency operation will go on to have a colectomy in the following year, with lowest rates in those rescued with biological therapy.[8,9]

The evidence-based medical management of ASC has previously been discussed.

Ideally patients with ASC should be managed under joint care with a surgical team. If initial response to steroids is not effective by day 3, then surgery or rescue therapy should be considered. Patients treated with rescue therapy should be reassessed on day 5 to determine response. Emergency colectomy is performed to control disease and prevent the life-threatening sequela of continued ASC. Patients referred for surgical opinion should be reassessed regularly by a member of the surgical team if an initial decision to continue with medical management is made. It should be noted that delayed surgery in those not responsive to medical therapy is associated with an increased risk of complications.[10]

An estimation of risk of colectomy can be made based on clinical criteria. Several algorithms have been suggested to assess the risk of colectomy in patients presenting with ASC.[11] The best known are Travis criteria, where on day 3 of corticosteroid treatment patients with more than eight stools per day and C-reactive protein (CRP) of greater than 45 mg/L had an 85% chance of requiring colectomy.[12] Other algorithms have similar predictive value.[13-15] It is important to remember that these algorithms predict the failure of medical management, but do not replace clinical judgment, regular review, and assessment.

Toxic Megacolon

Toxic megacolon occurs in 5% of patients with ASC.[16] Typically the patient will show signs of systemic inflammatory response, abdominal pain, and colonic dilatation of greater than 6 cm on plain abdominal X-ray. Diagnosis is usually made on admission, rather than progression on treatment. Medical treatment with steroids and antibiotics is indicated, but failure to progress in the first 12–24 hours represents an absolute indication for colectomy to prevent perforation. Mortality is relatively high in this group of patients, at approximately 8% in those with no perforation and over 40% in those with perforation.[16] Clinical suspicion should therefore be high, with a low threshold for colectomy.

Perforation

Perforation occurs in 2% of patients with UC and is almost always associated with toxic megacolon. Rapid diagnosis and surgical management are needed to avoid the severe complications associated with perforation. Patients who have been treated with long-term steroid or prolonged rescue therapy are at particular risk.

Bleeding

Severe colonic bleeding in patients with UC is rare, but usually associated with extensive disease.[17] Initial management with resuscitation and exclusion of other bleeding sources should be performed. Colectomy is inevitable in this group of patients.

Elective Indications

There are a variety of indications for elective surgery in patients with UC. Outcomes in patients undergoing elective surgery are generally better than in the emergency setting and surgery is more frequently performed by a colorectal specialist. Despite this, patients with UC are often nutritionally and immunologically compromised, and should be optimized before surgery.

Failure of Medical Management

Failure of medical management is the most common indication for surgical intervention and can manifest in several forms such as steroid dependency, acute relapsing episodes, and chronic unremitting symptomatology. Ultimately the decision to consider surgery should be made as part of a multidisciplinary process with the patient at the center of the decision making. Patients at particular risk of needing colectomy are those with absent clinical response to anti-TNF therapy or poor endoscopic and clinical response at 12 weeks.[18]

Malignant Transformation

Malignancy in patients with UC is associated with duration of disease, extent, and severity.[19] The cumulative risk of colorectal cancer is 2% at 10 years, 8% at 20 years, and 18% at 30 years.[20] Colonic carcinoma is an absolute indication for total colectomy. Patients with primary sclerosing cholangitis (PSC) have an additional risk up to fivefold compared to UC patients without PSC.[21] Regular colonoscopy reduces the risk of neoplasia and surveillance of patients with UC is recommended every 1–2 years commencing at 10 years post diagnosis.

As colonic carcinoma, the risk of colonic dysplasia is also increased in patients with UC. Management of patients with dysplasia is complex and should be performed in a multidisciplinary setting.

Low-grade dysplasia on colonic biopsy is a significant risk factor for malignant progression and also suggests the presence of high-grade dysplasia elsewhere in the colon in up to a quarter of patients. The presence of low-grade dysplasia is also as likely as the presence of high-grade dysplasia to be associated with an established occult malignancy on resected specimens.[22]

The recommendation to progress to total colectomy is therefore compelling.[22] The management of low-grade dysplasia is however an area of debate, and significant variations in management persist.[23] Progression to colectomy is generally low in this group and further research is needed.

High-grade dysplasia is associated with colorectal cancer in 45% of resected specimens and therefore total colectomy is recommended.[24]

Dysplasia-associated lesion or mass (DALM) is a raised dysplastic lesion, often associated with other areas of dysplasia. It should be distinguished from sporadic adenoma, which can also occur in patients with UC. Presence of DALM is an indication of total colectomy due to risk of malignancy.

Others Indications

There are several other indications for consideration of elective surgery. Control of extra-intestinal manifestations may occur, most markedly with erythema nodosum, arthralgia, and thromboembolic complication of the disease.[25] Growth retardation in children remains a theoretical indication, although a recent review of the natural history of pediatric onset UC in population-based studies did not demonstrate significant rates of growth retardation.[26]

Effect of Biological Therapy on Outcomes of Surgery

It is possible that the use of biological therapies for UC has affected colectomy rates, decision making with regards to type of operation, and outcomes in patients having surgery for UC.[27] Of greatest concern to the surgeon was the risk of increased rates of abdominal septic complications in early reports.[28] It has also been suggested that due to biological therapy, patients with UC are sicker, more complex, and require multiple procedures.[4] Meta-analysis of 13 studies involving nearly 3,000 patients however has showed that preoperative infliximab use does not increase the risk of early postoperative complications in UC patients undergoing major surgery. A more recent large population-based study has also suggested that anti-TNF therapy within both 12 and 4 weeks of surgery does not affect outcomes.[29] These findings are possibly in part due to the use of total colectomy and ileostomy as a primary procedure in patients with a suspected high risk of complications. If only patients undergoing ileal pouch anal anastomosis (IPAA) are considered there is evidence that outcome in those who have had treatment with anti-TNF have worse postoperative complication rates.[30,31] It has therefore been suggested that avoiding primary pouch formation in patients on anti-TNF medication is a sensible approach.

SURGICAL TECHNIQUE

Curative surgery for UC involves complete removal of the colon and rectum. This results in either permanent ileostomy or restoration of intestinal continuity by use of a restorative (pouch) procedure. Treatment can be staged, with initial removal of the colon with ileostomy, and then progression to either completion proctectomy or restorative procedure—with or without a defunctioning ileostomy. Removal of the colon in one stage with proctocolectomy or IPAA can also be performed. The main considerations for each procedure are outlined below.

The terminology in surgery for inflammatory bowel disease continues to be confusing with the use of the terms total colectomy, subtotal colectomy, proctocolectomy, and panproctocolectomy, being used, often interchangeably. There are also several terms used to describe the formation of an ileoanal pouch with anastomosis to the anus. For the purpose of this text, colectomy will describe removal of the colon, and proctectomy the removal of the rectum, with proctocolectomy the removal of the colon and rectum. IPAA will be used to describe ileal pouch procedures.

Colectomy and Ileostomy

Abdominal colectomy, leaving the rectum in situ, with end ileostomy, is the standard treatment of patients in the emergency setting. It removes the majority of the colon, allows the patients to recover, and avoids the morbidity of an emergency pelvic dissection. It also keeps options open regarding proceeding to restorative procedure at a later date. It is therefore also commonly performed as an elective procedure where patients may also be nutritionally and immunologically compromised, or unsure if a restorative procedure is appropriate.

It can be performed as an open or laparoscopic procedure, depending on competence of the surgical team. In patients undergoing laparoscopic surgery in the elective setting, there is a reduced incidence of wound infection, intra-abdominal abscesses, and also reduction in length of stay in pooled data.[32] Longer term outcomes appear unaffected.

Effective management of the rectal stump at the time of surgery can vary, but usually consists of rectal drainage using a rectal tube and intraperitoneal closure of the rectum without exteriorization. A mucous fistula should be in consideration in severe disease and the rectal stump can also be sutured subcutaneously to reduce the risk of rectal stump dehiscence.[33,34]

If malignancy is suspected then surgery should also include high ligation of lymphovascular pedicles to allow adequate staging.

Once recovered from colectomy, the patient has three options—(1) to proceed to IPAA, (2) completion proctectomy, or to avoid further surgical intervention, and (3) leave the rectum in situ. The latter option is not recommended due to the symptom burden associated with a retained diseased rectum and the risk of rectal malignancy. It may be appropriate, however, in selected patients.

The mortality rate from emergency resection remains relatively high at 5–6% and is considerably lower in elective surgery at around 1%.

Ileal Pouch Anal Anastomosis

Removal of the colon and rectum with formation of an ileoanal pouch with anastomosis is considered by many to be the gold standard surgical treatment for UC, but it is not suitable for all patients, particularly those with poor anal sphincters, low rectal tumors or significant comorbidity. It is also important to remember that the sole reason for performing IPAA rather than a proctocolectomy is to avoid a permanent stoma.

It may be performed as a one-, two- or three-staged procedure.

One stage procedure with removal of the colon and rectum, ileal pouch formation, and anastomosis without defunctioning ileostomy is rare and only appropriate in a select group of patients due to the risk of anastomotic leak.[35] More commonly, a two-stage procedure with IPAA and formation of loop ileostomy with subsequent reversal, or three stage following previous subtotal colectomy are performed. Surgery can be performed open, laparoscopically, and also robotically to aid pelvic dissection.[36,37]

The ileal pouch may be formed in a variety of configurations, but the standard J-pouch with stapled or hand sewn anastomosis remains the most commonly performed procedure, with no major difference in outcomes between techniques.[38]

It is important that patients undergoing IPAA understand both the complications and functional outcomes expected with the procedure as short- and long-term morbidity may be as high as 60%.[39]

Early complication includes pelvic sepsis due to anastomotic leak in between 5% and 18%, ileus, and wound infection.[40] Late complication of small bowel obstruction can occur in up to 30% of patients and pouchitis in 50% of patients on long-term follow-up. Pouch vaginal fistula is a rare but complex complication that is difficult to manage and usually will need specialist input as a re-do IPAA may be needed.[41] There is a well-documented rate of pouch failure resulting in excision or permanent defunctioning of around 10% at 10 years.[42] Rates are higher in patients who had pelvic sepsis following initial procedure.[42,43] Overall outcomes are thought to be worse as age increases, but IPAA can be performed safely in older patients with comparable complication rates to younger patient.[44]

Fertility rates in females are also reduced following pouch surgery and counseling regarding this is mandatory.[45,46] Consideration should be made to delaying IPAA until the patient does not desire future pregnancy. Laparoscopic surgery may reduce, but not negate the risk of infertility.[47]

Pouch function averages seven motions per day with one night time evacuation. Minor incontinence occurs in around 10%. Quality of life and patient satisfaction however remains high.[48,49] It has been demonstrated that outcomes are better in high volume centers, and that case selection differed significantly between high and low volume surgeons. It is therefore reasonable to consider referring patient to high volume centers for elective IPAA surgery.[6,42]

Proctocolectomy and Completion Proctectomy

Proctocolectomy or completion proctectomy following colectomy and ileostomy are indicated in patients who do not desire or who are not suitable for IPAA.

The rectum and anal canal are removed in their entirety and the pelvic floor defect is closed in layers. The result is a permanent ileostomy without the possibility of restoration of intestinal continuity in the future.

Complication rate is relatively low without the risk of anastomotic leak and subsequent pelvic sepsis, however, this is replaced with the possibility of stoma prolapse and stenosis.

Quality of life has also shown to be good in patients undergoing proctocolectomy with ileostomy, with comparable outcomes to patients who have IPAA surgery. It is therefore likely that the majority of benefit that is achieved in UC patients undergoing surgical intervention is derived from control of symptoms.[50]

REFERENCES

1. Targownik LE, Singh H, Nugent Z, Bernstein CN. The epidemiology of colectomy in ulcerative colitis: results from a population-based cohort. Am J Gastroenterol. 2012;107(8):1228-35.
2. Parragi L, Fournier N, Zeitz J, Scharl M, Greuter T, Schreiner P, et al. Colectomy rates in ulcerative colitis are low and decreasing: 10-year follow-up data from the Swiss IBD Cohort Study. J Crohns Colitis. 2018;12(7):811-8.
3. Leijonmarck CE, Persson PG, Hellers G. Factors affecting colectomy rate in ulcerative colitis: an epidemiologic study. Gut. 1990;31(3):329-33.
4. Abelson JS, Michelassi F, Mao J, Sedrakyan A, Yeo H. Higher surgical morbidity for ulcerative colitis patients in the era of biologics. Ann Surg. 2018;268(2):311-7.
5. Kaplan GG, McCarthy EP, Ayanian JZ, Korzenik J, Hodin R, Sands BE. Impact of hospital volume on postoperative morbidity and mortality following a colectomy for ulcerative colitis. Gastroenterology. 2008;134(3):680-7.
6. Burns EM, Bottle A, Aylin P, Clark SK, Tekkis PP, Darzi A, et al. Volume analysis of outcome following restorative proctocolectomy. Br J Surg. 2011;98(3):408-17.
7. Dinesen LC, Walsh AJ, Protic MN, Heap G, Cummings F, Warren BF, et al. The pattern and outcome of acute severe colitis. J Crohns Colitis. 2010;4(4):431-7.
8. Aratari A, Papi C, Clemente V, Moretti A, Luchetti R, Koch M, et al. Colectomy rate in acute severe ulcerative colitis in the infliximab era. Dig Liver Dis. 2008;40(10):821-6.
9. Narula N, Marshall JK, Colombel JF, Leontiadis GI, Williams JG, Muqtadir Z, et al. Systematic review and meta-analysis: Infliximab or cyclosporine as rescue therapy in patients with severe ulcerative colitis refractory to steroids. Am J Gastroenterol. 2016;111(4):477-91.
10. Randall J, Singh B, Warren BF, Travis SP, Mortensen NJ, George BD. Delayed surgery for acute severe colitis is associated with increased risk of postoperative complications. Br J Surg. 2010;97(3):404-9.

11. Ventham NT, Kalla R, Kennedy NA, Satsangi J, Arnott ID. Predicting outcomes in acute severe ulcerative colitis. Expert Rev Gastroenterol Hepatol. 2015;9(4):405-15.
12. Travis SP, Farrant JM, Ricketts C, Nolan DJ, Mortensen NM, Kettlewell MG, et al. Predicting outcome in severe ulcerative colitis. Gut. 1996;38(6):905-10.
13. Ho GT, Mowat C, Goddard CJ, Fennell JM, Shah NB, Prescott RJ, et al. Predicting the outcome of severe ulcerative colitis: development of a novel risk score to aid early selection of patients for second-line medical therapy or surgery. Aliment Pharmacol Ther. 2004;19(10):1079-87.
14. Lindgren SC, Flood LM, Kilander AF, Löfberg R, Persson TB, Sjödahl RI. Early predictors of glucocorticosteroid treatment failure in severe and moderately severe attacks of ulcerative colitis. Eur J Gastroenterol Hepatol. 1998;10(10):831-5.
15. Seo M, Okada M, Yao T, Ueki M, Arima S, Okumura M. An index of disease activity in patients with ulcerative colitis. Am J Gastroenterol. 1992;87(8):971-6.
16. Gan SI, Beck PL. A new look at toxic megacolon: an update and review of incidence, etiology, pathogenesis, and management. Am J Gastroenterol. 2003;98(11):2363-71.
17. Andersson P, Soderholm JD. Surgery in ulcerative colitis: indication and timing. Dig Dis. 2009;27(3):335-40.
18. Macaluso FS, Cavallaro F, Felice C, Mazza M, Armuzzi A, Gionchetti P, et al. Risk factors and timing for colectomy in chronically active refractory ulcerative colitis: a systematic review. Dig Liver Dis. 2019;51(5):613-20.
19. Yashiro M. Ulcerative colitis-associated colorectal cancer. World J Gastroenterol. 2014;20(44):16389-97.
20. Eaden JA, Abrams KR, Mayberry JF. The risk of colorectal cancer in ulcerative colitis: a meta-analysis. Gut. 2001;48(4):526-35.
21. Soetikno RM, Lin OS, Heidenreich PA, Young HS, Blackstone MO. Increased risk of colorectal neoplasia in patients with primary sclerosing cholangitis and ulcerative colitis: a meta-analysis. Gastrointest Endosc. 2002;56(1):48-54.
22. Thomas T, Abrams KA, Robinson RJ, Mayberry JF. Meta-analysis: cancer risk of low-grade dysplasia in chronic ulcerative colitis. Aliment Pharmacol Ther. 2007;25(6):657-68.
23. Thomas T, Nair P, Dronfield MW, Mayberry JF. Management of low and high-grade dysplasia in inflammatory bowel disease: the gastroenterologists' perspective and current practice in the United Kingdom. Eur J Gastroenterol Hepatol. 2005;17(12):1317-24.
24. Ullman T, Odze R, Farraye FA. Diagnosis and management of dysplasia in patients with ulcerative colitis and Crohn's disease of the colon. Inflamm Bowel Dis. 2009;15(4):630-8.
25. Goudet P, Dozois RR, Kelly KA, Ilstrup DM, Phillips SF. Characteristics and evolution of extraintestinal manifestations associated with ulcerative colitis after proctocolectomy. Dig Surg. 2001;18(1):51-5.
26. Fumery M, Duricova D, Gower-Rousseau C, Annese V, Peyrin-Biroulet L, Lakatos PL. Review article: the natural history of paediatric-onset ulcerative colitis in population-based studies. Aliment Pharmacol Ther. 2016;43(3):346-55.
27. Wong DJ, Roth EM, Feuerstein JD, Poylin VY. Surgery in the age of biologics. Gastroenterol Rep (Oxf). 2019;7(2):77-90.

28. Mor IJ, Vogel JD, da Luz Moreira A, Shen B, Hammel J, Remzi FH. Infliximab in ulcerative colitis is associated with an increased risk of postoperative complications after restorative proctocolectomy. Dis Colon Rectum. 2008;51(8):1202-7.
29. Ward ST, Mytton J, Henderson L, Amin V, Tanner JR, Evison F, et al. Anti-TNF therapy is not associated with an increased risk of post-colectomy complications, a population-based study. Colorectal Dis. 2018;20(5):416-23.
30. Kulaylat AS, Kulaylat AN, Schaefer EW, Tinsley A, Williams E, Koltun W, et al. Association of preoperative anti-tumor necrosis factor therapy with adverse postoperative outcomes in patients undergoing abdominal surgery for ulcerative colitis. JAMA Surg. 2017;152(8):e171538.
31. Selvaggi F, Pellino G, Canonico S, Sciaudone G. Effect of preoperative biologic drugs on complications and function after restorative proctocolectomy with primary ileal pouch formation: systematic review and meta-analysis. Inflamm Bowel Dis. 2015;21(1):79-92.
32. Bartels SA, Gardenbroek TJ, Ubbink DT, Buskens CJ, Tanis PJ, Bemelman WA. Systematic review and meta-analysis of laparoscopic versus open colectomy with end ileostomy for non-toxic colitis. Br J Surg. 2013;100(6):726-33.
33. Bedrikovetski S, Dudi-Venkata N, Kroon HM, Liu J, Andrews JM, Lewis M, et al. Systematic review of rectal stump management during and after emergency total colectomy for acute severe ulcerative colitis. ANZ J Surg. 2019;89(12):1556-60.
34. Lissel M, Omidy S, Myrelid P, Block M, Angenete E. The handling of the rectal stump does not affect severe morbidity after subtotal colectomy for ulcerative colitis: a retrospective cohort study. Scand J Surg. 2019:1457496919857269.
35. Weston-Petrides GK, Lovegrove RE, Tilney HS, Heriot AG, Nicholls RJ, Mortensen NJ. Comparison of outcomes after restorative proctocolectomy with or without defunctioning ileostomy. Arch Surg. 2008;143(4):406-12.
36. Anderson M, Lynn P, Aydinli HH, Schwartzberg D, Bernstein M, Grucela A. Early experience with urgent robotic subtotal colectomy for severe acute ulcerative colitis has comparable perioperative outcomes to laparoscopic surgery. J Robot Surg. 2019.
37. Hata K, Kazama S, Nozawa H, Kawai K, Kiyomatsu T, Tanaka J, et al. Laparoscopic surgery for ulcerative colitis: a review of the literature. Surg Today. 2015;45(8):933-8.
38. Lovegrove RE, Constantinides VA, Heriot AG, Athanasiou T, Darzi A, Remzi FH, et al. A comparison of hand-sewn versus stapled ileal pouch anal anastomosis (IPAA) following proctocolectomy: a meta-analysis of 4183 patients. Ann Surg. 2006;244(1):18-26.
39. Fazio VW, Kiran RP, Remzi FH, Coffey JC, Heneghan HM, Kirat HT, et al. Ileal pouch anal anastomosis: analysis of outcome and quality of life in 3707 patients. Ann Surg. 2013;257(4):679-85.
40. Freeha K, Bo S. Complications related to J-pouch surgery. Gastroenterol Hepatol (N Y). 2018;14(10):571-6.
41. Sapci I, Akeel N, DeLeon MF, Stocchi L, Hull T. What is the best surgical treatment of pouch-vaginal fistulas? Dis Colon Rectum. 2019;62(5):595-9.
42. Mark-Christensen A, Erichsen R, Brandsborg S, Pachler FR, Nørager CB, Johansen N, et al. Pouch failures following ileal pouch-anal anastomosis for ulcerative colitis. Colorectal Dis. 2018;20(1):44-52.

43. Fazio VW, Tekkis PP, Remzi F, Lavery IC, Manilich E, Connor J, et al. Quantification of risk for pouch failure after ileal pouch anal anastomosis surgery. Ann Surg. 2003;238(4):605-17.
44. Minagawa T, Ikeuchi H, Kuwahara R, Horio Y, Sasaki H, Chohno T, et al. Functional outcomes and quality of life in elderly patients after restorative proctocolectomy for ulcerative colitis. Digestion. 2019.
45. Pachler FR, Brandsborg SB, Laurberg S. Paradoxical impact of ileal pouch-anal anastomosis on male and female fertility in patients with ulcerative colitis. Dis Colon Rectum. 2017;60(6):603-7.
46. Hor T, Lefevre JH, Shields C, Chafai N, Tiret E, Parc Y. Female sexual function and fertility after ileal pouch-anal anastomosis. Int J Colorectal Dis. 2016;31(3):593-601.
47. Gorgun E, Cengiz TB, Aytac E, Aiello A, da Silva G, Goldberg JM, et al. Does laparoscopic ileal pouch-anal anastomosis reduce infertility compared with open approach? Surgery. 2019;166(4):670-7.
48. Somashekar U, Gupta S, Soin A, Nundy S. Functional outcome and quality of life following restorative proctocolectomy for ulcerative colitis in Indians. Int J Colorectal Dis. 2010;25(8):967-73.
49. Michelassi F, Lee J, Rubin M, Fichera A, Kasza K, Karrison T, et al. Long-term functional results after ileal pouch anal restorative proctocolectomy for ulcerative colitis: a prospective observational study. Ann Surg. 2003;238(3):433-41.
50. Murphy PB, Khot Z, Vogt KN, Ott M, Dubois L. Quality of life after total proctocolectomy with ileostomy or IPAA: a systematic review. Dis Colon Rectum. 2015;58(9):899-908.

CHAPTER

3

Microscopic Colitis

Catriona Scicluna, John Schembri, Pierre Ellul

INTRODUCTION

Microscopic colitis (MC) is an inflammatory bowel disorder, being more prevalent in females and in patients >50 years of age. It consists of two main subtypes—(1) collagenous colitis (CC) and (2) lymphocytic colitis (LC), and is characterized by watery nonbloody diarrhea, with no specific endoscopic features but typical histological features which are the gold standard for the diagnosis of the two different subtypes. Over time, the incidence of MC has been noted to be increasing and has now stabilized, which is attributed to an increase in investigations with colonoscopy and biopsies. Since there are no sensitive and specific diagnostic tests except for histological analysis, a high index of suspicion is needed to investigate such patients appropriately.

EPIDEMIOLOGY

Most of the data on the subject comes from developed countries, with very limited data from developing countries. CC has an annual incidence of 4.14 per 100,000 person-years, with an overall prevalence of 49.21 cases per 100,000 person-years. LC has an annual incidence of 4.85 per 100,000 person-years, with an overall prevalence of 63.05 cases per 100,000 person-years.[1] The female-to-male age-adjusted incidence ratios have been estimated to be 3.05 for CC and 1.92 for LC.[1,2] MC is more common in patients above the age of 60 years [Odds ratio (OR) 8.3 for age >65 years vs. <65 years)], with an overall mean age of diagnosis of 60.2 years.[2,3] Whilst the adjusted prevalence rate of MC was 107.1 cases per 100,000 residents [95% confidence interval (CI), 91.1–125.1], the adjusted rate of patients with active disease is 30.85 per 100,000 people (95% CI 22.6–41.1) reflecting the true burden of the disease.[4]

PATHOPHYSIOLOGY

The exact pathophysiology of MC is still largely unknown. However, several mechanisms have been proposed and it could also be that a multifactorial mechanism is responsible. The most common theory proposes that MC results from activation of the immune system in the colonic mucosa in response to exposure to different luminal antigenic factors, such as toxins, infections, bile acids, or drugs.[5]

Chronic mucosal inflammation, in turn, leads to reduced sodium chloride absorption, decreased passive permeability, and inhibition of chloride/bicarbonate exchange channels, all of which lead to secretory diarrhea that is observed in MC.[6] There is mucosal infiltration by CD8+ T lymphocytes, with a decrease in CD4+ T-cell levels in the lamina propria. This is in contrast to ulcerative colitis (UC) and Crohn's disease (CD) where there is mucosal infiltration with CD4+ lymphocytes.[7]

Another possible mechanism may be due to bile salt malabsorption, and bile acid sequestrants have been used successfully in the treatment of diarrhea in MC. A study by Ung et al. demonstrated that 44% (12/27) of patients with CC had abnormal bile acid absorption.[8]

Other mechanisms may involve both luminal contents and the antigens that may be present within. This is demonstrated by patients who undergo a diverting ileostomy. Stool diversion was found to lead to histologic improvement of MC, which later reoccurred upon stoma reversal.[9,10] The microbiome has also been implicated in the pathophysiology of MC, whereby an increase in the bacterial family of Desulfovibrionales and a decrease in *Coriobacteriaceae* were observed compared to healthy gastrointestinal tracts.[11] Bacterial toxins related to *Clostridium difficile* and *Yersinia* have also been associated with CC.[12-15] Improvement of symptoms with cholestyramine, which acts as a toxin binder, also supports this theory.[16]

Exogenous hormone (both the oral contraceptive pill and menopausal hormone therapy) use may also play a role in the pathophysiology of MC. In a pooled analysis, exogenous hormone therapy use was associated with the increased risk of MC.[17] In contrast, a recent study by Verhaegh et al. did not find any association between hormonal factors and the development of MC on multivariate analysis. However, the study groups, in this case, might not have been large enough to detect small differences.[18]

GENETIC FACTORS AND MICROSCOPIC COLITIS

Although there are reports of familial cases, genetic predisposition to MC seems to be relatively weak with only a few polymorphisms having been implicated with disease risk. Human leukocyte antigen (HLA) association between MC and HLA-DQ2/DQ1,3 and HLA-DR3-DQ2 haplotype has been reported. These genes also predispose to coeliac disease and may account for the epidemiological overlap between coeliac disease and MC.[19,20] Allelic variation in matrix metalloproteinase 9 (*MMP9*) gene has also been observed to increase the risk of MC.[21] Decreased expression of *PTEN* and *MACI1* in colonic mucosa may contribute to MC. There is also an indication that genetic variants of tight junction components are predisposing factors for MC.[22]

A genome-wide association study by Harry et al. that made use of genetic risk scoring found that there was an overlap in genetic risk factors for CD and inflammatory bowel disease (IBD) but not UC. The association occurred with single-nucleotide polymorphism (SNPs) on the major histocompatibility complex ancestral 8.1 haplotype. This also indicates an immune component to the pathogenesis of MC.[23]

ENVIRONMENTAL FACTORS

Prescribed Medications

Prescribed medications could account for up to 10% of all MC cases.[24] Nonsteroidal anti-inflammatory drugs (NSAIDs), selective serotonin reuptake inhibitors (SSRIs), proton-pump inhibitors (PPIs), statins, beta-blockers, angiotensin-converting enzyme inhibitors, and angiotensin receptor blockers, as well as novel chemotherapeutic agents and immune checkpoint inhibitors (ICPIs), have all been associated with MC **(Table 1)**.[25-32]

It is thought that NSAIDs inhibit prostaglandin synthesis, thus increasing intestinal permeability and allowing access of luminal contents into the lamina propria. This leads to inflammation and activation of pericryptal fibroblasts which in turn leads to thickening of the collagen layer.[26] PPIs cause growth inhibition and oxidative stress in CT26 cells, which express sodium–hydrogen exchanger genes, thus affecting water transport. PPIs also increase the expression of fibrosis-inducing factors and decrease the expression of replication factor C1 (a negative regulator of collagen production), leading to increased expression of collagen III and IV.[26]

Concomitant use of NSAIDs and PPIs poses the highest risk of MC.[27,28] Considering that these are commonly prescribed medications and relatively low incidence of MC, it is more likely that drug-induced cases are the result of an idiosyncratic reaction. In fact, MC was shown not to progress in a dose-dependent manner, and symptoms were reported even months after drug initiation.[28-30] Patients on ICPIs seem to develop a more aggressive disease course and very often require hospitalization, and treatment with corticosteroids, infliximab, or vedolizumab may have to be considered.[31] Meanwhile, anti-tumor necrosis factor α (TNFα) drugs have also been implicated in MC, albeit through a case series.[32]

Autoimmune Disorders

Concomitant autoimmune diseases are also present and have been associated with patients with MC, coeliac disease (2–20%), thyroid disease (10–20%), type 1 diabetes mellitus, rheumatoid arthritis, Sjogren's syndrome, and Raynaud's/CREST (calcinosis, Raynaud's phenomenon, esophageal dysmotility, sclerodactyly, and telangiectasia) syndrome being the main

Table 1: List of medications associated with the development of microscopic colitis.

Drug	Type of microscopic colitis	Reference	Odds ratio (OR)
Anti-TNFα	CC	Saad et al.[32]	Case reports
PPIs	CC and LC	Keszthelyi et al.[27]	OR 4.5 (2.0–9.5)
	CC	Verhaegh et al.[28] Bonderup et al.[29]	OR 4.00 (3.19–5.02) OR 6.98 (6.45–7.55)
	LC	Bonderup et al.[29]	OR 3.95 (3.60–4.33)
Lansoprazole	CC	Fernandez-Banares et al.[30] Bonderup et al.[29]	OR 6.4 OR 15.74 (14.12–17.55)
	LC	Bonderup et al.[29]	OR 6.87 (6.00–7.86)
Versus other PPIs	CC LC	Bonderup et al.[29] Bonderup et al.[29]	OR 5.04 (4.31–5.90) OR 2.38 (1.93–2.94)
Omeprazole	LC CC	Fernandez-Banares et al.[30] Bonderup et al.[29] Bonderup et al.[29]	OR 2.7 OR 3.01 (2.49–3.36) OR 3.14 (2.66–3.70)
Pantoprazole	CC LC	Bonderup et al.[29]	OR 3.01 (2.58–3.50) OR 2.60 (2.21–3.06)
Esomeprazole	CC LC	Bonderup et al.[29]	OR 3.75 (3.13–4.49) OR 2.93 (2.37–3.62)
NSAIDs	CC, LC CC LC	Keszthelyi et al.[27] Verhaegh et al.[28] Bonderup et al.[29]	OR 2.3 (0.8–6.5) OR 2.09 (1.78–2.46) OR 1.60 (1.45–1.76) OR 1.28 (1.14–1.43)
Aspirin	CC, LC	Fernandez-Banares et al.[30]	OR 3.8, 4.7 respectively
Concomitant NSAIDs and PPIs	CC LC	Verhaegh et al.[28] Bonderup et al.[29]	OR 5.40 (3.46–8.42) OR 7.45 (6.63–8.38) OR 3.54 (2.98–4.20)
H₂ receptor antagonist		Verhaegh et al.[28]	OR 2.40 (1.73–3.31)
Beta-blockers	CC	Fernandez-Banares et al.[30]	OR 3.6
SSRIs		Verhaegh et al.[28]	OR 2.03 (1.58–2.61)
Sertraline	LC	Fernandez-Banares et al.[30]	OR 17.5
ICPIs		Choi et al.[31]	Case reports
Anti-CTLA-4	LC		
Anti-PD-1	LC, CC		
Anti-PD-L1	LC		

(anti-CTLA-4: anti-cytotoxic T-lymphocyte-associated protein 4; anti-PD-1: anti-programmed cell death protein 1; anti-PD-L1: anti-programmed death-ligand 1; CC: collagenous colitis; ICPI: immune checkpoint inhibitor; LC: lymphocytic colitis; NSAIDs: nonsteroidal anti-inflammatory drugs; PPI: proton-pump inhibitor; SSRIs: selective serotonin reuptake inhibitors; TNFα: tumor necrosis factor α) associated disorders.[33-36] No association with autoimmune liver disease has been reported. Patients with coeliac disease have a 70-fold risk of developing MC, which is thought to be due to an association with HLA-DR3-DQ2, present in both diseases.[20,33] It has also been noted that an association is present between MC and lymphocytic disorders of the gut such as lymphocytic esophagitis, lymphocytic gastritis, and duodenal intraepithelial lymphocytosis.[37,38]

Smoking

Smoking is a significant risk factor for the development of MC, with smokers developing the condition 10 years earlier than nonsmokers. Smoking status, however, does not seem to influence the subsequent disease course.[39-41]

Other Risk Factors

While most cases of MC have negative stool cultures, certain infections have been linked with sudden-onset MC including *Yersinia*, *Campylobacter*, and *Clostridium difficile*.[14,15,42,43]

There have been reported cases of CC development after IBD onset. It is suggested that long-term TNFα inhibitors may lead to the development of CC in healing IBD mucosa. Two mechanisms are proposed. The first mechanism involves the overproduction of collagen in the extra-cellular matrix (ECM) by increased expression of α-smooth muscle actin and tenascin, increased connective tissue growth factor expression in fibroblasts, and decreased inhibition of TGF-β which leads to enhanced collagen deposition. Another proposed mechanism of action is the reduction of collagen degradation through prevention of induction of MMPs which would degrade and remodel collagen in the ECM.[33]

CLINICAL FEATURES

Microscopic colitis may develop acutely or progressively over a period of time. Symptoms may vary from mild to incapacitating chronic nonbloody watery diarrhea. Stool urgency and incontinence may also be present.

Associated symptoms may be abdominal pain, nocturnal symptoms, weight loss, arthralgia, and fatigue.[38,44-46] Due to symptoms overlapping with other gastrointestinal diseases, the diagnosis can be difficult to establish on clinical grounds and the differential diagnosis is broad. Severe complications are rare, with a few reports of colonic perforation either spontaneously or after a colonoscopy having been reported.[47,48]

Eighty-eight percent of patients reported a median stool form ≥6 on the Bristol Stool Scale while only 35% of patients' functional diarrhea had a Bristol Stool Scale of ≥6. Similarly, 81% of patients with bile acid diarrhea had a score of ≥6.[49]

Table 2: Predictors for microscopic colitis.

Predictors	Assigned points
Age >55 years of age	6
Duration of diarrhea <6 months	5
>5 bowel movements per day	3
Body mass index <30 kg/m^2	3
Current smoking	3
Current use of SSRIs/SNRIs	2
Current use of NSAIDs	2
Total score	

(NSAIDs: nonsteroidal anti-inflammatory drugs; SNRIs: serotonin-norepinephrine reuptake inhibitors; SSRIs: selective serotonin reuptake inhibitors)

Cotter et al. have suggested a scoring system for predicting MC in patients with chronic diarrhea. This makes the use of seven clinical variables: Age ≥55 years of age, duration of diarrhea ≤6 months, >5 bowel movements per day, body mass index <30 kg/m^2, current smoking, and current use of SSRIs/serotonin-norepinephrine reuptake inhibitors (SNRIs) and NSAIDs **(Table 2)**. A score of 10 or more yielded an area under the receiver operating characteristic (ROC) curve of 0.83 (93% sensitivity, 49% specificity), with a negative predictive value of 97.8%. Thus, this scoring system, having a high sensitivity, reasonable specificity, and a high negative predicted value (NPV), may be considered to determine which patients may benefit most from colonoscopy with biopsies.[50]

DIAGNOSIS

Blood Investigations and Stool Sampling

Blood investigations may show a mild rise in inflammatory markers, mild anemia, and positive autoantibodies (rheumatoid factor, antinuclear antibodies, antimitochondrial antibodies, antithyroid antibodies) in approximately 50% of patients.[51] Stool cultures are generally negative, and radiological studies do not have any role in the investigative and management algorithm. The diagnostic accuracy of fecal calprotectin (FCP) and lactoferrin is low and make them poor biomarkers for both the diagnosis and the follow-up of MC.[52,53] In IBD, an FCP > 50 μg/g has a sensitivity of 72.2%, a positive predictive value of 5.41%, and a negative predictive value of 98.9% for the disease.[54] Meanwhile, up to 38% of patients with MC have a normal calprotectin despite the active disease.[52,53,55] Thus, in MC, FCP has a limited or no role in the screening of patients with diarrhea as well as in its management.

Endoscopic Features and Sampling

Microscopic colitis was initially deemed to be invisible to the naked eye at endoscopy; however, more recent experience and evidence using high-definition and chromoendoscopy techniques have demonstrated otherwise. The first indication that MC could be macroscopically detected as abnormal surface patterns was from reports that employed the use of standard white-light imaging and indigo-carmine dye-spray chromoendoscopy. Over the years, thanks to the use of better equipment and increased endoscopist awareness, some changes have become visible during regular endoscopy, even without the use of endoscopic adjuncts.

Histological confirmation remains the benchmark for making a diagnosis of MC. Both CC and LC demonstrate increased lamina propria cellularity; however, in CC, this is also accompanied by a subepithelial collagen band thicker than 10 μm.[48] Inflammatory changes can be patchy and the severity of histological features tends to decline from proximal to the more distal colon; hence, a full colonoscopy is often advised. While a more limited sigmoidoscopy might miss up to 10% of cases, it remains a suitable alternative, especially in cases where the risks of colonoscopy might be particularly unacceptable.[47]

Macroscopic features that can be observed include slight edema, erythema, friability, exudative lesions, and scars.[56] These tend to be more common in CC than in LC **(Table 3)**. Furthermore, CC can also present with mucosal tears or hemorrhagic linear marks ("cat scratch" colon) induced by barotrauma and excessive stretching of the stiff nonpliable mucosa. Lacerations and tears may represent an increased risk of colonic perforation. If these lesions are recognized at intubation, it is advisable that the procedure is abandoned and biopsies are taken on withdrawal.[70] In one study, up to 30% of patients diagnosed with CC had macroscopic features detectable using white light standard definition endoscopy.[71]

Mucosal changes that can be accentuated by indigo-carmine dye-spray examination include disruption of the innominate grooves in turn leading to an irregular surface pattern, mucosal nodularity, and a mosaic pattern not unlike that observed in coeliac disease.[64] As a more convenient alternative to traditional dye-spray chromoendoscopy, all the main manufacturers of endoscopy equipment have devised their own patented image postprocessing technologies, termed electronic chromoendoscopy (ECE). Thanks to modern high-definition endoscopes with ECE capabilities, the same mucosal abnormalities observed with traditional chromoendoscopy can be detected without the need for extra resources or time expenditure.[68,70]

Fuji Intelligent Chromoendoscopy (FICE; Fujinon), iScan (Pentax), and Narrow Band Imaging (NBI; Olympus) have all shown their ability to pick up or enhance subtle mucosal changes of MC.[72,73] While histological confirmation remains the gold standard means of diagnosing MC, these techniques could

Table 3: Overview of studies reporting endoscopic findings in microscopic colitis.

Endoscopic modality		Author (Year of publication)	Microscopic colitis type	Study type	Number	Macroscopic changes Figure	Macroscopic changes Statistic
White light		Jobse et al.[57]	CC	Case series	83	24.1%*	Percentage
		Cimmino et al.[58]	CC	Case-control retrospective		19.4 (3.9–95.4)	Odds ratio (±95% CI)
		Simondi et al.[59]	LC	Retrospective observational	80	18.8%*	Percentage
		Saito et al.[60]	CC	Case series	25	44.0%*	Percentage
		Park et al.[56]	LC	Retrospective observational	14	71.4%*	Percentage
		Fumery et al.[61]	CC	Retrospective observational	87	29.0%*	Percentage
			LC		43	19.0%*	Percentage
		Mellander et al.[62]	CC	Retrospective observational	342	37.13%	Percentage
			LC		453	24.9%	Percentage
OGD (white light)		Koskela et al.[63]	CC	Case-control retrospective	27	2.4 (0.9–6.3)*	Odds ratio
			LC		48	0.3 (0.1–1.0)*	Odds ratio
Chromoendoscopy							
Dye spray		Suzuki et al.[64]	CC	Case series	10	NA	NA
			LC		3	NA	NA
		Narabayashi et al.[65]	CC	Case series	29	51.7%*	Percentage
Electronic	iScan (Pentax)	Iacucci et al.[66]	LC	Case report	1	NA	NA
	NBI (Olympus)	Kobayashi et al.[67]	CC	Case series	5	100%*	Percentage
	FICE (Fuji) (+NBI)	Yung et al.[68]	CC	Case series	8	NA	NA
iCLE		Zambelli et al.[69]	CC	Case series	7	75.0%*	Percentage

*Not calculated by original authors.
(CC: collagenous colitis; ICPI: immune checkpoint inhibitor; LC: lymphocytic colitis; CI: confidence interval; CLE: confocal laser endomicroscopy; OGD: oesophagogastroduodenoscopy)

help the endoscopist by guiding biopsies, thus employing a targeted biopsy approach rather than a random nontargeted approach.

An endoscopic technology that might be more effective at detecting MC, both CC and LC, might be integrated confocal laser endoscopy (iCLE); however, the lack of widespread availability of this technique outside of research settings limits its use in day-to-day practice.[73]

While all of this evidence comes from a small case series or from retrospective studies, it is clear that the term "microscopic colitis" is somewhat of a misnomer which might distract the endoscopist. On the contrary, increased awareness and a high index of suspicion are required in order to pick up the endoscopic signs of MC since these can often be subtle. In this regard, minimal change colitis which is the name used when the condition was first described might be more appropriate.[74]

The American Society of Gastrointestinal Endoscopy recommends two or more biopsies of the transverse, sigmoid, and descending colon if flexible sigmoidoscopy is performed and two or more biopsies of the right, transverse, descending, and sigmoid colon, if colonoscopy is performed as histologic changes, can be patchy in distribution and are usually more pronounced in the more proximal colon.[75] Though colonoscopy is usually recommended, flexible sigmoidoscopy can diagnose >90% of MC.[47]

Histology

Diagnosis relies on histology from colonic biopsies. CC is characterized by a subepithelial collagen band ≥10 μm in thickness (normally <3 μm), which may contain capillaries, red blood cells, and inflammatory cells. The mucosal epithelium may show vacuolization, flattening, mucin depletion, and focal detachment of the epithelium from the basement membrane. Increased numbers of intraepithelial lymphocytes (IELs), and lymphocytes, plasma cells and mast cells in the lamina propria, or cryptitis may also be seen. Hematoxylin and eosin (H&E) staining is usually sufficient, although tenascin immunostaining or Masson's trichrome may be used in unclear cases.[51,56]

Lymphocytic colitis is characterized by 20 or more IELs (normally <5). Vacuolization, flattening, and loss of mucin in the mucosa may also be seen with increased numbers of inflammatory cells. H&E stains are sufficient, although immunohistochemistry staining for CD3-positive IEL may be needed.[51,56]

In cases where the minimum criteria are not met for a diagnosis, a diagnosis of incomplete LC and incomplete CC may be made if there are >10 and <20 IELs per 100 surface epithelial cells and >5-μm and <10-μm thickness of the collagen band in colonic biopsies.[76]

MANAGEMENT

The current aim of treatment is symptomatic improvement, not histologic remission since MC does not impact mortality or pose an increased risk of colorectal cancer but affects the quality of life (QOL).[77] A large population-based study has proposed clinical remission as being <3 bowel movements per day, or <1 water stool daily for a week, which has correlated with a significant increase in health-related quality of life (HRQoL) and thus has been widely utilized.[78-80] This score is very easy to use and remember in daily clinical practice.

A more complex score has been proposed to determine disease activity. The Microscopic Colitis Disease Activity Index (MCDAI) has been proposed as a tool to assess disease activity and response to treatment.[81] A 1-unit decrease in disease activity (ΔMCDAI) has been associated with a 9-unit increase in QOL as measured using the IBD questionnaire **(Table 4)**.[81]

Lifestyle Modification

Elimination of risk factors such as medications that predispose to MC may induce remission. In a case of drug-induced MC, clinical and histological improvement, as well as recurrence after drug challenge, should be considered. However, on a daily clinical basis, rechallenging may be a difficult approach.[82] A decrease in caffeine, alcohol, and dairy products may also help

Table 4: Microscopic Colitis Disease Activity Index.

Scorecard item	Score-weighted coefficient	Total item score
The average number of unformed stools daily over the past week	× 0.31	
Nocturnal stools over past week (0 = absent, 1 = present)	× 0.78	
Maximum abdominal pain over the past week (score 1–10)	× 0.22	
Average weight loss per month (lbs*)	× 0.11	
Fecal urgency over past week (0 = absent, 1 = present)	× 0.93	
Number of episodes of fecal incontinence over the past month	× 0.01	

*kg × 2.2 = lbs
(6 item score + 1.1 is equal to total score)

control symptoms. Screening for celiac disease and bile acid malabsorption should also be performed and managed accordingly as they can be associated with MC. Loperamide may also be used to control symptoms. However, this does not improve the histological features.[51]

Medications

Budesonide

The 2016 American Gastroenterology Association (AGA) guideline on MC recommends budesonide as first-line therapy. Budesonide dissolves in a pH-dependent manner, and acts on the ileum and ascending colon, with minimal systemic absorption.[75] Initial treatment with budesonide 9 mg daily for 8 weeks is recommended and was shown to induce clinical remission at 8 weeks in 79% of patients versus 42% of patients who were administered a placebo. Histologic remission occurred in 68% of patients treated with budesonide versus 21% in the placebo arm. Budesonide 6 mg daily can maintain remission for 6 months.[82-84] However, high relapse rates of 40–81% as soon as 2 weeks on stopping treatment were noted.[85,86] A study by Münch et al. noted that remission was maintained at 1 year in 61.4% of patients (vs. 16.7% placebo) on low-dose (4.5 mg/day) budesonide maintenance therapy for 1 year.[83] In another study, it was noted that of those patients with relapse after withdrawal of budesonide, 21% needed budesonide >6 mg/day to maintain clinical remission while the rest needed 3 mg/day or alternate days for maintenance of remission. Consideration of alternative therapies should be considered in those needing >6 mg budesonide per day.[87]

Other Steroids

The use of prednisolone in MC has not been well studied, but small studies have shown decreased effectiveness when compared to budesonide (52.9% vs. 82.5% with budesonide) and higher relapse rates (HR 0.38; 95% CI 0.18–0.85, $p = 0.02$).[49,88] Overall, there is limited evidence for systemic corticosteroids and they may be considered in cases where patients have an adverse reaction to budesonide, patient preference, or the cost of budesonide is prohibitive.

Beclomethasone dipropionate, a synthetic corticosteroid with the topical colonic release, is another medication that can be considered. While beclomethasone does appear to induce remission (70% after 8 weeks), a 2010 trial demonstrated that only 26% of patients (from the 84% with initial response) maintained clinical remission at 1 year.[81,89]

Bismuth Salicylate, Mesalamine, and Cholestyramine

Bismuth salicylate or mesalamine are second-line therapies in cases where budesonide cannot be used. Bismuth was studied at a dose of eight to nine daily tablets (each tablet consists of 262 mg) administered in three divided doses, daily for 8 weeks. All studied patients (14) showed a clinical response (none in the placebo arm).[90] A retrospective study by Gentile et al. demonstrated a complete response in 53% of patients, with partial response in 28% of patients, with therapy being more effective in older patients and with milder symptoms.[88] Older age at diagnosis was associated with a better response to bismuth in both CC and LC (OR 1.76; 95% CI 1.21–2.56 for every 5-year increase).[91] Though the cost is low, concerns in terms of prescribing this drug are the risk of neurotoxicity and nephrological side effects with long-term use and the pill burden for the patients.

Another alternative to budesonide is mesalamine. This is recommended by the 2016 AGA guidelines, but not by the Spanish Microscopic Colitis Group and European Microscopic Colitis Group.[79] Two randomized placebo-controlled trials studying mesalamine 3 g/day showed no effect over placebo over 8 weeks. However, a study comparing mesalamine with mesalamine plus cholestyramine showed clinical and histological remission in 85.36% of LC patients and 91.3% in CC, with a better result in patients with CC treated with mesalamine and cholestyramine.[92] However, a randomized controlled trial where cholestyramine was also studied as an adjunct to mesalamine did not show any added benefit and the AGA guidelines recommended against combination therapy with cholestyramine.[75,92]

Bile acid malabsorption is thought to be involved in MC. Cholestyramine is a bile-acid binder and also adheres to bacterial toxins. In MC it may have a dual action, both by binding bile acids in patients with bile-acid malabsorption and by binding to toxins which may have a role in MC pathophysiology. In a small retrospective study ($n = 27$) by Ung et al., cholestyramine at a dose of 4 g, two to three times daily, showed rapid improvement in symptoms in 92% of patients with bile-acid malabsorption compared with 67% of patients without bile-acid malabsorption.[55] Two retrospective studies have shown response rates of 59–65% to cholestyramine in MC.[46,93] To date, no randomized clinical trials have been carried out to elucidate the appropriateness of cholestyramine monotherapy in MC.

Antibiotics and Probiotics

A small randomized controlled trial showed clinical improvement (though not statistically significant) in 44% of patients treated with *Boswellia serrata* probiotics (vs. 27% of patients with placebo).[94] A randomized placebo-controlled trial of *Lactobacillus acidophilus* LA-5 and *Bifidobacterium animalis* AB-Cap-10 showed no benefit in MC.[95] *Escherichia coli* Nissle 1917 was studied in an open-label trial and showed improvement in stool frequency (64%) and stool consistency (50%).[96] An open-label trial on 30 patients studying VSL#3 and mesalamine showed a 46% remission rate in the VSL#3 group compared to 8% remission on mesalamine.[96] Data is limited and products are not standardized or controlled, and improvements in these areas are needed before recommendations for use of such products can be made. The current guidelines recommend against treatment with probiotics, even if MC is not responsive to any other treatment.[75]

Although antibiotics have sometimes been used with some success, no controlled clinical trial data exists to support this. Data is also limited with regard to concomitant medication use and relapse rates.[24,46]

Immunomodulators

Azathioprine and 6-mercaptopurine may be used in refractory MC or steroid-dependent MC. A retrospective study showed an overall response rate of 41% when taking into consideration side effects secondary to thiopurines.[51,97,98] A Mayo Clinic case series showed a complete response in 43% of patients and a partial response in 22% of patients treated with thiopurines for 4 months. However, 35% of patients stopped treatment due to adverse effects.[99]

A study by Riddell et al. demonstrated a good or partial response to methotrexate in 16 patients with CC. Ten patients who had repeat colonoscopy after starting treatment showed normal histology in five patients, an improvement in two patients, and three patients had no histological improvement.[100] A small study by Münch et al. showed no improvement in nine patients with CC treated with methotrexate for 3 months.[101] A Mayo Clinic case series on 12 patients with MC treated with methotrexate showed a complete response in 58%, partial response in 17%, and no response in 25%. However, 75% of these were on concomitant budesonide treatment.[99] In view of these conflicting results, further studies are required.

Other immunosuppressants were reported to have been used, such as tacrolimus, which achieved a complete response in one patient, and cyclosporine.[99] Further studies are needed to elucidate the role of calcineurin inhibitors in MC.

Pentoxifylline

Pentoxifylline is a xanthine oxidase derivative with anti-TNFα properties. A case report of nine patients who were intolerant of or dependent on budesonide was then treated with pentoxifylline 400 mg three times daily for a median of 3 months. One patient had a complete response and three had a partial response.[99] Thus, such treatment may be considered in refractory cases.

Anti-TNFα Therapy

Anti-TNFα drugs may be considered in refractory cases of MC, which are rare and thus, evidence on the use of such treatment in these cases is limited. A case series of 10 patients with MC refractory to budesonide and immunomodulators were treated with adalimumab or infliximab at standard loading doses used for IBD. Eighty percent of patients achieved clinical and histologic remission with improved HRQoL.[79,102]

Vedolizumab was used in a case of refractory CC, where the patient was refractory to budesonide and dependent on steroids. Histologic remission was achieved after 3 months of treatment.[103] A case series of 11 patients with refractory MC immunosuppressants and/or anti-TNFα drugs were administered vedolizumab. Clinical remission was achieved in 5/11 patients treated with vedolizumab, and 75% of them had histologic remission.[104]

Fecal Transplant

A case report of a patient refractory to budesonide examined this treatment modality. The patient received three fecal transplants, with remission achieved after the last transplant, with remission maintained for 11 months, after which, despite relapse, MC became responsive to budesonide.[105]

Surgery

Surgical treatment options available for refractory cases of MC include ileostomy, subtotal colectomy, and ileal pouch-anal anastomosis. Individual case reports are available.[106,107]

CONCLUSION

Microscopic colitis remains the lesser well known of the inflammatory bowel disorders affecting the large bowel. Notwithstanding this, its incidence is relatively high, especially amongst the elderly. A less severe disease course together with the absence of endoscopic features or the presence of subtle endoscopic features means that it remains relatively underdiagnosed compared to the other disorders. However, a significant proportion of diagnosed patients require long-term maintenance treatment. A high index of suspicion is required by both clinicians and endoscopists alike in order to make a diagnosis, and while FCP has been widely promoted in the investigation of patients with loose stools, this is essentially normal in MC. Thus, the use of the seven-point risk score for predicting MC in patients with chronic diarrhea is useful as to correctly identify high-risk patients and correctly refer them for a colonoscopy with colonic biopsies.

REFERENCES

1. Tong J, Zheng Q, Zhang C, Lo R, Shen J, Ran Z. Incidence, prevalence, and temporal trends of microscopic colitis: a systematic review and meta-analysis. Am J Gastroenterol. 2015;110(2):265-76.
2. Bergman D, Clements MS, Khalili H, Agréus L, Hultcrantz R, Ludvigsson JF. A nationwide cohort study of the incidence of microscopic colitis in Sweden. Aliment Pharmacol Ther. 2019;49(11):1395-400.
3. Zabana Y, Ferrer C, Aceituno M, Salas A, Fernández-Bañares F. Advances for improved diagnosis of microscopic colitis in patients with chronic diarrhoea. Gastroenterol Hepatol. 2017;40(2):107-16.

4. Fernández-Bañares F, Zabana Y, Aceituno M, Ruiz L, Salas A, Esteve M. Prevalence and natural history of microscopic colitis: A population-based study with long-term clinical follow-up in Terrassa, Spain. J Crohn's Colitis. 2016;10(7):805-11.
5. Pisani LF, Tontini GE, Vecchi M, Pastorelli L. Microscopic colitis: what do we know about pathogenesis? Inflamm Bowel Dis. 2016;22:450-8.
6. Bürgel N, Bojarski C, Mankertz J, Zeitz M, Fromm M, Schulzke JD. Mechanisms of diarrhea in collagenous colitis. Gastroenterol. 2002;123(2):433-43.
7. Göranzon C, Kumawat AK, Hultgren-Hörnqvist E, Tysk C, Eriksson S, Bohr J, et al. Immunohistochemical characterisation of lymphocytes in microscopic colitis. J Crohns Colitis. 2013;7(10):e434-42.
8. Ung KA, Gillberg R, Kilander A, Abrahamsson H. Role of bile acids and bile acid binding agents in patients with collagenous colitis. Gut. 2000;46(2):170-5.
9. Järnerot G, Bohr J, Tysk C, Eriksson S. Faecal stream diversion in patients with collagenous colitis. Gut. 1996;38(1):154-5.
10. Daferera N, Kumar Kumawat A, Hultgren-Hörnqvist E, Ignatova S, Ström M, Münch A. Fecal stream diversion and mucosal cytokine levels in collagenous colitis: A case report. World J Gastroenterol. 2015;21(19):6065-71.
11. Millien V, Rosen D, Hou J, Shah R. Proinflammatory sulfur-reducing bacteria are more abundant in colonic biopsies of patients with microscopic colitis compared to healthy controls. Dig Dis Sci. 2019;64(2):432-8.
12. Khan MA, Brunt EM, Longo WE, Presti ME. Persistent Clostridium difficile colitis: a possible etiology for the development of collagenous colitis. Dig Dis Sci. 2000;45(5):998-1001.
13. Vesoulis Z, Lozanski G, Loiudice T. Synchronous occurrence of collagenous colitis and pseudomembranous colitis. Can J Gastroenterol. 2000;14(4):353-8.
14. Bohr J, Nordfelth R, Jarnerot G, Tysk C. Yersinia species in collagenous colitis: a serologic study. Scand J Gastroenterol. 2002;37(6):711-4.
15. Mäkinen M, Niemelä S, Lehtola J, Karttunen TJ. Collagenous colitis and Yersinia enterocolitica infection. Dig Dis Sci. 1998;43(6):1341-6.
16. Andersen T, Andersen JR, Tvede M, Franzmann MB. Collagenous colitis: are bacterial cytotoxins responsible? Am J Gastroenterol. 1993;88(3):375-7.
17. Burke KE, Ananthakrishnan AN, Lochhead P, Liu PH, Olen O, Ludvigsson JF, et al. Identification of menopausal and reproductive risk factors for microscopic colitis-results from the Nurses' Health study. Gastroenterology. 2018;155(6):1764-75.
18. Verhaegh BPM, Pierik MJ, Goudkade D, Cuijpers YSMT, Masclee AAM, Jonkers DMAE. Early life exposure, lifestyle, and comorbidity as risk factors for microscopic colitis: A case-control study. Inflamm Bowel Dis. 2017;23(6):1040-6.
19. Fine KD, Do K, Schulte K, Ogunji F, Guerra R, Osowski L, et al. High prevalence of celiac sprue-like HLA-DQ genes and enteropathy in patients with the microscopic colitis syndrome. Am J Gastroenterol. 2000;95(8):1974-82.
20. Koskela RM, Karttunen TJ, Niemelä SE, Lehtola JK, Ilonen J, Karttunen RA. Human leucocyte antigen and TNFα polymorphism association in microscopic colitis. Eur J Gastroenterol Hepatol. 2008;20(4):276-82.
21. Madisch A, Hellmig S, Schreiber S, Bethke B, Stolte M, Miehlke S. Allelic variation of the matrix metalloproteinase-9 gene is associated with collagenous colitis. Inflamm Bowel Dis. 2011;17(11):2295-8.

22. Nore E, Mellander M, Almer S, Soderman J. Genetic variation and gene expression levels of tight junction genes indicates relationships between PTEN as well as MAGI1 and microscopic colitis. Dig Dis Sci. 2018;63:105-12.
23. Green HD, Beaumont RN, Thomas A, Hamilton B, Wood AR, Sharp S, et al. Genome-wide association study of microscopic colitis in the UK Biobank confirms immune-related pathogenesis. J Crohns Colitis. 2019;13(12):1578-82.
24. Olesen M, Eriksson S, Bohr J, Jarnerot G, Tysk C. Lymphocytic colitis: a retrospective clinical study of 199 Swedish patients. Gut. 2004;53:536-41.
25. Shor J, Churrango G, Hosseini N, Marshall C. Management of microscopic colitis: challenges and solutions. Clin Exp Gastroenterol. 2019;12:111-20.
26. Kakar S, Pardi DS, Burgart LJ. Colonic ulcers accompanying collagenous colitis: implication of nonsteroidal anti-inflammatory drugs. Am J Gastroenterol. 2003;98(8):1834-7.
27. Keszthelyi D, Jansen SV, Schouten GA, de Kort S, Scholtes B, Engels L, et al. Proton pump inhibitor use is associated with an increased risk for microscopic colitis: a case-control study. Aliment Pharmacol Ther. 2010; 32:1124-8.
28. Verhaegh BP, deVries F, Masclee AA, Keshavarzian A, deBoer A, Souverein PC, et al. High risk of drug induced microscopic colitis with concomitant use of NSAIDs and proton pump inhibitors. Aliment Pharmacol Ther. 2016;43:1004-13.
29. Bonderup OK, Nielsen GL, Dall M, Pottegård A, Hallas J. Significant association between the use of different proton pump inhibitors and microscopic colitis: a nationwide Danish case-control study. Aliment Pharmacol Ther. 2018;48(6)1-8.
30. Fernández-Bañares F, de Sousa MR, Salas A, Beltrán B, Piqueras M, Iglesias E, et al. Epidemiological risk factors in microscopic colitis: a prospective case-control study. Inflamm Bowel Dis. 2013;19(2):411-7.
31. Choi K, Abu-Sbeih H, Samdani R, Nogueras Gonzalez G, Raju GS, Richards DM, et al. Can immune checkpoint inhibitors induce microscopic colitis or a brand new entity? Inflamm Bowel Dis. 2019;10;25(2):385-93.
32. Saad RE, Shobar RM, Jakate S, Mutlu EA. Development of collagenous colitis in inflammatory bowel disease: two case reports and a review of the literature. Gastroenterol Rep (Oxf). 2019;7(3):218-22.
33. Green PH, Yang J, Cheng J, Lee AR, Harper JW, Bhagat G. An association between microscopic colitis and celiac disease. Clin Gastroenterol Hepatol. 2009;7(11):1210-6.
34. Boland K, Nguyen GC. Microscopic colitis: A review of collagenous and lymphocytic colitis. Gastroenterol Hepatol. 2017;13(11):671-7.
35. Kao KT, Pedraza BA, McClune AC, Rios DA, Mao YQ, Zuch RH, et al. Microscopic colitis: a large retrospective analysis from a health maintenance organization experience. World J Gastroenterol. 2009;15(25):3122-7.
36. Vigren L, Tysk C, Strom M, Kilander AF, Hjortswang H, Bohr J, et al. Celiac disease and other autoimmune diseases in patients with collagenous colitis. Scand J Gastroenterol. 2013;48(8):944-50.
37. Sonnenberg A, Turner KO, Genta RM. Associations of microscopic colitis with other lymphocytic disorders of the gastrointestinal tract. Clin Gastroenterol Hepatol. 2018;16(11):1762-7.
38. Gentile N, Yen EF. Prevalence, pathogenesis, diagnosis, and management of microscopic colitis. Gut Liver. 2018;12(3):227-35.

39. Vigren L, Sjöberg K, Benoni C, Tysk C, Bohr J, Kilander A, et al. Is smoking a risk factor for collagenous colitis? Scand J Gastroenterol. 2011;46(11):1334-9.
40. Yen EF, Pokhrel B, Du H, Nwe S, Bianchi L, Witt B, et al. Current and past cigarette smoking significantly increase risk for microscopic colitis. Inflamm Bowel Dis. 2012;18(10):1835-41.
41. Fernández-Bañares F, de Sousa MR, Salas A, Beltrán B, Piqueras M, Iglesias E, et al. Impact of current smoking on the clinical course of microscopic colitis. Inflamm Bowel Dis. 2013;19(7):1470-6.
42. Erim T, Alazmi WM, O'Loughlin CJ, Barkin JS. Collagenous colitis associated with Clostridium difficile: a cause effect? Dig Dis Sci. 2003;48(7):1374-5.
43. Perk G, Ackerman Z, Cohen P, Eliakim R. Lymphocytic colitis: a clue to an infectious trigger. Scand J Gastroenterol. 1999;34(1):110-2.
44. Nyhlin N, Wickbom A, Montgomery SM, Tysk C, Bohr J. Long-term prognosis of clinical symptoms and health-related quality of life in microscopic colitis: a case-control study. Aliment Pharmacol Ther. 2014;39(9):963-72.
45. Kane JS, Irvine AJ, Derwa Y, Ford AC. Fatigue and its associated factors in microscopic colitis. Therap Adv Gastroenterol. 2018;11:175628481879959.
46. Bohr J, Tysk C, Eriksson S, Abrahamsson H, Järnerot G. Collagenous colitis: a retrospective study of clinical presentation and treatment in 163 patients. Gut. 1996;39(6):846-51.
47. Macaigne G, Lahmek P, Locher C, Boivin JF, Lesgourgues B, Yver M, et al. Over 90% of cases of microscopic colitis can be diagnosed by performing a short colonoscopy. Clin Res Hepatol Gastroenterol. 2017;41(3):333-40.
48. Langner C, Aust D, Ensari A, Villanacci V, Becheanu G, Miehlke S, et al. Histology of microscopic colitis review with a practical approach for pathologists. Histopathology. 2015;66(5):613-26.
49. Stotzer PO, Abrahamsson H, Bajor A, Kilander A, Sadik R, Sjövall H, et al. Are the definitions for chronic diarrhoea adequate? Evaluation of two different definitions in patients with chronic diarrhoea. United European Gastroentrol J. 2015;3(4):381-6.
50. Cotter TG, Binder M, Harper EP, Smyrk TC, Pardi, DS. Optimization of a scoring system to predict microscopic colitis in a cohort of patients with chronic diarrhea. J Clin Gastroenterol. 2017;51:228-34.
51. Bohr J, Wickbom A, Hegedus A, Nyhlin N, Hultgren Hornquist E, Tysk C. Diagnosis and management of microscopic colitis: current perspectives. Clin Exp Gastroenterol. 2014;8:273-84.
52. Wildt S, Nordgaard-Lassen I, Bendtsen F, Rumessen JJ. Metabolic and inflammatory faecal markers in collagenous colitis. Eur J Gastroenterol Hepatol. 2007;19(7):567-74.
53. Fine KD, Ogunji F, George J, Niehaus MD, Guerrant RL. Utility of a rapid fecal latex agglutination test detecting the neutrophil protein, lactoferrin, for diagnosing inflammatory causes of chronic diarrhea. Am J Gastroenterol. 1998;93(8):1300-5.
54. Conroy S, Hale MF, Cross SS, Swallow K, Sidhu RH, Sargur R, et al. Unrestricted faecal calprotectin testing performs poorly in the diagnosis of inflammatory bowel disease in patients in primary care. J Clin Pathol. 2018;71(4):316-22.
55. Batista L, Ruiz L, Ferrer C, Zabana Y, Aceituno M, Arau B, et al. Usefulness of fecal calprotectin as a biomarker of microscopic colitis in a cohort of patients with chronic watery diarrhoea of functional characteristics. Dig Liver Dis. 2019;51(12):1641-51.

56. Park HS, Han DS, Ro YO, Eun CS, Yoo KS. Does lymphocytic colitis always present with normal endoscopic findings? Gut Liver. 2015;9:197.
57. Jobse P, Flens MJ, Loffeld RJ. Collagenous colitis: description of a single centre series of 83 patients. Eur J Intern Med. 2009;20(5):499-502.
58. Cimmino DG, Mella JM, Pereyra L. A colorectal mosaic pattern might be an endoscopic feature of collagenous colitis. J Crohns Colitis. 2010;4:139-43.
59. Simondi D, Pellicano R, Reggiani S, Pallavicino F, David E, Squazzini C, et al. A retrospective study on a cohort of patients with lymphocytic colitis. Revista Española de Enfermedades Digestivas. 2010;102(6):381-4.
60. Saito S, Tsumura T, Nishikawa H, Takeda H, Nakajima J, Kanesaka T, et al. Clinical characteristics of collagenous colitis with linear ulcerations. Digestive Endoscopy. 2014;26(1):69-76.
61. Fumery M, Kohut M, Gower-Rousseau C, Duhamel A, Brazier F, Thelu F, et al. Incidence, clinical presentation, and associated factors of microscopic colitis in Northern France: A population-based study. Dig Dis Sci. 2017;62(6):1571-9.
62. Mellander MR, Ekbom A, Hultcrantz R, Löfberg R, Öst A, Björk J. Microscopic colitis: a descriptive clinical cohort study of 795 patients with collagenous and lymphocytic colitis. Scand J Gastroenterol. 2016;51(5):556-62.
63. Koskela RM, Niemelä SE, Lehtola JK, Bloigu RS, Karttunen TJ. Gastroduodenal mucosa in microscopic colitis. Scand J Gastroenterol. 2011;46(5):567-76.
64. Suzuki G, Meliander MR, Suzuki A, Rubio CA, Lambert R, Björk J, et al. Usefulness of colonoscopic examination with indigo carmine in diagnosing microscopic colitis. Endoscopy. 2011;43:1100-4.
65. Narabayashi K, Murano M, Egashira Y, Noda S, Kawakami K, Ishida K, et al. Endoscopic and histopathological evaluation of collagenous colitis. Digestion. 2012;85(2):136-40.
66. Iacucci M, Urbanski S. Recognition of microscopic colitis at colonoscopy. Can J Gastroenterol. 2012;26(4):183-4.
67. Kobayashi M, Hoshi T, Morita S, Kanefuji T, Suda T, Hasegawa G, et al. Magnifying image-enhanced endoscopy for collagenous colitis. Endosc Int Open. 2017;05: 1069-73.
68. Yung DE, Koulaouzidis A, Fineron P, Plevris JN. Microscopic colitis: a misnomer for a clearly defined entity? Endoscopy. 2015;47(8):754-7.
69. Zambelli A, Villanacci V, Buscarini E, Bassotti G, Albarello L. Collagenous colitis: a case series with confocal laser microscopy and histology correlation. Endoscopy. 2008;40:606-8.
70. Koulaouzidis A, Saeed AA. Distinct colonoscopy findings of microscopic colitis: not so microscopic after all? World J Gastroenterol. 2011;17(37):4157-65.
71. Koulaouzidis A, Yung DE, Nemeth A, Sjoberg K, Giannakou A, Qureshi R, et al. Macroscopic findings in collagenous colitis: a multi-center, retrospective, observational cohort study. Ann Gastroenterol. 2017;30:309-14.
72. Grassia R, Capone P, Villanacci V, Tanzi GP, Buffoli F. Endoscopic features of microscopic colitis: The "grid-like" pattern detected with HD+ colonoscopy plus i-scan. Dig Liver Dis. 2017;49(3):318-9.
73. East JE, Vleugels JL, Roelandt P, Bhandari P, Bisschops R, Dekker E, et al. Advanced endoscopic imaging: European Society of Gastrointestinal Endoscopy (ESGE) Technology Review. Endoscopy. 2016;48(11):1029-45.

74. Elliott PR, Williams CB, Lennard-Jones JE, Dawson AM, Bartram CI, Thomas BM, et al. Colonoscopic diagnosis of minimal change colitis in patients with a normal sigmoidoscopy and normal air-contrast barium enema. Lancet. 1982;1(8273):650-1.
75. Sharaf RN, Shergill AK, Odze RD, Krinsky ML, Fukami N, Jain R, et al. Endoscopic mucosal tissue sampling. Gastrointest Endosc. 2013;78(2):216-24.
76. Guagnozzi D, Landolfi S, Vicario M. Towards a new paradigm of microscopic colitis: Incomplete and variant forms. World J Gastroenterol. 2016;22(38):8459-71.
77. Levy A, Borren NZ, Maxner B, Tan W, Bellavance D, Staller K, et al. Cancer risk in microscopic colitis: a retrospective cohort study. BMC Gastroenterol. 2019;19(1):1.
78. O'Toole A. Optimal management of collagenous colitis: a review. Clin Exp Gastroenterol. 2016;9:31-9.
79. Fernández-Bañares F, Casanova MJ, Arguedas Y, Beltrán B, Busquets D, Fernández JM, et al. Current concepts on microscopic colitis: evidence-based statements and recommendations of the Spanish microscopic colitis group. Aliment Pharmacol Ther. 2016;43(3):400-26.
80. Hjortswang H, Tysk C, Bohr J, Benoni C, Kilander A, Larsson L, et al. Defining clinical criteria for clinical remission and disease activity in collagenous colitis. Inflamm Bowel Dis. 2009;15(12):1875-81.
81. Cotter TG, Binder M, Loftus EV Jr, Abboud R, McNally MA, Smyrk TC, et al. Development of a Microscopic Colitis Disease Activity Index: a prospective cohort study. Gut. 2018;67(3):441-6.
82. Münch A, Langner C. Microscopic colitis: clinical and pathologic perspectives. Clin Gastroenterol Hepatol. 2015;13(2):228-36.
83. Münch A, Bohr J, Miehlke S, Benoni C, Olesen M, Öst A, et al. BUC-63 investigators. Lowdose budesonide for maintenance of clinical remission in collagenous colitis: a randomised, placebo-controlled, 12-month trial. Gut. 2016;65(1):47-56.
84. Miehlke S, Aust D, Mihaly E, Armerding P, Böhm G, Bonderup O, et al. Efficacy and safety of budesonide, vs mesalazine or placebo, as induction therapy for lymphocytic colitis. Gastroenterol. 2018;155(6):1795-804.
85. Bonderup OK, Hansen JB, Teglbjaerg PS, Christensen LA, Fallingborg JF. Long-term budesonide treatment of collagenous colitis: a randomised, double-blind, placebo-controlled trial. Gut. 2009;58:68-72.
86. Gentile NM, Abdalla AA, Khanna S, Smyrk TC, Tremaine WJ, Faubion WA, et al. Outcomes of patients with microscopic colitis treated with corticosteroids: a population-based study. Am J Gastroenterol. 2013;108(2):256-9.
87. Fernandez-Bañares F, Piqueras M, Guagnozzi D, Robles V, Ruiz-Cerulla A, Casanova MJ, et al. Collagenous colitis: requirement for high-dose budesonide as maintenance treatment. Dig Liver Dis. 2017;49(9):973-97.
88. Chande N, Al Yatama N, Bhanji T, Nguyen TM, McDonal WJ, MacDonal JK. Interventions for treating lymphocytic colitis. Cochrane Database Syst Rev. 2017;7:CD006096.
89. Fine K, Lee E, Lafon G. Randomized double-blind, placebo-controlled trial of bismuth subsalicylate for microscopic colitis. Gastroenterology. 1999;116:A880.
90. Colussi D, Salari B, Stewart KO, Lauwers GY, Richter JR, Chan AT, et al. Clinical characteristics and patterns and predictors of response to therapy in collagenous and lymphocytic colitis. Scand J Gastroenterol. 2015;50(11):1382-8.
91. Calabrese C, Fabbri A, Areni A, Zahlane D, Scialpi C, Di Febo G. Mesalazine with or without cholestyramine in the treatment of microscopic colitis: randomized controlled trial. J Gastroenterol Hepatol. 2007;22(6):809-14.

92. Pardi DS, Ramnath VR, Loftus EV, Tremaine WJ, Sandborn WJ. Lymphocytic colitis: clinical features, treatment, and outcomes. Am J Gastroenterol. 2002;97(11):2829-33.

93. Madisch A, Miehlke S, Eichele O, Mrwa J, Bethke B, Kuhlisch E, et al. Boswellia serrata extract for the treatment of collagenous colitis. A double-blind, randomized, placebo-controlled, multicenter trial. Int J Colorectal Dis. 2007;22(12):1445-51.

94. Wildt S, Munck LK, Vinter-Jensen L, Hanse BF, Nordgaard-Lassen I, Christensen S, et al. Probiotic treatment of collagenous colitis: a randomized, double-blind, placebo-controlled trial with Lactobacillus acidophilus and Bifidobacterium animalis subsp. lactis. Inflamm Bowel Dis. 2006;12(5):395-401.

95. Tromm A, Niewerth U, Khoury M, Baestlein E, Wilhelms G, Schulze J, et al. The probiotic E. coli strain Nissle 1917 for the treatment of collagenous colitis: first results of an open-label trial. Z Gastroenterol. 2004;42(5):365-9.

96. Rohatgi S, Ahuja V, Makharia GK, Rai T, Das P, Dattagupta S, et al. VSL#3 induces and maintains short-term clinical response in patients with active microscopic colitis: a two-phase randomised clinical trial. BMJ Open Gastroenterol. 2015;2(1):e000018.

97. Münch A, Fernandez-Banares F, Munck LK. Azathioprine and mercaptopurine in the management of patients with chronic, active microscopic colitis. Aliment Pharmacol Ther. 2013;37(8):795-8.

98. Cotter TG, Kamboj AK, Hicks SB, Tremaine WJ, Loftus EV, Pardi DS. Immune modulator therapy for microscopic colitis in a case series of 73 patients. Aliment Pharmacol Ther. 2017;46(2):169-74.

99. Riddell J, Hillman L, Chiragakis L, Clarke A. Collagenous colitis: oral low-dose methotrexate for patients with difficult symptoms: long-term outcomes. J Gastroenterol Hepatol. 2007;22(10):1589-93.

100. Münch A, Bohr J, Vigren L, Tysk C, Ström M. Lack of effect of methotrexate in budesonide-refractory collagenous colitis. Clin Exp Gastroenterol. 2013;6:149-52.

101. Esteve M, Mahadevan U, Sainz E, Rodriguez E, Salas A, Fernández-Bañares F. Efficacy of anti-TNF therapies in refractory severe microscopic colitis. J Crohns Colitis. 2011;5(6):612-8.

102. Cushing KC, Mino-Kenudson M, Garber J, Lochhead P, Khalili H. Vedolizumab as a novel treatment for refractory collagenous colitis: a case report. Am J Gastroenterol. 2018;113(4):632-3.

103. Rivière P, Münch A, Michetti P, Chande N, de Hertogh G, Schoeters P, et al. Vedolizumab in refractory microscopic colitis: an international case series. J Crohns Colitis. 2019;26(13):337-40.

104. Günaltay S, Rademacher L, Hultgren Hörnquist E, Bohr J. Clinical and immunologic effects of faecal microbiota transplantation in a patient with collagenous colitis. World J Gastroenterol. 2017;23(7):1319-24.

105. Varghese L, Galandiuk S, Tremaine WJ, Burgart LJ. Lymphocytic colitis treated with proctocolectomy and ileal J-pouch-anal anastomosis: report of a case. Dis Colon Rectum. 2002;45(1):123-6.

106. Yusuf TE, Soemijarsih M, Arpaia A, Goldberg SL, Sottile VM. Chronic microscopic enterocolitis with severe hypokalemia responding to subtotal colectomy. J Clin Gastroenterol. 1999;29(3):284-8.

107. Cotter TG, Pardi DS. Current approach to the evaluation and management of microscopic colitis. Curr Gastroenterol Rep. 2017;19(2):8.

CHAPTER

4

Eosinophilic Gastroenteritis: Eosinophilic Gastrointestinal Disorders Distal to the Esophagus

Her Hsin Tsai

INTRODUCTION

Eosinophilic gastrointestinal disorders (EGID) are a group of gastrointestinal (GI) conditions that are characterized by often dense eosinophilic infiltration of the GI tract. Depending on the site involved, it may be variously referred to in the literature as eosinophilic esophagitis (EoE), eosinophilic gastritis (EG), eosinophilic gastroenteritis, enteritis (EGE), and eosinophilic colitis (EC). While gastric, small and large bowel involvement have been recognized for over 80 years, EoE is a more recently recognized clinical entity and is well reviewed in the literature. This review will thus focus on gastrointestinal eosinophilic diseases distal to the esophagus. For the purpose of this review, EGID is the umbrella term covering all the different parts of the GI tract affected.

CLASSIFICATION

Eosinophilic gastroenteritis was first described by Kaijser in 1937 on surgical resection specimens who correctly referred to it as an "allergic affection".[1] Attempts to classify it were made by Klein et al. in 1970.[2] Aside from the site of disease, they classified the condition into three distinct groups:
- *Type 1* has a predominantly mucosal disease only without muscularis infiltration or serosal disease
- *Type 2* has infiltration of the muscularis but without serosal disease or ascites
- *Type 3* involves the serosa as well as presence of ascites.

There is some degree of correlation between the histological type and clinical manifestation of the disease. Mucosal disease might result in diarrhea but does not result in obstructive symptoms. Type 2 would result in narrowing of the gut and obstructive symptoms while type 3 would have both obstructive symptoms and ascites. The exact symptoms would also depend on site—dysphagia in esophageal disease, vomiting if gastric outlet narrowing occurs, and more classical obstructive symptoms if the small bowel is affected. Mucosal disease in colonic involvement would manifest itself as diarrheal disease.

EPIDEMIOLOGY

Eosinophilic gastrointestinal disorder is relatively rare. Based on pediatric survey, it is estimated to have a prevalence of around 22–28 per 100,000 of the population.[3] This figure is likely to be underrepresented and if we include adult cases, the figure is likely to be higher. It still remains a rare disease. Another study estimated the prevalence of EG, EGE, and colitis to be 6.3/100,000, 8.4/100,000, and 3.3/100,000, respectively in United States.[4] EG/EGE can affect patients of any age, but in adults typically presents in the third through fifth decades and has a peak age of onset in the third decade.[5]

PATHOGENESIS

The etiology and pathogenesis of EGID are not fully understood. However, there is good epidemiologic evidence of an allergic component. As with many allergic conditions like asthma, there are raised IgE levels and peripheral eosinophilia.[6,7] In the GI tract, the role of food as possible allergens is based on reports of elimination diets being of benefit in patients with EGID. There is involvement of interleukin-5 (IL-5) which is pivotal in expressing food allergen-specific T-helper 2 (Th2) response.[8] A detailed discussion of eosinophils in the gut in health and disease is available in Chapter 5.

CLINICAL FEATURES

A history of atopic conditions is frequently encountered. There may be defined food allergies, eczema, asthma, and rhinitis.[8]

The clinical manifestation of eosinophilic GI disorders will depend on site affected and class (depth) of eosinophilic infiltration. Hence in the esophagus, the main feature is dysphagia. If the inflammation affects the body and antrum of stomach, it may result in epigastric symptoms of pain and nausea/vomiting. If the small bowel is affected, there would be pain and perhaps small bowel obstruction as well. Colonic involvement would typically result in diarrhea. Mucosal involvement may result in malabsorption while muscularis involvement may lead to dysmotility of the area affected. In the esophagus, it will result in dysmotility, reflux, and dysphagia. Thickening of the antrum of the stomach or wall of the small bowel may result in gastric outlet obstruction or small bowel obstruction. One study suggested a predominance of duodenal, ileal, and colonic involvement with gastric involvement less frequently encountered.[9] If the serosa is affected then there may be ascites. Very occasionally, pleural effusion may occur. In both abdominal ascitic fluid and pleural effusion, the aspirate will be teeming with eosinophils.[10]

CLINICAL ASSESSMENT

As with any patient with a GI complaint, history is paramount in elucidating the problem. A drug history is essential (both prescription and nonprescription medication). Drug-induced eosinophilia syndromes are not uncommon. There may be a rash associated. History of atopy and any food intolerances should be evaluated. Ingestion of poorly cooked meats from endemic areas should raise concern of parasitic infestations and history of travel to areas where parasitic infestations are prevalent should be noted.

A full physical examination should focus on the abdomen. There may be palpable mass which may or may not be tender. If there is gastric obstruction, a succession splash may be heard and bowel sounds may be active in small bowel hold-up. Look for signs of other organs being involved (skin, eyes, and lymph glands) that may suggest an alternative diagnosis.

Laboratory Findings

Table 1 lists the number (not exhaustive) of useful laboratory investigations. The most common finding is raised peripheral eosinophil count found in over 70% of presentations. The eosinophil count can fluctuate and historic results if available could also be helpful. Counts are usually over 500/μL, typically 500–3,500/μL. On average, levels of 1,000/μL are usual.

IgE levels are raised in children but less often in adults.[6] Stool examination is essential to exclude a variety of parasitic infestations. Serology for HIV, *Strongyloides*, and *Toxocara* may be useful. Iron deficiency is a common feature. Celiac antibody may be helpful. In patients presenting with diarrheal illness, fecal calprotectin is frequently requested. It is helpful in distinguishing between function bowel problems and organic ones. There are few studies in EGID but calprotectin levels are modestly raised, to levels of 50–100 mg/kg but not to the very high levels encountered in inflammatory bowel diseases which tend to be over 500 mg/kg in active disease.[11]

Imaging

A plain abdominal film is often performed if the patient presents to an emergency department. This may show some mucosal thickening in the form of "islands" or "nodules". These reflect areas of the gut with infiltrative disease. Occasionally there is evidence of subacute small bowel obstruction with dilated loops of bowel with fluid levels. Perforation is extremely rare but has been documented.

Table 1: Laboratory investigation.

Full blood count film examination	Biochemistry profile
Immunoglobulins, IgE	Iron studies
HIV serology	Tryptase (mastocytosis/hypereosinophilia syndromes)
Stool examination (cysts, ova)	Parasite serology (strongyloides, toxocara)
C-reactive protein (CRP)	Fecal calprotectin

Computed tomography (CT) scan is widely performed in patients with abdominal symptoms. Magnetic resonance imaging (MRI) is also very helpful in investigating these patients. These imaging modalities will show the affected part of the GI tract with gut wall thickening. This can be very dramatic as seen in the antrum of the stomach in **Figures 2 and 3**. The appearance will depend on the depth of eosinophilic involvement. Mucosal disease may show thickening and nodularity of antrum and duodenum **(Fig. 4)** or a saw-tooth mucosa **(Fig. 7)**. Muscular involvement would reveal luminal narrowing especially in the antrum **(Figs. 2 and 3)** with marked thickening and signs of gastric hold-up with food remnants. In the small bowel, there may be irregular thickening and signs of small bowel hold-up.

Endoscopy

If the site of EGID involvement is accessible to an endoscope, it should be performed and mucosal biopsy specimen obtained. Thus esophageal, gastric, and duodenal diseases are amiable to an upper GI endoscopy and colonic and terminal ileal disease can be accessed with a colonoscope. The appearances can vary from mucosal edema to frank ulceration, but is usually more subtle **(Figs. 1, 5 and 6)**. In the stomach there may be thickening of the folds and in the antrum, mild reddening and thickening. The appearances may mimic *linitis plastica* which is caused by infiltrative tumor of the stomach. Biopsy (sometimes deep mucosal biopsies) will be required to differentiate the two. In the duodenum, there may be raised nodular lesions. In the colon, the inflammation is often patchy and subtle, frank ulceration and spontaneous bleeding or contact bleeding is uncommon.[12] Biopsies should be obtained from any inflamed looking mucosa. In general, mucosal biopsies would suffice. Deep mucosal biopsies are rarely needed and fine-needle aspiration (FNA) is seldom required to establish diagnosis.

Laparoscopy

It is rare to require laparoscopic biopsy. If there is lymph node involvement or suspicion of lymphoma then a laparoscopic examination and a full-thickness biopsy can be performed.

Ascitic Tap

In patients with ascites, ascitic fluid analysis should include cell count with differential, Gram stain, culture, acid-fast bacillus stain, fungal and mycobacterial cultures, and cytology. Although there are no established criteria for ascitic fluid eosinophilia, studies have reported markedly elevated eosinophil counts in patients with EGID with ascites.

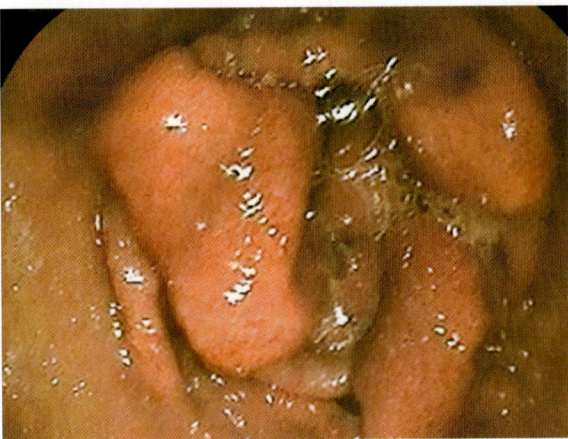

Fig. 1: Eosinophilic gastritis with thickened pylorus.

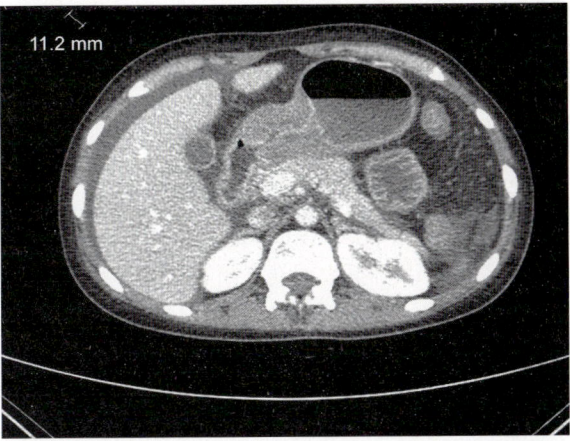

Fig. 2: CT scan showing marked antral thickening of the stomach.

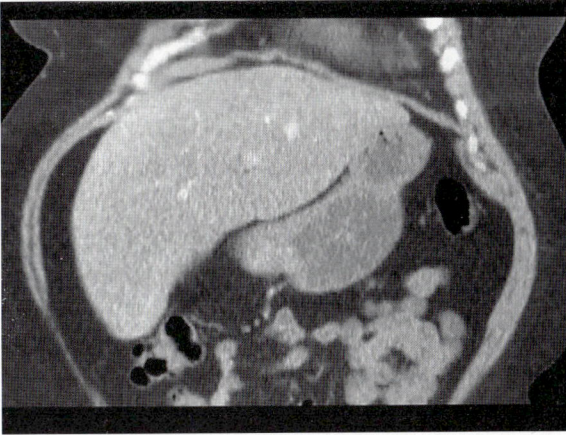

Fig. 3: CT scan of the above coronal view.

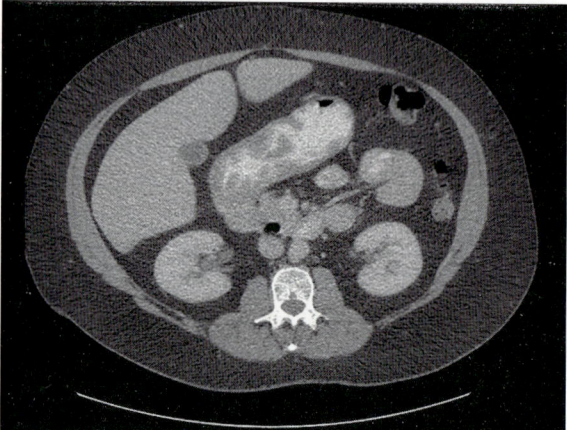

Fig. 4: Duodenal involvement with nodular appearance on CT.

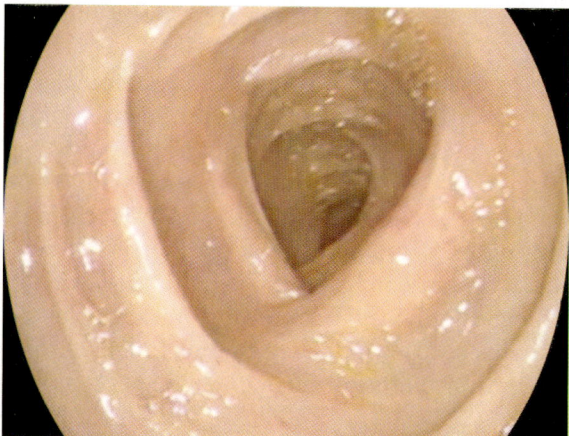

Fig. 5: Eosinophilic colitis affecting the transverse colon.

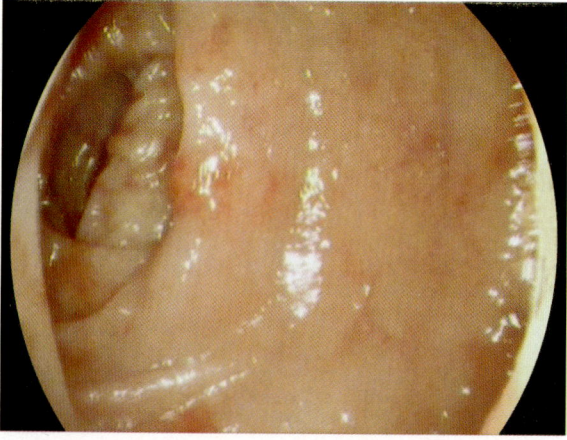

Fig. 6: Colonoscopic appearance of sigmoid eosinophilic colitis.

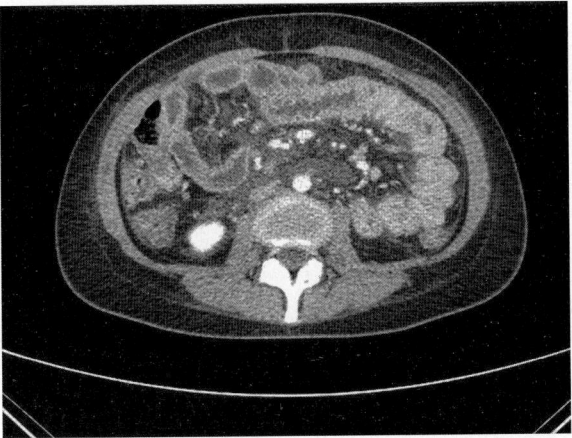

Fig. 7: Small bowel involvement of eosinophilic gastroenteritis.

DIAGNOSIS

Diagnosis is made on histological examination of affected tissue. With the exception of the esophagus, eosinophils can be present in normal physiologic states throughout the rest of the GI tract. Thus the diagnosis of mucosal EGID is established by the presence of more than the number of expected eosinophils on microscopic examination of biopsies of the GI tract. There is no agreed number of eosinophils per microscopic field to make the diagnosis. It depends largely on an experienced histopathologist's call. Many other inflammatory conditions such as inflammatory bowel disease and drug-induced changes may show an excess of eosinophils in the biopsy.

Conventional staining is with hematoxylin and eosin stain (HE) staining **(Fig. 8A to C)** with the eosinophils staining bright pink. It is readily recognized by cell morphology and staining counts made per high power field. Collins had suggested cut-off numbers of eosinophils that would suggest a diagnosis of EGID **(Table 2)**.[13]

Ultimately the diagnosis is made on the combination of clinical presentation, radiological features, and endoscopic and histological correlation. This is best achieved in a multidisciplinary team meeting and presentation of all the evidence together and reaching the most appropriate diagnosis.

DIFFERENTIAL DIAGNOSIS

Many conditions can mimic eosinophilic GI disorders. These include conditions where peripheral eosinophilia is present.

Malignancy

Many malignant conditions are associated with raised peripheral eosinophil count.[14] In addition, the radiological features may show thickening of the

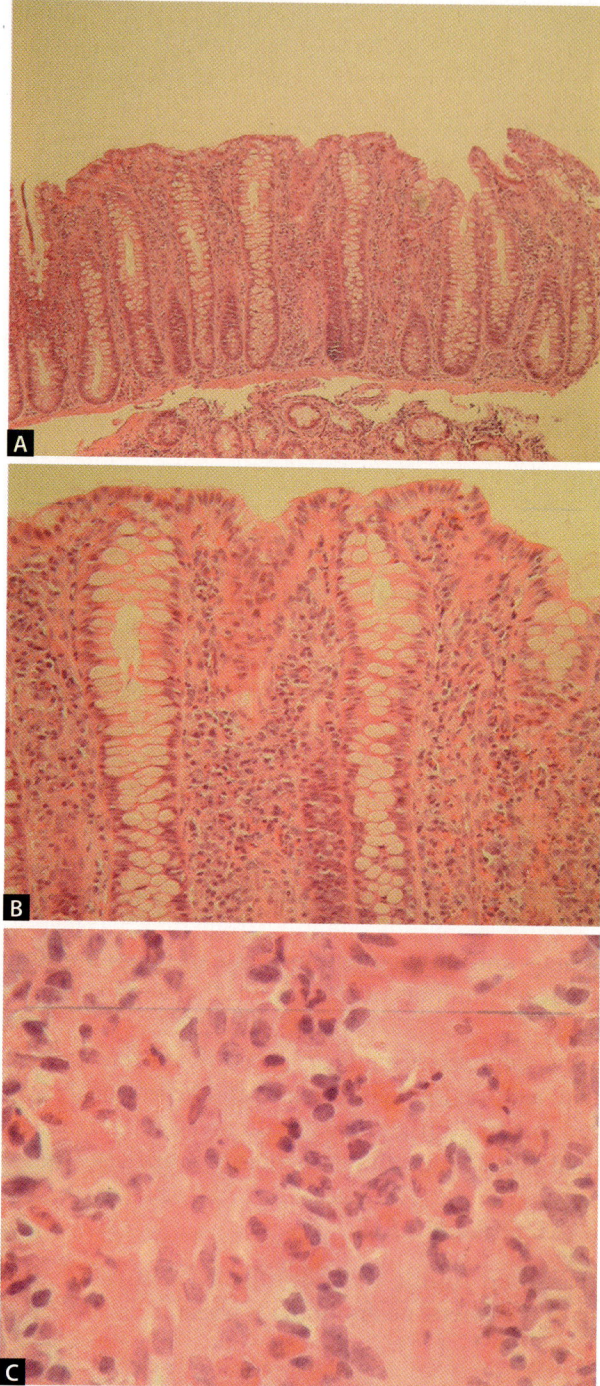

Figs. 8A to C: Histology of EGID. (A) Low magnification power; (B) Higher magnification; (C) High magnification.
Courtesy: Dr L Karsai.

Table 2: Suggested cut-off levels of eosinophils in biopsies.	
	Eosinophils per high-power field (HPF) in 5 HPF
Stomach	≥30 eosinophils
Duodenum	≥30 eosinophils
Ileum	>56 per HPF in the ileum
Right colon	>100 per HPF
Transverse and descending colon	>84 per HPF
Rectosigmoid colon	>64 per HPF

gut wall. They may also present with obstructive symptoms. In the stomach, infiltrative gastric cancer (*linitis plastica*) can have very similar appearance on CT. Obstruction or localized thickening of colon may more likely be cancer than an esoteric condition like EGID. Endoscopy should be possible in most cases and biopsy readily establishes the diagnosis. Lymphoma may be more difficult and may require laparoscopy node or full thickness biopsy of affected bowel.

Inflammatory Bowel Disease

Symptoms of abdominal pain and diarrhea similarly occur in initial presentation of inflammatory bowel diseases. Crohn's disease can affect the upper GI tract but most commonly the terminal ileum. Ulcerative colitis will tend to produce more confluent inflammation and biopsy obtained at colonoscopy should show crypt abscesses and distortion suggesting a chronic inflammatory bowel disease and granuloma may be seen in Crohn's disease biopsies. Occasionally, there may be an excess of eosinophils in histological samples of the colonic biopsies and it is important to consult an experienced histopathologist.

Parasitic Infestations

Infection with *Ancylostoma, Anisakis, Ascaris, Basidiobolomycosis, Capillaria, Strongyloides, Toxocara, Trichiura*, and *Trichinella* can all cause GI symptoms and peripheral eosinophilia. Infection with the dog hookworm, *Ancylostoma caninum*, can mimic EGID clinically and pathologically with eosinophilic infiltration of the gut wall and ascites.[15] However, a parasitic infection can be excluded by examination of the stool for ova or parasites and/or serologic testing. In addition, stool examination in patients with a parasitic infection may reveal Charcot-Leyden crystals, which are the product of eosinophil granules.

Hypereosinophilic Syndrome

Hypereosinophilic syndrome (HES) is an idiopathic condition associated with marked peripheral eosinophilia and may rarely present with GI symptoms as well. Many EGID patients may fulfill the diagnostic criterion for HES (absolute eosinophil count ≥ 1,500 cells/mL present for over 6 months). However, in contrast with EGID, HES involves multiple organ systems (e.g., heart, lungs, brain, and kidneys).[16]

Other Rare Conditions

Polyarteritis nodosa (PAN) is associated with peripheral eosinophilia and abdominal pain. Nodular masses may also be visualized in the stomach, but, in contrast with EGID, patients with PAN have systemic manifestations, a markedly elevated erythrocyte sedimentation rate, and on biopsy, the eosinophilia is perivascular. Eosinophilic granulomatosis with polyangiitis (Churg-Strauss syndrome) is a vasculitis condition which can affect the bowel with abdominal pain, diarrhea, gastrointestinal bleeding, and colitis. Asthma is the cardinal feature of this disorder (occurring in >95% of patients) and usually precedes the vasculitic phase by approximately 8 to 10 years. Eosinophilic granuloma (Langerhans cell histiocytosis), such as EG, can present as a gastric antral mass. However, it can be differentiated from EGID by its typical granulomatous appearance on biopsy.[17]

NATURAL HISTORY AND CLINICAL COURSE

The natural history and clinical course of EGID are not fully elucidated. However, there is a French study of 43 patients whom they followed up for a mean of 13 years. They found that disease phenotype can be classified as mucosal, subserosal, or muscular in 44%, 39%, and 12%, respectively. Disease location was mostly duodenal (62%), ileal (72%), or colonic (88%); it was less frequently esophageal (30%) or gastric (38%). Blood eosinophilia (numbers > 500/mm^3) was observed in 74% of cases. Spontaneous remission occurred in 40% of patients; the majority of treated patients (74%) received oral corticosteroids, which were effective in most cases. After a median follow-up period of 13 years (0.8–29 years), they identified three different courses of disease progression—18 patients (42%; 9 with subserosal disease) had an initial flare of the disease without relapse, 16 (37%) had multiple flares that were separated by periods of full remission (recurring disease), and 9 (21%) had chronic disease.[9]

MANAGEMENT

There are few controlled trials to base our evidence of best treatment practice. The few trials that are available are on EoE and many of the recommendations below are based on these studies and extended to cover other sites. Treatments that work for EoE may not necessarily apply to other sites. Efforts are now gathering pace to have a consortium to tackle the critical issues of best treatment for these patients. One such consortium is the Consortium of Eosinophilic Gastrointestinal Disease Researchers.[18] One of their projects

"The Outcome Measures for Eosinophilic Gastrointestinal Diseases across Ages (OMEGA)" is an observational, prospective, multicenter study of the clinical, endoscopic, histologic, molecular, and patient-reported outcomes (PROs) in pediatric and adult patients with EGIDs, namely, EoE, EG, and EC, and is focused on defining the natural history of EGIDs. The results of this study are eagerly awaited.

Dietary Therapy

The mainstay of treatment is either dietary or drugs. The rationale behind dietary therapy is the hypothesis that food is the main trigger of the allergic response. However specific testing for food allergens such as skin testing has consistently been less than useful with fewer than 20% having any proven allergies. However, trials have shown benefit from dietary therapy.[19] There are three different dietary approaches to the management of EGID—(1) the elemental diet, (2) the removal of foods based on allergy testing, and (3) the removal of the foods that are most commonly blamed for eosinophilic gastroenteritis.

Elemental diet in its complete form consists of amino acids, short chain fatty acids, and carbohydrates. As such it has no food allergens. However, to have a complete diet of elemental feeds is expensive and unpleasant to take. In most cases and in pediatric practice, a nasogastric tube is usually required to deliver the feeds. The second strategy does not appear to work. Food testing rarely identifies the incriminating allergen or food. The most practical approach is the removal of foods most commonly associated with allergic conditions. A combination approach may also be practical, with the use of elemental diets and transitioning or weaning to an exclusion diet.

There had been a few small studies of dietary therapy in EoE. A retrospective observational study assessed the short-term clinical and histologic responses of two cohorts of children with EE evaluated during two different time periods—one was treated with the standard six-food elimination diet (SFED) and the other was treated with elemental diet (ELED). Of the 60 children who met the inclusion criteria and were compliant with the dietary protocol, 35 were treated with a diet excluding cow-milk protein, soy protein, wheat, egg, peanut, and seafood while allowing all other table foods and 25 were treated exclusively with ELED. Repeat esophageal biopsy specimens were obtained at least 6 weeks later. 26 of 35 (74%) in the SFED group and 22 of 25 (88%) in the ELED group achieved significant improvement of esophageal inflammation (≤10 eosinophils/high-power field). The pretreatment and post-treatment peak eosinophil counts for the SFED were 80.2 ± 44.0 and 13.6 ± 23.8 ($p < 0.0001$) and 58.8 ± 31.9 and 3.7 ± 6.5 ($p < 0.001$) for the ELED group, respectively.[20]

Compliance is the main limitation of dietary therapy. Even highly motivated patients may find elemental diets unpleasant and exclusion diets hard to adhere to. Careful coaching from a dietitian would be necessary to consolidate patient education. Avoidance of proscribed foods while maintaining adequate nutrition may be difficult, especially in children. Supplementation with vitamins and other micronutrients may be necessary.

If the patient is adherent to the dietary therapy, it has to be continued for at least 6 weeks before reintroducing foods. The patient can be monitored using peripheral eosinophil counts. A response is a reduction of eosinophils by 50%. In patients without a peripheral eosinophilia, the clinical response may be based on symptom improvement. A simple PRO may be all that is necessary which may vary according to disease site. In some cases, histological monitoring may be justified. If endoscopic samples are easily obtained, then a follow-up biopsy at 6 weeks may be obtained. There is a disconnect between reported symptom severity and histological appearance, so such an approach has its merits.

In another study, 50 adults with EoE underwent esophagogastroduodenoscopies (EGDs), biopsies, and skin-prick tests for food and aeroallergens. After 6 weeks of SFED, patients underwent repeat EGD and biopsies. The mean peak eosinophil counts in the proximal and distal esophagus were reduced significantly after the SFED ($p < 0.0001$). After the SFED, 64% of patients had peak counts ≤5 eosinophils/high-power field and 70% had peak counts of ≤10 eosinophils/high-power field. Symptom scores decreased in 94% ($p < 0.0001$). After food reintroduction, esophageal eosinophil counts returned to pretreatment values ($p < 0.0001$). Based on reintroduction, the foods most frequently associated with EoE were wheat (60% of cases) and milk (50% of cases). Skin-prick testing predicted only 13% of foods associated with EoE.[21]

The success of dietary therapy depends on motivation of the patient, good dietetic support, and careful individualizing of therapy.

Adrenocorticosteroids

Corticosteroids have been extensively used in eosinophilic and allergic disorders like asthma. Its use in EGID is logical and intuitive. However, there are few trials to base our evidence on. It is usual to start steroids if dietary therapy fails or compliance is difficult. A dose of prednisolone 20–40 mg/day should suffice. Response usually is apparent within 2 weeks and then a rapid taper over the following 2 weeks can be initiated. The goal of therapy is to induce clinical response while avoiding the toxic effects of corticosteroids.[22]

Monitoring of response is usually by symptoms as peripheral eosinophilia does not accurately predict tissue response. Steroids can quite rapidly reduce peripheral eosinophilia. If response is poor, then further clinical evaluation may be necessary.

In the majority of cases, the patient responds to therapy, and successfully tapered. If they do flare up again, then the same therapy should work. Many patients stay in remission for many months or even years so this strategy of intermittent therapy is sound.

In a few patients, the standard oral therapy with prednisolone is ineffective or if they have difficulty taking oral medication or in sick patients with bowel hold-up, then intravenous steroids may be indicated. The equivalent dose of 100 mg hydrocortisone intravenously a day is usually adequate and as soon as able, a switch to oral product is instituted.

In a few patients, steroid taper is rapidly met with recurrence of symptoms. These patients may be regarded as steroid-dependent. Prolonged use of steroids is best avoided. If the dose is low (below 10 mg prednisolone a day) then it may be considered after individualizing risks/benefits of such a strategy. Alternatively, one can use budesonide, which has a high first-pass metabolism by the liver and hence reducing the systemic side effects of steroids. One such preparation is a controlled-release version budesonide (3–9 mg/day) in which the drug is released into the terminal ileum. It would be appropriate with disease affecting the terminal ileum and colon. In this situation, the drug may be used for up to 3–6 months if necessary. Some systemic toxicity occurs in the higher doses of the drug. For the proximal gut, it may be possible to use budesonide preparations. These have been studied in EoE and both budesonide slurry and triamcinolone are equally effective.[23] There is little reason to imagine that it will not work in gastric and duodenal disease as well. If the slurry is not available, breaking a slow-release budesonide tablet may be an option for proximal disease.

Other Drug Therapies

The use of azathioprine as immunomodulatory and steroid-sparing agent is widespread in inflammatory bowel disease but there are no reports of its use in EGID except a single case report. Hence at the present moment, its use cannot be recommended.[24]

Sodium cromoglycate (cromolyn) (800 mg/day in four divided doses) is a mast cell stabilizer and has been tried in EGID.[25] This drug prevents the release of inflammatory chemicals such as histamine from mast cells. It is reasonably safe to try as a long-term alternative to steroids. However, there is the usual paucity of information about its efficacy.

The leukotriene inhibitor montelukast has been reportedly of benefit in a few case reports.[26] Furthermore, a clinical response to suplatast tosilate, which is a novel antiallergic drug that suppresses cytokine production, including interleukin (IL)-4 and IL-5 from T-helper 2 cells, was described in a single patient.[27]

There has been intriguing reports of the successful use of clarithromycin (500 mg bd) in EGE.[12,28] It is unlikely to be due to its antibiotic effects but perhaps more likely through its anti-inflammatory and immunomodulatory properties. Treatment with macrolides significantly reduces the secretion of proinflammatory cytokines, ILs, and tumor necrotic factors in both sputum and plasma[29] and macrolide triggers the eosinophil apoptosis by the suppression of the IL-5-induced prolongation of eosinophil survival.[30]

Biologic therapies of specific antibodies against target cytokines have promised much but unfortunately failed to deliver consistent results. One such is the use of humanized anti-IL-5 antibody treatment. IL-5 is pivotal in eosinophil biology and as such would seem an obvious target. However, to date, two such antibodies (mepolizumab and reslizumab) have been disappointing. Despite a demonstrable reduction in esophageal eosinophilia, only a minority of patients have a complete histological response in EoE. The maximal effect of anti-IL-5 on esophageal eosinophilia appears to reach a plateau within weeks, at which point no further improvements can be achieved by increasing the dosing regimen.[31,32] The effect of treatment on symptoms is also inconsistent. Furthermore, rebound eosinophilia has been observed after treatment is discontinued.[33]

Omalizumab is an anti-IgE monoclonal antibody that has been associated with a significant improvement in symptoms and measures of IgE-mediated allergy in an open label, single arm, unblinded study on patients with EoE. Omalizumab was administered for 12 weeks to 15 subjects with longstanding EoE.[34] The results of a more rigorous randomized controlled trial are awaited.

Eosinophilic gastrointestinal disorders are rare and challenging conditions to the GI physician. Understanding the biology of eosinophils and their role in these conditions will help equip the GI physicians to more adequately meet the challenges of management of these patients.[12]

SUMMARY

- Eosinophilic gastrointestinal diseases are a group of conditions characterized by dense infiltration of eosinophils in the GI tract.
- It can occur in any part of the GI tract and can be mucosal only, muscularis or transmural with serosal disease.
- Clinical manifestations depend on the site and depth (class) of disease.
- Diagnosis is made by histological findings of appropriate biopsy sample.
- Treatment is dietary elimination and the use of short courses of steroids.

REFERENCES

1. Kaijser R. Zur Kenntnis der allergischen Affektionen des Verdauungs-Kanals vom Standpunkt des Chirurgien aus. Arch Klin Chir. 1937;188:36-64.
2. Klein NC, Hargrove RL, Sleisenger MH, Jeffries GH. Eosinophilic gastroenteritis. Medicine (Baltimore). 1970;49(4):299-319.
3. Spergel JM, Book WM, Mays E, Song L, Shah SS, Talley NJ, et al. Variation in prevalence, diagnostic criteria, and initial management options for eosinophilic gastrointestinal diseases in the United States. J Pediatr Gastroenterol Nutr. 2011;52(3):300-6.
4. Jensen ET, Martin CF, Kappelman MD, Dellon ES. Prevalence of eosinophilic gastritis, gastroenteritis, and colitis: estimates from a national administrative database. J Pediatr Gastroenterol Nutr. 2016;62(1):36-42.

5. Talley NJ, Shorter RG, Phillips SF, Zinsmeister AR. Eosinophilic gastroenteritis: a clinicopathological study of patients with disease of the mucosa, muscle layer, and subserosal tissues. Gut. 1990;31(1):54-8.
6. Caldwell JH, Tennenbaum JI, Bronstein HA. Serum IgE in eosinophilic gastroenteritis. Response to intestinal challenge in two cases. N Engl J Med. 1975;292(26):1388-90.
7. Min KU, Metcalf DD. Eosinophilic gastroenteritis. Immunol Allergy Clin North Am. 1991;11:799-813.
8. Pineton de Chambrun G, Dufour G, Tassy B, Rivière B, Bouta N, Bismuth M, et al. Diagnosis, natural history, and treatment of eosinophilic enteritis: a review. Curr Gastroenterol Rep. 2018;20(8):37.
9. Pineton de Chambrun G, Gonzalez F, Canva JY, Gonzalez S, Houssin L, Desreumaux P, et al. Natural history of eosinophilic gastroenteritis. Clin Gastroenterol Hepatol. 2011;9(11):950-6.
10. Cello JP. Eosinophilic gastroenteritis—a complex disease entity. Am J Med. 1979;67(6):1097-104.
11. Komraus M, Wos H, Wiecek S, Kajor M, Grzybowska-Chlebowczyk U. Usefulness of faecal calprotectin measurement in children with various types of inflammatory bowel disease. Mediators Inflamm. 2012;2012:608249.
12. Phaw NA, Tsai HH. Eosinophilic gastroenteritis: a challenge to diagnose and treat. BMJ Case Rep. 2016;2016:bcr2016215964.
13. Collins MH. Histopathologic features of eosinophilic esophagitis and eosinophilic gastrointestinal diseases. Gastroenterol Clin North Am. 2014;43(2):257-68.
14. Viola MV, Chung E, Mukhopadhyay MG. Eosinophilia and metastatic carcinoma. Med Ann Dist Columbia. 1972;41(1):1-3.
15. Walker NI, Croese J, Clouston AD, Parry M, Loukas A, Prociv P. Eosinophilic enteritis in northeastern Australia. Pathology, association with *Ancylostoma caninum*, and implications. Am J Surg Pathol. 1995;19(3):328-37.
16. Fauci AS, Harley JB, Roberts WC, Ferrans VJ, Gralnick HR, Bjornson BH. NIH conference. The idiopathic hypereosinophilic syndrome. Clinical, pathophysiologic, and therapeutic considerations. Ann Intern Med. 1982;97(1):78-92.
17. Blackshaw AJ, Levison DA. Eosinophilic infiltrates of the gastrointestinal tract. J Clin Pathol. 1986;39(1):1-7.
18. Gupta SK, Falk GW, Aceves SS, Chehade M, Collins MH, Dellon ES, et al. Consortium of Eosinophilic Gastrointestinal Disease Researchers: Advancing the field of eosinophilic GI disorders through collaboration. Gastroenterology. 2019;156(4):838-42.
19. Spergel JM, Shuker M. Nutritional management of eosinophilic esophagitis. Gastrointest Endosc Clin N Am. 2008;18(1):179-94.
20. Kagalwalla AF, Sentongo TA, Ritz S, Hess T, Nelson SP, Emerick KM, et al. Effect of six-food elimination diet on clinical and histologic outcomes in eosinophilic esophagitis. Clin Gastroenterol Hepatol. 2006;4(9):1097-102.
21. Gonsalves N, Yang GY, Doerfler B, Ritz S, Ditto AM, Hirano I. Elimination diet effectively treats eosinophilic esophagitis in adults; food reintroduction identifies causative factors. Gastroenterology. 2012;142(7):1451-9.

22. Chen MJ, Chu CH, Lin SC, Shih SC, Wang TE. Eosinophilic gastroenteritis: clinical experience with 15 patients. World J Gastroenterol. 2003;9(12):2813-6.
23. Dellon ES, Woosley JT, Arrington A, McGee SJ, Covington J, Moist SE, et al. Efficacy of budesonide vs fluticasone for initial treatment of eosinophilic esophagitis in a randomized controlled trial. Gastroenterology. 2019;157(1):65-73.
24. Netzer P, Gschossmann JM, Straumann A, Sendensky A, Weimann R, Schoepfer AM. Corticosteroid-dependent eosinophilic oesophagitis: azathioprine and 6-mercaptopurine can induce and maintain long-term remission. Eur J Gastroenterol Hepatol. 2007;19(10):865-9.
25. Perez-Millan A, Martin-Lorente JL, Lopez-Morante A, Yuguero L, Saez-Royuela F. Subserosal eosinophilic gastroenteritis treated efficaciously with sodium cromoglycate. Dig Dis Sci. 1997;42(2):342-4.
26. Vanderhoof JA, Young RJ, Hanner TL, Kettlehut B. Montelukast: use in pediatric patients with eosinophilic gastrointestinal disease. J Pediatr Gastroenterol Nutr. 2003;36(2):293-4.
27. Shirai T, Hashimoto D, Suzuki K, Osawa S, Aonahata M, Chida K, et al. Successful treatment of eosinophilic gastroenteritis with suplatast tosilate. J Allergy Clin Immunol. 2001;107(5):924-5.
28. Ohe M, Hashino S. Successful treatment of eosinophilic gastroenteritis with clarithromycin. Korean J Intern Med. 2012;27(4):451-4.
29. Pukhalsky AL, Shmarina GV, Kapranov NI, Kokarovtseva SN, Pukhalskaya D, Kashirskaja NJ. Anti-inflammatory and immunomodulating effects of clarithromycin in patients with cystic fibrosis lung disease. Mediators Inflamm. 2004;13(2):111-7.
30. Adachi T, Motojima S, Hirata A, Fukuda T, Kihara N, Kosaku A, et al. Eosinophil apoptosis caused by theophylline, glucocorticoids, and macrolides after stimulation with IL-5. J Allergy Clin Immunol. 1996;98(Pt 2):S207-15.
31. Straumann A, Conus S, Grzonka P, Kita H, Kephart G, Bussmann C, et al. Anti-interleukin-5 antibody treatment (mepolizumab) in active eosinophilic oesophagitis: a randomised, placebo-controlled, double-blind trial. Gut. 2010;59(1):21-30.
32. Spergel JM, Rothenberg ME, Collins MH, Furuta GT, Markowitz JE, Fuchs G 3rd, et al. Reslizumab in children and adolescents with eosinophilic esophagitis: results of a double-blind, randomized, placebo-controlled trial. J Allergy Clin Immunol. 2012;129(2):456-63.
33. Kim YJ, Prussin C, Martin B, Law MA, Haverty TP, Nutman TB, et al. Rebound eosinophilia after treatment of hypereosinophilic syndrome and eosinophilic gastroenteritis with monoclonal anti-IL-5 antibody SCH55700. J Allergy Clin Immunol. 2004;114(6):1449-55.
34. Loizou D, Enav B, Komlodi-Pasztor E, Hider P, Kim-Chang J, Noonan L, et al. A pilot study of omalizumab in eosinophilic esophagitis. PLoS ONE. 2015;10(3):e0113483.

CHAPTER
5

Eosinophils and the Gut: Eosinophils in the Human Intestinal Tract in Normal Conditions and Major Colorectal Diseases

Alexandre Loktionov

INTRODUCTION

Eosinophils constitute a subtype of granulocyte leukocytes that had been identified over 150 years ago, but for many years, they were regarded as terminally differentiated effector cells mostly involved in cytotoxic action against helminths and exertion of allergic reactions. Recent investigations, however, revealed multiple previously unknown roles performed by eosinophils, and such important functions as control of inflammatory responses, maintenance of epithelial barriers, tissue remodeling, and coordination of innate and adaptive immunity are now proven to be among them.[1-3] Human eosinophils are permanently generated in the bone marrow, and eosinophilopoiesis with its complex regulatory mechanisms was comprehensively described in a few recent reviews.[4-6] Eosinophil maturation occurs in the bone marrow under the influence of eosinophil-promoting hematopoietic cytokines that include interleukins IL-5 and IL-3 and granulocyte–macrophage colony-stimulating factor.[6,7] It is now postulated that terminally differentiated eosinophils formed in the bone marrow are no longer able to proliferate and possess all typical characteristics of mature cells of this lineage. A simplified scheme of eosinophil development is shown in the bottom part of **Figure 1**.

STRUCTURAL AND FUNCTIONAL CHARACTERISTICS OF MATURE EOSINOPHILS

Human eosinophils are easily identifiable microscopically by conventional histological staining with hematoxylin and eosin. Typical bilobed nuclei and large specific granules stained red by eosin make them easy to distinguish from leukocytes of other types. The specific cytoplasmic granules of eosinophils are organelles possessing a unique structure. Electron microscopy allowed establishing that they have a dense crystalline core, which is surrounded by a less dense outer matrix and enclosed in a trilaminar membrane.[2,8] Cytotoxic cationic proteins (major basic proteins 1 and 2, eosinophil cationic protein, eosinophil-derived neurotoxin, eosinophil peroxidase and Charcot–Leyden crystal protein) constitute the main component of the specific granules, but

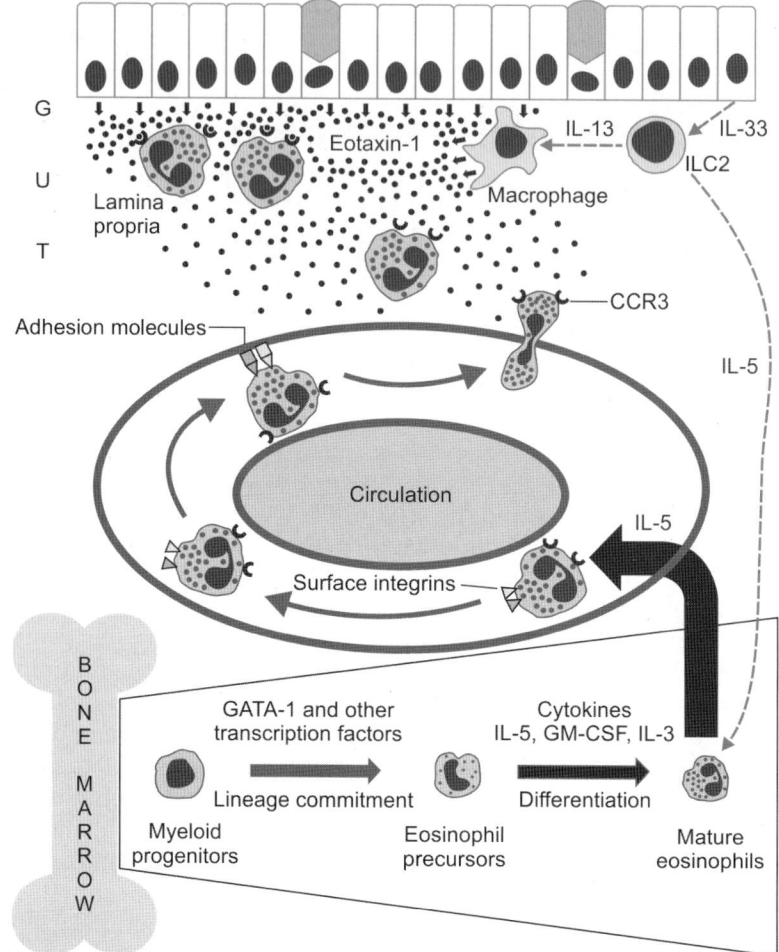

Fig. 1: Eosinophilopoiesis and migration of mature eosinophils to the gut.
(ILC2: type 2 innate lymphoid cells; GM-CSF: granulocyte-macrophage colony-stimulating factor)

these organelles also store a plethora of other pre-formed biologically active substances comprising cytokines, growth factors, chemokines, and enzymes readily available for extremely rapid stimulus-triggered release.[2,6,9,10] Other eosinophil-specific organelles include lipid bodies involved in the production of lipid mediators of inflammation[11] and pleomorphic vesiculotubular carriers often called eosinophil sombrero vesicles.[12]

Secretion of biologically active products stored in the granules (or degranulation) constitutes the core of all functional activities of eosinophils. Recent studies suggest that the piecemeal degranulation (PMD) is the most common secretory mechanism used by these cells.[2,3,10] In PMD, specific granule-derived proteins are differentially packaged into spherical or tubular secretory vesicles that are transported through the cytoplasm to the cell membrane. These vesicles are then fused with the membrane, releasing their contents to the extracellular space. Importantly, PMD leaves specific granules intact and only partially emptied, thus repetitive rounds of this process are possible.[10] In humans, PMD is a highly specific receptor-mediated process typically employed by eosinophils for rapid release of pre-formed cytokines involved in inflammatory and allergic responses.[3,10] Another commonly observed mechanism of eosinophil degranulation is cytolysis, which is associated with rapid cell death accompanied by chromatin decondensation, dissolution of nuclear and plasma membranes, and the release of intact cell-free specific granules that preserve their functionality extracellularly.[10,13] Interestingly, eosinophil cytolysis often results in the formation of "extracellular traps," net-like structures formed by the released histone-coated DNA strands and initially described in neutrophils.[14] This phenomenon was later observed in other innate immune cells,[15] and in case of eosinophils, the released intact specific granules are associated with the nets formed by DNA, thus combining bactericidal and cytotoxic properties of histone-coated DNA and cationic proteins of the granules.[16] Moreover, an alternative nonlethal mechanism of extracellular trap formation (ETosis) involving mitochondrial DNA release combined with PMD and associated with antibacterial action was also described for eosinophils.[17] These features of ETosis and cytolytic degranulation of eosinophils may be especially important for gastrointestinal (GI) barrier maintenance and major colorectal diseases.

Secretory functions of eosinophils depend on their ability to respond to a variety of molecular signals, and these cells were demonstrated to express numerous surface markers including receptors for adhesion molecules, cytokines, chemokines, growth factors, lipid mediators, as well as pattern recognition receptors and Fc receptors.[3,18] Receptors for cytokines and chemokines were also found to be located on the surface of the specific granules,[13,19] thus confirming their functional autonomy. Comprehensive recent reviews[3,18] provide us detailed information on eosinophil surface markers.

MIGRATION OF EOSINOPHILS TO THE GUT

It is generally accepted that GI tract is the main destination of the mature eosinophils leaving the bone marrow and entering the circulation. Early experiments of Mishra et al. allowed establishing that these granulocytes are already detectable in the intestinal *lamina propria* of 19-day-old mouse embryos,[20] which indicates that eosinophil migration to the gut does not depend on the subsequent colonization of the colonic lumen by microbiota. In the normal conditions, the esophagus is the only segment of the GI tract devoid of eosinophils.[20] The process of eosinophil egress from the bone marrow is believed to be primarily regulated by IL-5 that causes their trafficking into the peripheral circulation. Human eosinophils stay in the circulation for about 25 hours[21] before eventual extravasation at destination sites followed by amoeboid movement in the interstitial space.[22] Eosinophil transendothelial crossing in the gut is governed by interactions between cell surface integrins expressed by eosinophils and endothelial adhesion molecules (VCAM-1, MadCAM-1 and ICAM-1) of capillaries located in the gut mucosa.[23] Extravasated eosinophils continue their journey to the *lamina propria*, being chemotactically attracted by chemokine eotaxin-1 (CCL-11) that interacts with eosinophil surface CCR3 receptor.[6,24] It was shown that eotaxin-1 production in the intestinal mucosa is exerted by intestinal macrophages and epithelial cells.[25] Notably, it emerges that the regulation of eosinophil trafficking largely depends on long-lived type 2 innate lymphoid cells (ILC2) residing in peripheral tissues including the gut. ILC2 cells secrete IL-5, thus maintaining its serum levels, and are also able to co-express IL-13, which stimulates eotaxin-1 production by macrophages of the *lamina propria*.[26] In its turn, IL-13 expression appears to depend on the availability of IL-33.[27] These regulatory mechanisms are schematically shown in **Figure 1**. It should, however, be noted that Fu et al. have recently reported that human intestinal allografts from adult donors contain functional hematopoietic stem cells and progenitor cells.[28] If confirmed, this finding may considerably change the existing views on the genesis of immune cells residing in the gut, in particular, eosinophils.

FUNCTIONS OF EOSINOPHILS IN THE NORMAL GUT

In the *lamina propria* of the normal human GI tract, the most significant presence of eosinophils is observed in the colon (especially cecum and ascending colon), with a gradual decrease throughout small intestine and stomach to almost complete absence in the esophagus.[29,30] For this reason, eosinophil role in the normal intestine and colon is clearly more pronounced than in the stomach and esophagus. It is also remarkable that eosinophils isolated from mouse small intestine have a much longer lifetime compared with their counterparts from blood or lung.[31] Recent reinterpretation of the paradigms describing activities of gut-dwelling eosinophils[1,2] resulted in proposing a few major functional areas briefly considered below.

Sustenance of the Integrity and Functionality of the Intestinal Mucosal Barrier

The key element of the mucosal protective barrier is the gut epithelium made up of several cell types exerting specific activities related to absorptive, secretory, and immunosurveillance functions.[32] Alongside selectively absorbing nutrients, water and electrolytes, this epithelium through its goblet cells produces abundant protective mucus overlaying the epithelial surface. In the normal conditions, the epithelial surface throughout the gut is covered by the glycocalyx of enterocytes and colonocytes and well-structured mucin *MUC2*-rich mucus that forms two (inner dense and outer loose) layers in the colon and a single loose layer in the small intestine.[33] This recently characterized gut mucus system is considered in detail in a Chapter 6.

In the normal conditions, the presence of the permanently renewing mucus effectively excludes any contact between microbiota populating the gut lumen and the epithelial surface.[33] The protective action of the mucus is enhanced by the presence of antibacterial α-defensins and lysozyme released by Paneth cells of the small intestine[34] as well as IgA secreted by subepithelial plasma cells of the *lamina propria*.[35,36] The role of immune cells located in the *lamina propria* clearly makes the latter structure an additional layer of the protective intestinal barrier, and gut eosinophils certainly contribute to maintaining mucosal homeostasis. The presence of eosinophils appears to be an important factor for goblet cell development and mucus production since these processes were found to be suppressed in eosinophil-deficient mice.[37] Moreover, eosinophils are likely to be involved in the intestinal permeability regulation, as eosinophil depletion induced by high-fat diet resulted in an increase in intestinal permeability probably reflecting alterations in the integrity of the intestinal protective barrier.[37] Also, there may be links between gut eosinophils and Paneth cells since the both cell types are able to produce antibacterial α-defensins,[38] but these links remain to be investigated. The role of eosinophils in antibacterial action of the gut mucus is further corroborated by the necessity of their presence for maintaining mucosal IgA production by plasma cells of the *lamina propria*.[35,36,39]

Participation in Immunosurveillance of Pathogenic Microbiota of the Gut

Human gut lumen is the home of an immense number of microorganisms, hence constant surveillance and rapid elimination of occasional contacts between bacteria and the mucosal surface is the key task of the GI immune system. It is believed that the main mechanism of immune surveillance in the gut is luminal antigen sampling carried out by immune cells belonging to the gut-associated lymphoid tissue (GALT) that consists of the Peyer's patches of the small intestine, lymphoid aggregates of the colon, and immune cells diffusely distributed throughout the lamina propria. Although it has recently been shown that eosinophils in the *lamina propria* of mice express surface markers (MHCII and CD80) consistent with antigen presentation functions,[40] there is no clarity on their participation in this process in the normal gut. It is suggested that eosinophils are more likely to perform this function as "amateur" antigen-presenting cells in type 2 inflammatory responses.[41] Other immunity-stimulating functions of gut eosinophils include Peyer's patch development promotion[36] and control of CD103(+) dendritic cell activation and migration.[42] In this context, it is also worth recalling already highlighted link between eosinophils and mucosal goblet cells,[36] as goblet cells were shown to be strongly involved in the immune system's exposure to luminal antigens through goblet cell-associated antigen passages.[43]

Impact in the Maintenance of Gut Immune System and Coordination of its Innate and Adaptive Arms

Although innate and adaptive immunity were traditionally regarded as distinct entities, it is now becoming clear that their coordinated interaction provides the most effective immune response.[44] Recent progress in the investigation of innate lymphoid cells (ILCs) allowed suggesting that these cells may bridge the gap between the innate and adaptive immune responses by sensing environmental changes and releasing a wide range of regulatory cytokines.[45] In the gut, ILC2 are known to support the gut-residing eosinophil population[26] and they closely interact with dendritic cells and Th2 lymphocytes.[44] In their turn, gut eosinophils were shown to release Th2-inducing cytokines IL-4 and IL-13 associated with type 2 immune responses,[46] however they were also reported to produce cytokines-targeting Th1 cells.[47] Active interactions of eosinophils with other immune cells residing in the *lamina propria* are already well documented, but it should be admitted that further intense research is required to achieve full understanding of their place in the immune system of the normal gut.

Interactions with the Enteric Nervous System

Intense research of eosinophil involvement in asthma allowed establishing that major basic proteins released from eosinophil granules act as antagonists of inhibitory M_2 muscarinic receptors, thus activating sensory nerves and triggering parasympathetic nerve-mediated responses.[48] It was also demonstrated that eosinophils can produce neurotrophins that stimulate neuron growth,[49] and co-culturing of eosinophils with neuroblastoma cells resulted in an increased expression of cholinergic genes in the nerve cells.[50] Although direct interactions of eosinophils with nerves are certainly possible, it seems to be more probable that in their communication with the enteric nervous system, eosinophils act in concert with mast cells of the *lamina propria*.[51] Paracrine and membrane interactions between eosinophils and mast cells lead to active release of soluble mediators[52] that may stimulate nociceptive enteric nerves as eosinophils and mast cells are typically located in the vicinity of sensory nerve fibers.[51,53] This mechanism is likely to contribute to an increased visceral pain perception in patients with functional GI disorders, especially irritable bowel syndrome that also involves intestinal motility alterations accompanied by diarrhea or constipation.[51] In addition, interaction of eosinophils and mast cells is extremely important for the pathogenesis of GI allergic conditions and infections, but interested readers can find detailed information on these topics elsewhere.[54]

EOSINOPHILS IN THE MAJOR COLORECTAL DISEASES

Eosinophils constitute the dominant pathogenetic element of several hypereosinophilic syndromes often associated with severe GI manifestations that can affect any segment of the GI tract. However, these conditions, often referred to as eosinophilic gastrointestinal diseases, are relatively rare, and specifically focused reviews,[55-57] as well as other chapters of this book describe them in detail. Therefore, further discussion in this chapter is focused on such highly prevalent chronic conditions as inflammatory bowel disease (IBD) and colorectal cancer (CRC).

Eosinophils in IBD

There are two major chronic diseases that account for the majority of IBD cases. Ulcerative colitis (UC) is an inflammatory condition usually confined to the colonic mucosa,[58] and Crohn's disease (CD) is defined as a segmental, asymmetrical, and transmural inflammation that can involve the entire GI tract, but is most commonly limited to the terminal ileum and colon.[59] The pathogenesis of IBD is complex and remains to be completely elucidated, but dysregulated immune responses driving disease development are believed to be triggered by a combination of genetic predisposition, susceptibility to environmental factors, impacts of gut microbiota and deterioration of the intestinal protective barrier.[58-62] The developing inflammatory process eventually leads to inflammation-associated damage to the enteric nervous system that results in abnormal neurotransmission causing such symptoms as severe alterations of bowel motility and abdominal pain.[7,52] Intestinal barrier dysfunction and eventual dysregulation of immune responses can be directly affected by eosinophils accumulating in the gut mucosa of patients with IBD,[6,7,63] particularly in those with UC.[6,64,65] This influx of eosinophils to the *lamina propria* is primarily driven by a considerably increased production of eotaxin-1 by colonocytes[25,66] as well as macrophages[25,67] and B-lymphocytes.[68] It was also demonstrated that eotaxin-2 and eotaxin-3 were produced by colonic epithelial cells alongside eotaxin-1 in both UC and CD, but especially in UC.[69] The eotaxins interact with CCR3 receptor on the surface of eosinophils, but CCR3+ T-lymphocytes were also abundantly present in UC patients and apparently contributed to the mucosal inflammation.[69] Moreover, eosinophil accumulation in the gut of IBD patients is strongly promoted by IL-33, which is associated with the development of Th2 immune responses.[70,71] Again, the IL-33 influence is more pronounced in UC cases.[72,73] The difference between UC and CD is further highlighted by persisting activation of *lamina propria* eosinophils during remission in UC patients, which was not observed in CD cases.[63,66] In general, the distinct patterns of eosinophil involvement in UC and CD pathogenesis are likely to be defined by the difference in prevailing immune response types driving these conditions. While CD is characterized by inflammatory cytokine profile consistent with Th1 immune response combined with Th17 involvement,[74-76] Th2-specific pattern is typical for UC.[44,75-77]

Although gut eosinophils normally have a range of homeostasis-maintaining functions discussed above, these cells start combining this regulatory role with effector behavior once inflammatory reaction is initiated in the intestinal mucosa. Once the protective barrier formed by intestinal or colonic mucus (*see* Chapter 6) is damaged, gut microbiota comes into direct contact with the epithelial surface, and bacterial antigen interactions with the elements of GALT trigger abnormal immune responses resulting in inflammatory disease development. In these conditions, activated eosinophils accumulated in the gut mucosa[63-66] start degranulating, thus releasing cytotoxic granule proteins that aggravate alterations of the epithelium.[78] A plethora of other factors, including proinflammatory cytokines, is simultaneously released by eosinophils as well. It is currently difficult to precisely locate specific targets of eosinophil-derived cytokines within complex cytokine-regulated cascades associated with CD and UC and involving multiple immune cell lineages. Cytokine impacts in IBD pathogenesis are reviewed elsewhere.[75,79] Already mentioned interaction between the enteric nervous system, eosinophils, and mast cells was also shown to contribute to mucosal barrier disruption in UC. Cholinergic signals were demonstrated to activate muscarinic receptors expressed by eosinophils and induce these cells to produce corticotropin-releasing factor that provoked neighboring mast cell degranulation, which increased permeability of colonic epithelial cells to protein antigens.[80] Moreover, concerted action of eosinophils and mast cells may cause neuronal damage and contribute to enhanced nociception and aberrant gut muscle contractility altering peristalsis.[7,53] Another example of inflammation promotion by eosinophils in both CD and UC is the excessive production of IL-22-binding protein (IL-22BP) that inhibits anti-inflammatory cytokine IL-22.[81] In addition, in vitro experiments showed that eosinophils can act in concert with epithelial cells in producing a range of neutrophil attractants that jointly with activated macrophage-generated signaling stimulate neutrophil migration to the intestinal/colonic mucosa when inflammation develops.[82] Dense infiltration of the colonic mucosa with neutrophils is a characteristic feature of UC, where its degree reflects disease activity.[83] In contrast, neutrophil influx into the gut of CD patients seems to be less pronounced, probably due to deficient production of chemotactic mediators by macrophages[84] that were demonstrated to dominate the *lamina propria* in patients with CD.[85]

Pathogenetic mechanisms of IBD were until recently considered mostly at the level of phenomena occurring within the intestinal or colonic wall. Although crypt abscess formation is a typical feature of IBD, the significance of inflammatory cell movement through the epithelial barrier remained poorly understood despite the existing knowledge regarding mechanisms of transepithelial migration of neutrophils.[86,87] It was shown that following transmigration, neutrophils release microparticles that are rich in matrix metalloproteinase 9, which cleaves desmoglein-2, thus disrupting epithelial intercellular adhesions and facilitating further transepithelial migration.[88] Transepithelial migration of other immune cells, including eosinophils, in the gut remains to be investigated. However, experiments in mice have shown that eosinophils rapidly migrate from tracheobronchial mucosa into the airway lumen,[89] and in vitro models of eosinophil migration through cultured airway[90] and intestinal[91] epithelium were successfully applied. Furthermore, detection of both neutrophil- and eosinophil-derived biomarkers in stool is well documented.[92,93] Studies of our group clearly demonstrated the abundant presence of well-preserved inflammatory cells in colorectal mucus samples noninvasively collected from patients with IBD.[94-96] Eosinophils were easily identifiable in these samples, especially in cases of active UC **(Fig. 2)**,[95] and dramatically increased eosinophil-derived neurotoxin (EDN) concentrations correlated with disease activity.[96] The author of this chapter also hypothesized that both neutrophils and eosinophils present in colorectal mucus frequently undergo ETosis resulting in extracellular DNA trap formation that may be both protective from luminal bacteria and damaging for intestinal or colonic epithelium.[6] Interestingly, neutrophil ETosis was previously described within crypt abscesses developing in UC patients.[97] It is also noteworthy that eosinophil-derived extracellular DNA traps released into airway mucus were previously demonstrated to injure epithelial cells in chronic obstructive pulmonary disease[98] and chronic rhinosinusitis.[99] One can assume that intense ETosis within gut mucus can lead to the accumulation of released DNA strands, increasing mucus viscosity and possibly compensating for disease-associated degradation of *MUC2*. Furthermore, colon biopsy sample analysis allowed detecting extracellular DNA traps in both UC[100,101] and CD[101] patients, providing evidence of ETosis occurring in the mucosa. Although the impact of eosinophils in the observed IBD-associated ETosis remains to be elucidated, it is currently impossible to exclude that extracellular histone-coated DNA strands derived from eosinophils during ETosis in the colonic mucus may be abundant in UC patients. These structures are likely

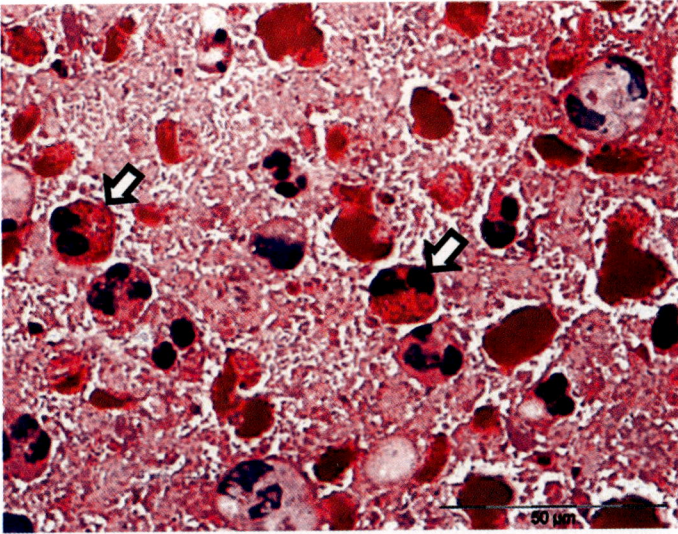

Fig. 2: Eosinophils (marked by arrows) present in colorectal mucus noninvasively collected from a patient with active ulcerative colitis. Neutrophils (including apoptotic cells), macrophages, and erythrocytes are present as well.

to be loaded with entrapped eosinophil granules releasing cytotoxic cationic proteins. Such eosinophil-generated ETosis may cause additional damage to colorectal mucosa, thus contributing to sustained ulceration and constituting a previously unexplored pathogenetic factor in UC and, possibly, in colonic CD.[6]

Transepithelial migration of immune cells is also recognized as an important mechanism involved in disease (or disease flare-up) resolution. This mechanism is known to operate in airway diseases,[102] but we were able to see that in colorectal mucus samples collected from patients with active IBD both inflammatory cell numbers and levels of biomarkers associated with them (including EDN) rapidly declined following successful treatment of disease flare-ups.[96] This phenomenon can be interpreted as a sign of colonic barrier restoration probably accompanied by the inhibition of transepithelial trafficking of immune cells and gradual elimination of dead or obsolete cells by distally moving colorectal mucus.[103]

It is apparent that eosinophils exert a wide range of regulatory functions important for the development of IBD-associated immune responses, but these responses often become inadequate and often host-damaging, especially when effector cytotoxic action of eosinophils becomes excessive and indiscriminate. It appears that structural and functional alterations of the protective barrier of the gut may be induced by eosinophil-derived substances released by these cells on the both sides of this barrier. Although eosinophil role in the pathogenesis of UC seems to be more significant and better understood than in the context of CD, serious gaps in our knowledge of diverse functions of these cells in IBD remain.

Eosinophils in Colorectal Cancer

Cancer, in general, is a multifactorial disease characterized by an extremely complex and incompletely understood pathogenesis that involves a strong immune component that certainly contributes to creating the "tumor microenvironment".[104] Although several types of immune cells (e.g., cytotoxic T-cells, macrophages, dendritic cells) are intensely investigated in relation to neoplasia, the role of other immune cells, in particular eosinophils, surprisingly, remains a conundrum.[105] Both abundant eosinophil presence in tumor tissue and blood eosinophilia are often described in tumors of different sites, but these phenomena were associated with either favorable or unfavorable prognoses that appeared to be site-dependent.[1,2,105,106] The latter feature may reflect specific characteristics of eosinophil populations in different tumor microenvironments.[1,105] In the context of CRC, blood eosinophilia is usually associated with a reduced disease risk[107] and more favorable prognosis.[108,109] Similarly, more pronounced eosinophil infiltration either within the CRC tissue[110,111] or observed peritumorally[112] predicted a better prognosis. However, these descriptive clinical observations did not allow making any conclusions regarding anti-cancer effects of eosinophils in CRC patients.

Although only limited information regarding mechanisms attracting eosinophils to colorectal tumors is available, several possible explanations emerge. Early in vitro experiments demonstrated that necrotic epithelial cells derived from cultured human colorectal adenocarcinoma could induce a positive chemotaxis of human eosinophils, whereas this effect was absent when viable cultured cells were used.[113] It was suggested that eosinophil chemotaxis could be often caused by damage-associated molecular patterns (DAMPs) including the nuclear protein high mobility group box protein 1 (HMGB1).[114] Likewise, IL-33 was shown to be released by damaged and necrotic tissues and is now regarded as alarmin,[115] which can contribute to eosinophil chemotaxis induction. A strong eosinophil-attractant ecalectin was shown to be expressed by human colorectal carcinoma cell lines[116] and eotaxin-1 protein levels were demonstrated to be significantly higher in CRC tissue compared with normal colonic tissue.[117] Moreover, eotaxin-1 and eotaxin-2 expression in the epithelial cells of colorectal adenomas and adenocarcinomas correlated with the degree of eosinophil infiltration within tumor tissue, and tumor progression was associated with significant parallel reductions of eotaxin expression and infiltrating eosinophil numbers.[118] Regulation of eotaxin-1 generation by tumors was recently analyzed by Hollande et al., who demonstrated that tumor-derived IL-33 stimulated eotaxin-1 production, attracting eosinophils, degranulation of which resulted in tumor growth reduction.[119] This study has also shown that eosinophil-mediated anti-tumor action can be enhanced by inhibiting the dipeptidyl peptidase DPP4 (CD26), which downregulates eotaxin-1. Interestingly, DPP4 inhibitor sitagliptin used by the authors is a drug that has already been approved by the US Food and Drug Administration for the treatment of hyperglycemia, thus it could potentially be re-purposed as a novel anti-tumor agent enhancing tumoricidal effect of eosinophils.[120] At the same time, the role of alarmin IL-33 as an important modulator of eosinophil-driven anti-cancer responses in CRC is also becoming clear. In vitro experiments revealed that IL-33 both stimulates eosinophil degranulation and increases their survival.[121] In addition, IL-33-deficient mice were highly susceptible to developing colitis and colitis-associated cancer,[122] and it is impossible to exclude that this could be linked to impaired protective action of eosinophils. Other cytokines secreted by various elements of tumor microenvironment, such as IL-5 produced by ICL2 cells or Th2 lymphocytes may also contribute to eosinophil recruitment to CRC, however this possible mechanism remains to be elucidated.

As eosinophils are known to act as effector cells in type 2 immune responses,[1-3] it is logical to expect that the abundance of these cells in the *lamina propria* greatly facilitates their recruitment in tumor-associated inflammation, which is now recognized as a major cancer-promoting factor.[104] In these circumstances, eosinophils are likely to release both cytotoxic granule proteins and a wide range of pre-formed cytokines, chemokines, growth factors, enzymes, and lipid mediators.[1-3,105] The release of these substances appears to be regulated by interactions with other cells within tumor microenvironment and can be lethal for malignant cells. Tumoricidal activity of eosinophils was proven in vitro when the death of cultured human colon cell carcinoma cells was associated with the release of eosinophil cationic protein, eosinophil-derived neurotoxin, TNFα and proteolytic granzyme A by co-cultured human eosinophils.[123] This anticancer effect also depended on a better contact between eosinophils and malignant cells that depended on the presence of adhesion molecules, LFA-1 and ICAM1, which appeared to be upregulated by IL-18.[124] It is also remarkable that direct tumoricidal effect of eosinophils in vivo was observed in genetically modified mice during experimental induction of inflammation-associated CRC, when massive tumor infiltration with degranulating eosinophils led to tumor rejection.[125] Another eosinophil-generated factor potentially affecting neoplastic growth is ETosis of eosinophils. ETosis is usually interpreted only as a neutrophil-associated phenomenon, and recent experimental study results implicate neutrophil extracellular traps (NETs) produced during inflammation in extracellular matrix remodeling and awakening dormant cancer cells.[126] It is, however, likely that eosinophil ETosis may exert a similar effect. ETosis remains poorly investigated in the context of CRC, but the presence of NETs in colorectal tumors has already been demonstrated.[127] In vitro experiments have also shown that these NETs impeded growths of cultured cancer cells by inducing apoptosis and inhibiting proliferation.[127] As it is usually impossible to distinguish between extracellular DNA traps generated by eosinophils and neutrophils, there is a strong possibility of eosinophil ETosis being an additional mechanism of cancer cell killing by eosinophils, especially given that the histone-coated DNA strands formed during ETosis of eosinophils are associated with the specific granules able to quickly release highly cytotoxic proteins.[16] It is also highly likely that eosinophils transmigrating to the colonic mucus layer may undergo ETosis and constitute an important causative factor in frequent surface ulceration of colorectal malignancies. Nevertheless, as it was discussed earlier in this chapter, this hypothetic mechanism can be a major factor in the development of UC, which is clearly associated with elevated CRC risk.[128] For this reason, eosinophil Etosis possibly may act both as a cancer-promoting and as an anti-cancer factor, depending on pathobiological contexts.

In addition to directly suppressing colorectal tumor growth, eosinophils seem to be able to promote either Th2 or Th1 immune response and influence other effector cells, depending on cytokine profiles in the tumor microenvironment.[47,129] Notably, experiments using xenograft-bearing mice allowed demonstrating that eosinophils infiltrating tumors were able to produce chemoattractants that attracted CD8+ effector T-cells into the tumor, thus facilitating tumor rejection.[130] That study has also shown that tumor-associated eosinophils initiated detectable prognostically favorable changes in the tumor microenvironment, causing macrophage polarization and normalization of the tumor vasculature.[130] Indeed, it is now accepted that the factors produced by eosinophils contribute to tissue repair and remodeling[1-3] and can affect angiogenesis.[1,3,131] It is, however, interesting that eosinophil-derived MBP was shown to stimulate angiogenesis in vitro only at noncytotoxic low concentrations.[131] Intense infiltration of tumor tissue with degranulating eosinophils often observed in CRC patients is most probably associated with high MBP concentrations, not supporting new blood vessel generation. Indeed, MBP was shown to be associated with necrotic areas of solid tumors as experiments with melanoma cell injection model demonstrated.[132] Mechanisms involved in eosinophil attraction to colorectal tumor site and anti-cancer action of these cells are schematically shown in **Figure 3**.

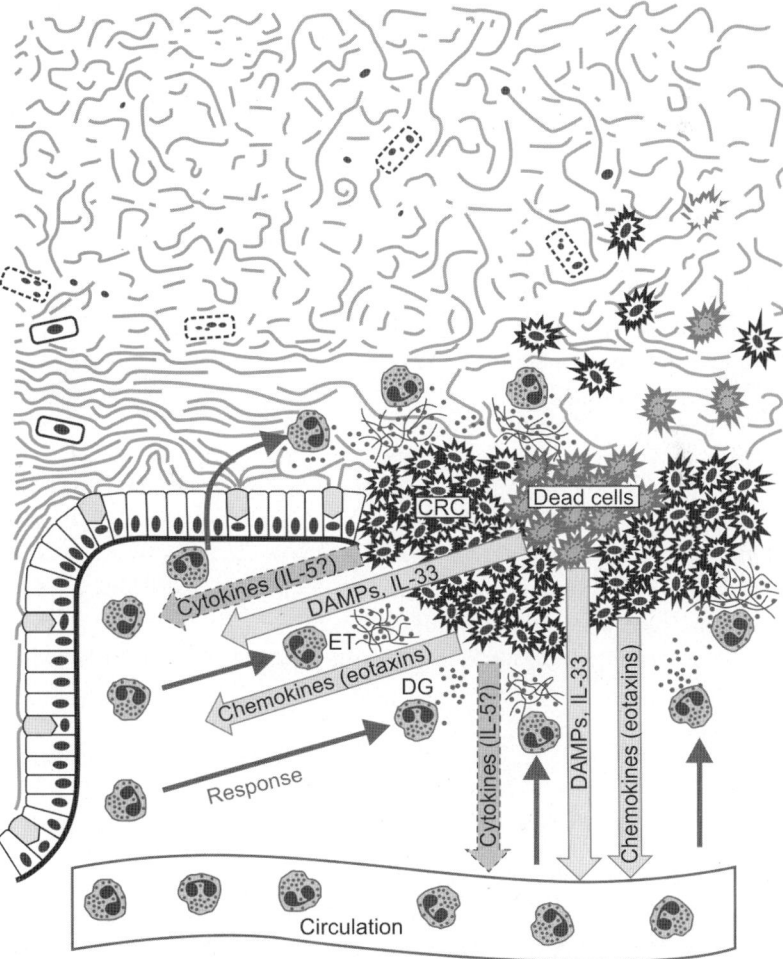

Fig. 3: Eosinophil trafficking to colorectal cancer (CRC) site and their possible direct anti-cancer action.
[DAMPs: damage-associated molecular patterns; DG: degranulation; ET: extracellular DNA trap formation (ETosis)]

It should be admitted that despite several impressive recent studies discussed above, the role of eosinophils in CRC pathogenesis remains only partially understood. This lack of understanding does not allow efficiently developing new eosinophil-targeting methods of CRC treatment today. Only further intense research in the area will provide the required knowledge.

CONCLUSION

Recent advances in eosinophil research have significantly expanded our understanding of multiple biological roles performed by these versatile cells, which uniquely combine protective effector duties and a plethora of varying regulatory functions. Eosinophils are especially important for the gut, being intimately involved in both maintaining homeostasis of this tissue in the normal conditions and contributing to a wide range of immune responses involved in the pathogenesis of such major chronic diseases as IBD and CRC. Despite impressive progress achieved in the last two decades, further research efforts are needed for clarifying highly complex networks of interactions between eosinophils, immune system and other tissue elements of the gut. It can be anticipated that these efforts will result in developing new therapeutic approaches specifically targeting eosinophils.

REFERENCES

1. Lee JJ, Jacobsen EA, McGarry MP, Schleimer RP, Lee NA. Eosinophils in health and disease: the LIAR hypothesis. Clin Exp Allergy. 2010;40(4):563-75.
2. Shamri R, Xenakis JJ, Spencer LA. Eosinophils in innate immunity: an evolving story. Cell Tissue Res. 2011;343(1):57-83.
3. Rosenberg HF, Dyer KD, Foster PS. Eosinophils: changing perspectives in health and disease. Nat Rev Immunol. 2013;13:9-22.
4. Willebrand R, Voehringer D. Regulation of eosinophil development and survival. Curr Opin Hematol. 2017;24(1):9-15.
5. Fulkerson PC. Transcription factors in eosinophil development and as therapeutic targets. Front Med (Lausanne). 2017;4:115.
6. Loktionov A. Eosinophils in the gastrointestinal tract and their role in the pathogenesis of major colorectal disorders. World J Gastroenterol. 2019;25(27):3503-26.
7. Filippone RT, Sahakian L, Apostolopoulos V, Nurgali K. Eosinophils in inflammatory bowel disease. Inflamm Bowel Dis. 2019;25(7):1140-51.
8. Muniz VS, Weller PF, Neves JS. Eosinophil crystalloid granules: structure, function, and beyond. J Leukoc Biol. 2012;92(2):281-8.
9. Hogan SP, Rosenberg HF, Moqbel R, Phipps S, Foster PS, Lacy P, et al. Eosinophils: biological properties and role in health and disease. Clin Exp Allergy. 2008;38(5):709-50.
10. Weller PF, Spencer LA. Functions of tissue-resident eosinophils. Nature Rev Immunol. 2017;17(12):746-60.

11. Melo RC, Weller PF. Unraveling the complexity of lipid body organelles in human eosinophils. J Leukoc Biol. 2014;96:703-12.
12. Melo RC, Spencer LA, Dvorak AM, Weller PF. Mechanisms of eosinophil secretion: large vesiculotubular carriers mediate transport and release of granule-derived cytokines and other proteins. J Leukoc Biol. 2008;83:229-36.
13. Neves JS, Perez SA, Spencer LA, Melo RC, Reynolds L, Ghiran I, et al. Eosinophil granules function extracellularly as receptor-mediated secretory organelles. Proc Natl Acad Sci USA. 2008;105:18478-83.
14. Brinkmann V, Reichard U, Goosmann C, Fauler B, Uhlemann Y, Weiss DS, et al. Neutrophil extracellular traps kill bacteria. Science. 2004;303:1532-5.
15. Daniel C, Leppkes M, Muñoz LE, Schley G, Schett G, Herrmann M, et al. Extracellular DNA traps in inflammation, injury and healing. Nat Rev Nephrol. 2019;15:559-75.
16. Mukherjee M, Lacy P, Ueki S. Eosinophil extracellular traps and inflammatory pathologies—untangling the web! Front Immunol. 2018;9:2763.
17. Yousefi S, Gold JA, Andina N, Lee JJ, Kelly AM, Kozlowski E, et al. Catapult-like release of mitochondrial DNA by eosinophils contributes to antibacterial defense. Nat Med. 2008;14:949-53.
18. Gangwar RS, Landolina N, Arpinati L, Levi-Schaffer F. Mast cell and eosinophil surface receptors as targets for anti-allergic therapy. Pharmacol Ther. 2017;170:37-63.
19. Neves JS, Weller PF. Functional extracellular eosinophil granules: novel implications in eosinophil immunology. Curr Opin Immunol. 2009;21:694-9.
20. Mishra A, Hogan SP, Lee JJ, Foster PS, Rothenberg ME. Fundamental signals that regulate eosinophil homing to the gastrointestinal tract. J Clin Invest. 1999;103:1719-27.
21. Farahi N, Singh NR, Heard S, Loutsios C, Summers C, Solanki CK, et al. Use of 111-Indium-labeled autologous eosinophils to establish the in vivo kinetics of human eosinophils in healthy subjects. Blood. 2012;120:4068-71.
22. Weninger W, Biro M, Jain R. Leukocyte migration in the interstitial space of non-lymphoid organs. Nat Rev Immunol. 2014;14:232-46.
23. Fulkerson PC, Rothenberg ME. Origin, regulation and physiological function of intestinal oeosinophils. Best Pract Res Clin Gastroenterol. 2008;22:411-23.
24. Rothenberg ME. The eosinophil. Annu Rev Immunol. 2006;24:147-74.
25. Ahrens R, Waddell A, Seidu L, Blanchard C, Carey R, Forbes E, et al. Intestinal macrophage/epithelial cell-derived CCL11/eotaxin-1 mediates eosinophil recruitment and function in pediatric ulcerative colitis. J Immunol. 2008;182:7390-9.
26. Nussbaum JC, Van Dyken SJ, von Moltke J, Cheng LE, Mohapatra A, Molofsky AB, et al. Type 2 innate lymphoid cells control eosinophil homeostasis. Nature. 2013;502:245-8.
27. Hung LY, Lewkowich IP, Dawson LA, Downey J, Yang Y, Smith DE, et al. IL-33 drives biphasic IL-13 production for noncanonical Type 2 immunity against hookworms. Proc Natl Acad Sci USA. 2013;110:282-7.
28. Fu J, Zuber J, Martinez M, Shonts B, Obradovic A, Wang H, et al. Human intestinal allografts contain functional hematopoietic stem and progenitor cells that are maintained by a circulating pool. Cell Stem Cell. 2019;24:227-39.

29. DeBrosse CW, Case JW, Putnam PE, Collins MH, Rothenberg ME. Quantity and distribution of eosinophils in the gastrointestinal tract of children. Pediatr Dev Pathol. 2006;9:210-8.
30. Matsushita T, Maruyama R, Ishikawa N, Harada Y, Araki A, Chen D, et al. The number and distribution of eosinophils in the adult human gastrointestinal tract: a study and comparison of racial and environmental factors. Am J Surg Pathol. 2015;39:521-7.
31. Carlens J, Wahl B, Ballmaier M, Bulfone-Paus S, Förster R, Pabst O, et al. Common γ-chain-dependent signals confer selective survival of eosinophils in the murine small intestine. J Immunol. 2009;183:5600-7.
32. Parikh K, Antanaviciute A, Fawkner-Corbett D, Jagielowicz M, Aulicino A, Lagerholm C, et al. Colonic epithelial cell diversity in health and inflammatory bowel disease. Nature. 2019;567:49-55.
33. Johansson ME, Sjövall H, Hansson GC. The gastrointestinal mucus system in health and disease. Nat Rev Gastroenterol Hepatol. 2013;10:352-61.
34. Clevers HC, Bevins CL. Paneth cells: maestros of the small intestinal crypts. Annu Rev Physiol. 2013;75:289-311.
35. Chu VT, Beller A, Rausch S, Strandmark J, Zänker M, Arbach O, et al. Eosinophils promote generation and maintenance of immunoglobulin-A-expressing plasma cells and contribute to gut immune homeostasis. Immunity. 2014;40:582-93.
36. Jung Y, Wen T, Mingler MK, Caldwell JM, Wang YH, Chaplin DD, et al. IL-1β in eosinophil-mediated small intestinal homeostasis and IgA production. Mucosal Immunol. 2015;8:930-42.
37. Johnson AMF, Costanzo A, Gareau MG, Armando AM, Quehenberger O, Jameson JM, et al. High fat diet causes depletion of intestinal eosinophils associated with intestinal permeability. PLoS One. 2015;10:e0122195.
38. Driss V, Legrand F, Hermann E, Loiseau S, Guerardel Y, Kremer L, et al. TLR2-dependent eosinophil interactions with mycobacteria: role of alpha-defensins. Blood. 2009;113:3235-44.
39. Berek C. Eosinophils: important players in humoral immunity. Clin Exp Immunol. 2016;183:57-64.
40. Xenakis JJ, Howard ED, Smith KM, Olbrich CL, Huang Y, Anketell D, et al. Resident intestinal eosinophils consistently express antigen presentation markers and include two phenotypically distinct subsets of eosinophils. Immunology. 2018;154:298-308.
41. Schuijs MJ, Hammad H, Lambrecht BN. Professional and 'amateur' antigen-presenting cells in type 2 immunity. Trends Immunol. 2019;40:22-34.
42. Chu DK, Jimenez-Saiz R, Verschoor CP, Walker TD, Goncharova S, Llop-Guevara A, et al. Indigenous enteric eosinophils control DCs to initiate a primary Th2 immune response in vivo. J Exp Med. 2014;211:1657-72.
43. Knoop KA, Newberry RD. Goblet cells: multifaceted players in immunity at mucosal surfaces. Mucosal Immunology. 2018;11:1551-7.
44. Lloyd CM, Snelgrove RJ. Type 2 immunity: expanding our view. Sci Immunol. 2018;3.
45. Symowski C, Voehringer D. Interactions between innate lymphoid cells and cells of the innate and adaptive immune system. Front Immunol. 2017;8:1422.
46. Spencer LA, Weller PF. Eosinophils and Th2 immunity: contemporary insights. Immunol Cell Biol. 2010;88:250-6.

47. Travers J, Rothenberg ME. Eosinophils in mucosal immune responses. Mucosal Immunology. 2015;8:464-75.
48. Drake MG, Lebold KM, Roth-Carter QR, Pincus AB, Blum ED, Proskocil BJ, et al. Eosinophil and airway nerve interactions in asthma. J Leukoc Biol. 2018;104:61-7.
49. Kobayashi H, Gleich GJ, Butterfield JH, Kita H. Human eosinophils produce neurotrophins and secrete nerve growth factor on immunologic stimuli. Blood. 2002;99:2214-20.
50. Durcan N, Costello RW, McLean WG, Blusztajn J, Madziar B, Fenech AG, et al. Eosinophil-mediated cholinergic nerve remodeling. Am J Respir Cell Mol Biol. 2006;34:775-86.
51. Wouters MM, Vicario M, Santos J. The role of mast cells in functional GI disorders. Gut. 2016;65:155-68.
52. Elishmereni M, Alenius HT, Bradding P, Mizrahi S, Shikotra A, Minai-Fleminger Y, et al. Physical interactions between mast cells and eosinophils: a novel mechanism enhancing eosinophil survival in vitro. Allergy. 2011;66:376-85.
53. Bernardazzi C, Pêgo B, de Souza HS. Neuroimmunomodulation in the gut: focus on inflammatory bowel disease. Mediators Inflamm. 2016;2016:1363818.
54. Robida PA, Puzzovio PG, Pahima H, Levi-Schaffer F, Bochner BS. Human eosinophils and mast cells: Birds of a feather flock together. Immunol Rev. 2018;282:151-67.
55. Rothenberg ME. Molecular, genetic, and cellular bases for treating eosinophilic esophagitis. Gastroenterology. 2015;148:1143-57.
56. Nanagas VC, Kovalszki A. Gastrointestinal manifestations of hypereosinophilic syndromes and mast cell disorders: a comprehensive review. Clin Rev Allergy Immunol. 2018;57(2):194-212.
57. Gonsalves N. Eosinophilic gastrointestinal disorders. Clin Rev Allergy Immunol. 2019;57(2):272-85.
58. Ungaro R, Mehandru S, Allen PB, Peyrin-Biroulet L, Colombel JF. Ulcerative colitis. Lancet. 2017;389:1756-70.
59. Torres J, Mehandru S, Colombel JF, Peyrin-Biroulet L. Crohn's disease. Lancet. 2017;389:1741-55.
60. Cader MZ, Kaser A. Recent advances in inflammatory bowel disease: mucosal immune cells in intestinal inflammation. Gut. 2013;62:1653-64.
61. de Souza HS, Fiocchi C. Immunopathogenesis of IBD: current state of the art. Nat Rev Gastroenterol Hepatol. 2016;13:13-27.
62. Vancamelbeke M, Vermeire S. The intestinal barrier: a fundamental role in health and disease. Expert Rev Gastroenterol Hepatol. 2017;11:821-34.
63. Lampinen M, Backman M, Winqvist O, Rorsman F, Rönnblom A, Sangfelt P, et al. Different regulation of eosinophil activity in Crohn's disease compared with ulcerative colitis. J Leukoc Biol. 2008;84:1392-9.
64. Zezos P, Patsiaoura K, Nakos A, Mpoumponaris A, Vassiliadis T, Giouleme O, et al. Severe eosinophilic infiltration in colonic biopsies predicts patients with ulcerative colitis not responding to medical therapy. Colorectal Dis. 2014;16:O420-30.
65. Park S, Abdi T, Gentry M, Laine L. Histological disease activity as a predictor of clinical relapse among patients with ulcerative colitis: systematic review and meta-analysis. Am J Gastroenterol. 2016;111:1692-701.

66. Lampinen M, Rönnblom A, Amin K, Kristjansson G, Rorsman F, Sangfelt P, et al. Eosinophil granulocytes are activated during the remission phase of ulcerative colitis. Gut. 2005;54:1714-20.

67. Lampinen M, Waddell A, Ahrens R, Carlson M, Hogan SP. CD14$^+$CD33$^+$ myeloid cell-CCL11-eosinophil signature in ulcerative colitis. J Leukoc Biol. 2013;94:1061-70.

68. Rehman MQ, Beal D, Liang Y, Noronha A, Winter H, Farraye FA, et al. B-cells secrete eotaxin-1 in human inflammatory bowel disease. Inflamm Bowel Dis. 2013;19:922-33.

69. Manousou P, Kolios G, Valatas V, Drygiannakis I, Bourikas L, Pyrovolaki K, et al. Increased expression of chemokine receptor CCR3 and its ligands in ulcerative colitis: the role of colonic epithelial cells in in vitro studies. Clin Exp Immunol. 2010;162:337-47.

70. De Salvo C, Wang XM, Pastorelli L, Mattioli B, Omenetti S, Buela KA, et al. IL-33 drives eosinophil infiltration and pathogenic type 2 helper T-cell immune responses leading to chronic experimental ileitis. Am J Pathol. 2016;186:885-98.

71. Lampinen M, Fredriksson A, Vessby J, Martinez JF, Wanders A, Rorsman F, et al. Downregulated eosinophil activity in ulcerative colitis with concomitant primary sclerosing cholangitis. J Leukoc Biol. 2018;104:173-83.

72. Pastorelli L, Garg RR, Hoang SB, Spina L, Mattioli B, Scarpa M, et al. Epithelial-derived IL-33 and its receptor ST2 are dysregulated in ulcerative colitis and in experimental Th1/Th2 driven enteritis. Proc Natl Acad Sci USA. 2010;107:8017-22.

73. Beltrán CJ, Nuñez LE, Diaz-Jiménez D, Farfan N, Candia E, Heine C, et al. Characterization of the novel ST2/IL-33 system in patients with inflammatory bowel disease. Inflamm Bowel Dis. 2010;16:1097-107.

74. Brand S. Crohn's disease: Th1, Th17 or both? The change of a paradigm: new immunological and genetic insights implicate Th17 cells in the pathogenesis of Crohn's disease. Gut. 2009;58:1152-67.

75. Strober W, Fuss IJ. Proinflammatory cytokines in the pathogenesis of inflammatory bowel diseases. Gastroenterology. 2011;140:1756-67.

76. Li J, Ueno A, Fort Casia M, Luider J, Wang T, Hirota C, et al. Profiles of lamina propria T helper cell subsets discriminate between ulcerative colitis and Crohn's disease. Inflamm Bowel Dis. 2016;22:1779-92.

77. Heller F, Florian P, Bojarski C, Richter J, Christ M, Hillenbrand B, et al. Interleukin-13 is the key effector Th2 cytokine in ulcerative colitis that affects epithelial tight junctions, apoptosis, and cell restitution. Gastroenterology. 2005;129:550-64.

78. Furuta GT, Nieuwenhuis EE, Karhausen J, Gleich G, Blumberg RS, Lee JJ, et al. Eosinophils alter colonic epithelial barrier function: role for major basic protein. Am J Physiol Gastrointest Liver Physiol. 2005;289:G890-7.

79. Neurath MF. Cytokines in inflammatory bowel disease. Nat Rev Immunol. 2014;14:329-42.

80. Wallon C, Persborn M, Jönsson M, Wang A, Phan V, Lampinen M, et al. Eosinophils express muscarinic receptors and corticotropin-releasing factor to disrupt the mucosal barrier in ulcerative colitis. Gastroenterology. 2011;140:1597-607.

81. Martin JC, Bériou G, Heslan M, Bossard C, Jarry A, Abidi A, et al. IL-22BP is produced by eosinophils in human gut and blocks IL-22 protective actions during colitis. Mucosal Immunol. 2016;9:539-49.

82. Dent G, Loweth SC, Hasan AM, Leslie FM. Synergic production of neutrophil chemotactic activity by colonic epithelial cells and eosinophils. Immunobiology. 2014;219:793-7.
83. Bressenot A, Salleron J, Bastien C, Danese S, Boulagnon-Rombi C, Peyrin-Biroulet L, et al. Comparing histological activity indexes in UC. Gut. 2015;64:1412-8.
84. Segal AW. The role of neutrophils in the pathogenesis of Crohn's disease. Eur J Clin Invest. 2018;48(Suppl 2):e12983.
85. Thiesen S, Janciauskene S, Uronen-Hansson H, Agace W, Högerkorp CM, Spee P, et al. $CD14^{(hi)}HLA-DR^{(dim)}$ macrophages, with a resemblance to classical blood monocytes, dominate inflamed mucosa in Crohn's disease. J Leukoc Biol. 2014;95:531-41.
86. Matthews JD, Weight CM, Parkos CA. Leukocyte-epithelial interactions and mucosal homeostasis. Toxicol Pathol. 2014;42:91-8.
87. Parkos CA. Neutrophil-epithelial interactions: a double-edged sword. Am J Pathol. 2016;186:1404-16.
88. Butin-Israeli V, Houser MC, Feng M, Thorp EB, Nusrat A, Parkos CA, et al. Deposition of microparticles by neutrophils onto inflamed epithelium: a new mechanism to disrupt epithelial intracellular adhesions and promote transepithelial migration. FASEB J. 2016;30:4007-20.
89. Erjefält JS, Uller L, Malm-Erjefält M, Persson C. Rapid and efficient clearance of airway tissue granulocytes through transepithelial migration. Thorax. 2004;59:136-43.
90. Yuan Q, Campanella GS, Colvin RA, Hamilos DL, Jones KJ, Mathew A, et al. Membrane-bound eotaxin-3 mediates eosin transepithelial migration in IL-4-stimulated epithelial cells. Eur J Immunol. 2006;36:10.
91. Michail S, Abernathy F. A new model for studying eosinophil migration across cultured intestinal epithelial monolayers. J Pediatr Gastroenterol Nutr. 2004;39:56-63.
92. Wagner M, Peterson CG, Stolt I, Sangfelt P, Agnarsdottir M, Lampinen M, et al. Fecal eosinophil cationic protein as a marker of active disease and treatment outcome in collagenous colitis: a pilot study. Scand J Gastroenterol. 2011;46:849-54.
93. Di Ruscio M, Vernia F, Ciccone A, Frieri G, Latella G, et al. Surrogate fecal biomarkers in inflammatory bowel disease: rivals or complementary tools of fecal calprotectin? Inflamm Bowel Dis. 2017;24:78-92.
94. Loktionov A, Chhaya V, Bandaletova T, Poullis A. Assessment of cytology and mucin 2 in colorectal mucus collected from patients with inflammatory bowel disease: results of a pilot trial. J Gastroenterol Hepatol. 2016;31:326-33.
95. Bandaletova T, Chhaya V, Poullis A, Loktionov A. Colorectal mucus non-invasively collected from patients with inflammatory bowel disease and its suitability for diagnostic cytology. APMIS. 2016;124:160-8.
96. Loktionov A, Chhaya V, Bandaletova T, Poullis A. Inflammatory bowel disease detection and monitoring by measuring biomarkers in non-invasively collected colorectal mucus. J Gastroenterol Hepatol. 2017;32:992-1002.
97. Savchenko AS, Inoue A, Ohashi R, Jiang S, Hasegawa G, Tanaka T, et al. Long pentraxin 3 (PTX3) expression and release by neutrophils in vitro and in ulcerative colitis. Pathol Int. 2011;61:290-7.
98. Uribe Echevarria L, Leimgruber C, García González J, Nevado A, Álvarez R, García LN, et al. Evidence of eosinophil extracellular trap cell death in COPD: does it

represent the trigger that switches on the disease? Int J Chron Obstruct Pulmon Dis. 2017;12:885-96.

99. Ueki S, Tokunaga T, Fujieda S, Honda K, Hirokawa M, Spencer LA. Eosinophil ETosis and DNA traps: a new look at eosinophilic inflammation. Curr Allergy Asthma Rep. 2016;16:54.

100. Bennike TB, Carlsen TG, Ellingsen T, Bonderup OK, Glerup H, Bøgsted M, et al. Neutrophil extracellular traps in ulcerative colitis: a proteome analysis of intestinal biopsies. Inflamm Bowel Dis. 2015;21:2052-67.

101. Gottlieb Y, Elhasid R, Berger-Achituv S, Brazowski E, Yerushalmy-Feler A, Cohen S. Neutrophil extracellular traps in pediatric inflammatory bowel disease. Pathol Int. 2018;68:517-23.

102. Persson C, Uller L. Resolution of leukocyte-mediated mucosal diseases. A novel in vivo paradigm for drug development. Br J Pharmacol. 2012;165:2100-9.

103. Loktionov A. Cell exfoliation in the human colon: myth, reality and implications for colorectal cancer screening. Int J Cancer. 2007;120:2281-9.

104. Hanahan D, Weinberg RA. Hallmarks of cancer: the next generation. Cell. 2011;144: 646-74.

105. Reichman H, Karo-Atar D, Munitz A. Emerging roles for eosinophils in the tumor microenvironment. Trends Cancer. 2016;11:664-75.

106. Davis BP, Rothenberg ME. Eosinophils and cancer. Cancer Immunol Res. 2014;2:1-8.

107. Prizment AE, Anderson KE, Visvanathan K, Folsom AR. Inverse association of eosinophil count with colorectal cancer incidence: atherosclerosis risk in communities study. Cancer Epidemiol Biomarkers Prev. 2011;20:1861-4.

108. Yalcin AD, Kargi A, Gumuslu S. Blood eosinophil and platelet levels, proteomic patterns of trail and CXCL8 correlated with survival in bevacizumab treated metastatic colon cancers. Clin Lab. 2014;60:339-40.

109. Wei Y, Zhang X, Wang G, Zhou Y, Luo M, Wang S, et al. The impacts of pretreatment circulating eosinophils and basophils on prognosis of stage I-II colorectal cancer. Asia Pac J Clin Oncol. 2018;14:e243-51.

110. Moezzi J, Gopalswamy N, Haas RJ, Markert RJ, Suryaprasad S, Bhutani MS. Stromal eosinophiliain colonic epithelial neoplasms. Am J. Gastroenterol. 2000;95:520-3.

111. Prizment AE, Vierkant RA, Smyrk TC, Tillmans LS, Lee JJ, Sriramarao P, et al. Tumor eosinophil infiltration and improved survival of colorectal cancer patients: Iowa Women's Health Study. Mod Pathol. 2016;29:516-27.

112. Harbaum L, Pollheimer MJ, Kornprat P, Lindtner RA, Bokemeyer C, Langner C. Peritumoral eosinophils predict recurrence in colorectal cancer. Mod Pathol. 2015;28:403-13.

113. Stenfeldt AL, Wennerås C. Danger signals derived from stressed and necrotic epithelial cells activate human eosinophils. Immunology. 2004;112:605-14.

114. Lofti R, Lee JJ, Lotze MT. Eosinophilic granulocytes and damage-associated molecular pattern molecules (DAMPs): role in the inflammatory response within tumors. J Immunother. 2007;30:16-28.

115. Larsen KM, Minaya MK, Vaish V, Peña MMO. The role of IL-33/ST2 pathway in tumorigenesis. Int J Mol Sci. 2018;19:E2676.

116. Lahm H, Hoeflich A, Andre S, Sordat B, Kaltner H, Wolf E, et al. Gene expression of galectin-9/ecalectin, a potent eosinophil chemoattractant, and/or the insertional

isoform in human colorectal carcinoma cell lines and detection of frame-shift mutations for protein sequence truncations in the second functional lectin domain. Int J Oncol. 2000;17:519-24.
117. Wågsäter D, Löfgren S, Hugander A, Dienus O, Dimberg J. Analysis of single nucleotide polymorphism in the promoter and protein expression of the chemokine eotaxin-1 in colorectal cancer patients. World J Surg Oncol. 2007;5:84.
118. Cho H, Lim SJ, Won KY, Bae GE, Kim GY, Min JW, et al. Eosinophils in colorectal neoplasms associated with expression of CCL11 and CCL24. J Pathol Transl Med. 2016;50:45-51.
119. Hollande C, Boussier J, Ziai J, Nozawa T, Bondet V, Phung W, et al. Inhibition of the dipeptidyl peptidase DPP4 (CD26) reveals IL-33-dependent eosinophil-mediated control of tumor growth. Nat Immunol. 2019;20:257-64.
120. Munitz A, Hogan SP. Alarming eosinophils to combat tumors. Nat Immunol. 2019;20:250-2.
121. Cherry WB, Yoon J, Bartemes KR, Iijima K, Kita H. A novel IL-1 family cytokine, IL-33, potently activates human eosinophils. J Allergy Clin Immunol. 2008;121:1484-90.
122. Malik A, Sharma D, Zhu Q, Karki R, Guy CS, Vogel P, et al. IL-33 regulates the IgA-microbiota axis to restrain IL-1α-dependent colitis and tumorigenesis. J Clin Invest. 2016;126:4469-81.
123. Legrand F, Driss V, Delbeke M, Loiseau S, Hermann E, Dombrowicz D, et al. Human eosinophils exert TNFα and granzyme A-mediated tumoricidal activity toward colon carcinoma cells. J Immunol. 2010;185:7443-51.
124. Gatault S, Delbeke M, Driss V, Sarazin A, Dendooven A, Kahn JE, et al. IL-18 is involved in eosinophil-mediated tumoricidal activity against a colon carcinoma cell line by upregulating LFA-1 and ICAM-1. J Immunol. 2015;195:2483-92.
125. Reichman H, Itan M, Rozenberg P, Yarmolovski T, Brazowski E, Varol C, et al. Activated eosinophils exert antitumorigenic activities in colorectal cancer. Cancer Immunol Res. 2019;7:388-400.
126. Albrengues J, Shields MA, Ng D, Park CG, Ambrico A, Poindexter ME, et al. Neutrophil extracellular traps produced during inflammation awaken dormant cancer cells in mice. Science. 2018;361:eaao4227.
127. Arelaki S, Arampatzioglou A, Kambas K, Papagoras C, Miltiades P, Angelidou I, et al. Gradient infiltration of neutrophil extracellular traps in colon cancer and evidence for their involvement in tumour growth. PLoS One. 2016;11:e0154484.
128. Choi CR, Bakir IA, Hart AL, Busse WW, Bertics PJ, Kelly EA, et al. Clonal evolution of colorectal cancer in IBD. Nat Rev Gastroenterol Hepatol. 2017;14:218-29.
129. Liu LY, Bates ME, Jarjour NN, Busse WW, Bertics PJ, Kelly EAB. Generation of Th1 and Th2 chemokines by human eosinophils: evidence for a critical role of TNF-alpha. J Immunol. 2007;179:4840-8.
130. Carretero R, Sektioglu IM, Garbi N, Salgado OC, Beckhove P, Hämmerling GJ, et al. Eosinophils orchestrate cancer rejection by normalizing tumor vessels and enhancing infiltration of CD8(+) T cells. Nat Immunol. 2015;16:609-17.
131. Puxeddu I, Berkmman N, Nissim Ben Efraim AH, Davies D, Ribatti D, Gleich GJ, et al. The role of eosinophil major basic protein in angiogenesis. Allergy. 2009;64:368-74.
132. Cormier SA, Taranova AG, Bedient C, Nguyen T, Protheroe C, Ralph P, et al. Pivotal Advance: eosinophil infiltration of solid tumors is an early and persistent inflammatory host response. J Leukoc Biol. 2006;79:1131-9.

CHAPTER

6

Gut Mucus and its Functional Significance in Health and Disease

Alexandre Loktionov

INTRODUCTION

It is well known that the inner cavities of the human body are overlaid by protective mucus possessing specific properties in different organs.[1] In the gastrointestinal tract, the largest surface of contact between the body and the external world, gut mucus constitutes the interface between the epithelial tissue and the gut contents, which is overwhelmingly dominated by microbiota in the distal part of the gut. In addition, gastrointestinal tract lumen contains potentially harmful endogenous molecules produced by the organism and comprising proteolytic, nucleolytic, and lipolytic digestive enzymes; bile acids; and gastric hydrochloric acid.[2] It is thus evident that the epithelial surface of the gastrointestinal tract should be efficiently protected; however, neither the structure nor the role of the protective mucus could be perceived until the beginning of this century.[1] This chapter addresses this important issue with a special emphasis on its impact in the pathogenesis of major colorectal diseases comprising inflammatory bowel disease (IBD) and colorectal cancer (CRC).

MUCUS COMPOSITION AND STRUCTURE THROUGHOUT THE GASTROINTESTINAL TRACT

In the normal physiological conditions, gastrointestinal mucus is perfectly transparent as >95% of this substance is composed of water.[1] This characteristic feature partially explains the surprisingly late discovery of gut mucus structure. Although the existence of distinct surface mucus layers in surgically resected specimens of the human colon was described in 1997,[3] the first convincing evidence of the structural organization of the colonic mucus was obtained in a mouse model and published by Johansson et al. only in 2008.[4] They reported the existence of two colonic mucus layers, the inner one being dense and impenetrable for bacteria[4] whereas the outer loose one presenting a good habitat for commensal microbiota.[5] Further studies of the same Swedish group headed by GC Hansson soon revealed that mouse stomach and colon had this two-layer organization.[6] Notably, the inner mucus in the stomach was fully penetrable to microbeads comparable to bacteria in size. In contrast, the mucosa of the small intestine and domes of Peyer patches had only one thick layer of loose and penetrable mucus.[6] It is now known that the normal thickness of the inner mucus layer in the distal human colon is 200–300 μm, and the outer layer is approximately twice as thick.[2] The mucus structure in the stomach, small intestine, and colon is schematically shown in **Figure 1**. Studies of Hanson's group have also established that gel-forming mucin *MUC2* secreted by goblet cells of the intestinal or colonic epithelium[2,7] constitutes the main component of both inner and outer mucus layers.[1,5] One distinctive feature of *MUC2* is its large PTS (rich in proline, threonine and serine) domain that is densely *O*-glycosylated in goblet cell Golgi apparatus. The resulting *O*-glycan-decorated structures form "mucin domains" contributing to high water-binding capacity and gel-forming properties. In addition, N- and C-terminal parts of *MUC2* protein frequently form dimers that facilitate the creation of disulfide bonds and eventual generation of net-like structures upon *MUC2* secretion. A more detailed description of these molecular mechanisms is available elsewhere,[5,8] but it should be noted that the main mucin in the stomach mucus is *MUC5AC*.[9]

MUC2 polymers are densely packed in the secretory granules of the goblet cells, where low pH and high calcium concentration are preserved. Immediately following secretion, these structures expand over than 1,000-fold and form large net-like planar sheets[7,8] assembled in porous lamellar networks.[10] In the normal conditions, *MUC2* synthesis is a continuous active process maintaining fast mucus renewal (inner mucus layer turnover is about 1 hour) from underneath as was clearly demonstrated for the distal colon of mice.[11] The highly organized inner mucus layer in the colon is stratified and remains securely attached to the goblet cells producing it. In contrast, *MUC2* synthesized in the small intestine is proteolytically cleaved

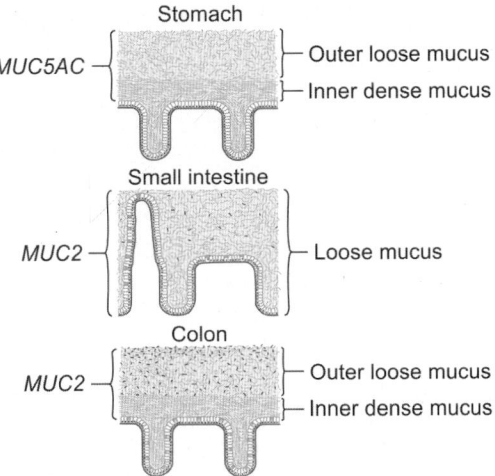

Fig. 1: Gastrointestinal mucus structure in the stomach, small intestine and colon.

by the metalloproteinase meprin β abundantly expressed by enterocytes.[12] This mechanism is likely to be responsible for the loosening of the resulting substance and the absence of the two-layered mucus structure in the small intestine. In the normal conditions, the inner mucus layer in the colon is completely free from bacteria, but mucus sheets becoming more distant from the epithelial surface are then gradually converted to the looser outer layer, probably via proteolytic cleavage of *MUC2* by the host enzymes or gut bacteria.[5] As mentioned above, the commensal bacteria in the colon are abundantly present in the outer mucus layer **(Fig. 1)**, where they may use *MUC2*-associated glycans as an important source of energy, gradually breaking the loose mucus down.[5] It should, however, be noted that the utilization of mucus glycoproteins as nutrients for bacteria is apparently an additional compensatory mechanism that may be activated by a limited availability of other sources of polysaccharides digestible by gut microbiota. Experimentally induced dietary fiber deficiency was shown to result in a largely enhanced use of mucus glycoproteins by bacteria, which lead to colonic mucus deterioration.[13]

MUCUS AS A COMPONENT OF THE INTESTINAL PROTECTIVE BARRIER

Gut mucus constitutes an important element of the intestinal barrier, but underlying epithelial cells are charged with both mucus production and provision of a continuous physical barrier formed by apical surfaces of enterocytes or colonocytes. These cells are linked by intracellular tight junctions and covered with a complex apical glycocalyx formed by the transmembrane mucins *MUC3*, *MUC12*, and *MUC17* that are anchored to the epithelial cell surface.[2,14] Under the mucus, distinct types of terminally differentiated epithelial cells exert either absorptive (enterocytes, colonocytes) or secretory (goblet cells, Paneth cells, and enteroendocrine cells) functions, but there are also chemosensory tuft cells and microfold (M) cells associated with gut lymphoid tissue and responsible for immunosurveillance.[15] In addition, progenitor cells located in the crypts permanently produce new cells rapidly renewing gut epithelium. It has recently been shown that the degree of colonic epithelial cell diversity is even higher, because functionally diverse subpopulations of conventionally defined cell types could be identified.[16] Goblet cells play a pivotal role in the maintenance of the mucus barrier, being specialized in mucus synthesis and secretion, and it is now suggested that there may be several functionally different subtypes of goblet cells,[17] some of which are also able to take part in delivering low molecular weight soluble antigens from the intestinal lumen to the underlying CD103$^+$ dendritic cells of the intestinal *lamina propria*.[18] It is evident that goblet cells are the key players in maintaining rapid mucus renewal, and mechanisms of their activity regulation are only starting to become clear. Patel et al. revealed the necessity of autophagy proteins and endosome formation that causes reactive oxygen species' generation for controlling goblet cell mucin granule accumulation.[19] It was later shown that the NLRP6 inflammasome controls autophagy in colonic goblet cells, thus acting as a key regulator of mucin secretion.[20] Finally, Birchenough et al. were able to identify "sentinel" goblet cells localized at colonic crypt entrance.[21] The sentinel cells respond to the presence of microbe-derived soluble products in the gut lumen by NLRP6 inflammasome activation followed by enhanced *MUC2* production.[21] In addition, these cells trigger an intercellular gap junction signal provoking *MUC2* secretion from the adjacent goblet cells as well.[21] This defensive cascade appears to co exist with the above-mentioned alternative phenomenon, when soluble luminal antigens are transferred by goblet cells to the underlying dendritic cells of the *lamina propria*.[18] The latter mechanism was also demonstrated to function in colonic epithelium.[22] The role of goblet cells as monitors of extracellular environment closely linked with the immune system is currently actively discussed[17,23] but remains to be entirely elucidated.

In addition to the main *MUC2*, goblet cells secrete several other mucus components.[7] In the small intestine, mucus also contains a range of antimicrobial peptides (AMPs) secreted by Paneth cells located in the crypts. Human AMPs include two α-defensins (HD5 and HD6), lysozyme, secretory phospholipase A2, RegIIIα, cathelicidin LL-37[24] and, possibly, DMBT1.[25] Other AMPs detectable in colonic mucus from healthy individuals are defensins HBD1 and HBD3, ubiquitin, histones H2A and H2B, ubiquicitidin, protein *HMGN2*, and ribosomal proteins L30 and L39.[26] Moreover, gut mucus is rich in IgA produced by plasma cells of the *lamina propria* and transported to the mucus by transcytosis through epithelial cells.[27] Interestingly, it was shown that in the colon IgA is predominantly concentrated in the outer mucus layer accessible for microbiota.[28] Finally, it should not be forgotten that gut mucus close to the mucosal surface is relatively well-oxygenated,[29] and this factor further prevents anaerobic luminal bacteria from reaching the epithelium. In addition, gut mucus is a dynamic system also charged with mechanically eliminating unwelcome luminal bacteria and food-derived debris[1] as well as exfoliated cells or cell remnants occasionally released from the epithelial surface.[30] As the small intestinal mucus is not anchored to the epithelium, it permanently moves distally with the peristaltic waves, being replaced by fresh mucus generated by the goblet cells,[2] and this process continues in the colon;[30,31] however, only the outer mucus layer may be able to move in the distal gut in the normal conditions.

The presented information leaves no doubt about the importance of gut mucus as an integral element of the intestinal protective barrier, but unanswered questions remain. Recent experimental studies indicating that mucus restructuring may occur due to dietary influences or therapeutic interventions[32] or be modulated by the presence and consistency of the colonic content[33] deserve close attention and further research.

GUT MUCUS AND MICROBIOME

The loose mucus of the distal small intestine and the outer loose layer of colonic mucus can serve as both energy sources and habitats for the colonic microflora. Although the discrimination between mucosa-associated (i.e., mucus-dwelling) and luminal bacterial communities is often difficult, it is generally recognized that in humans Firmicutes and Bacteroidetes are the dominant phyla in the both locations, but bacteria such as *Ruminococcus gnavus*, *Ruminococcus torques*, *Bacteroides thetaiotaomicron*, *Bacteroides fragilis*, *Bacteroides vulgatus*, *Akkermansia muciniphila*, and *Desulfovibrio desulfuricans* were found to be associated with the mucosal surface.[34,35] Intriguingly, several commensals known to possess probiotic properties, including *Lactobacillus reuteri*, *Lactobacillus plantarum*, *Lactobacillus rhamnosus*, *Lactobacillus johnsonii*, *Bifidobacterium breve*, and *Bifidobacterium longum*, were also shown to belong to healthy mucosa microbiome.[34] As already noted above, *MUC2* molecules are rich in O-glycans, which specifically interact with bacteria and regulate microbial community composition in the outer colonic mucus layer.[36] It was suggested that, under the normal conditions, microbiota can establish microcolonies there.[37] O-glycan formation on *MUC2* is mediated by multiple glycosyltransferases, and interesting associations were revealed between the presence of some O-glycan-modifying enzymes and alterations in mucus-associated bacterial community.[38] Experiments of Staubach et al. in genetically modified mice lacking the β1,4-N-acetylgalactosaminyltransferase 2 have demonstrated that these animals significantly differed from their wild-type counterparts in the proportions of specific bacterial phyla.[39] In humans, microbial community composition in the gut was shown to depend on the presence of a functional *FUT2* gene, which encodes galactoside 2-alpha-L-fucosyltransferase 2 (*FUT2*) that modifies mucus O-glycans and is responsible for the expression of ABO histo-blood group antigen precursors in gut mucus.[36,38,40] Individuals with at least one functional *FUT2* allele are termed as "secretors," whereas homozygosity for the loss-of-function mutations (found in about 20% of Caucasians) defines "nonsecretors."[40] Notably, by investigating mucosal bacterial profiles in colonic biopsy samples, Rausch et al. found that, while in samples from healthy "secretors," the presence of the probiotic *Lactobacillus* genus was more prominent, there was a clear association of healthy "nonsecretors" with the genus *Prevotella*.[40] Other groups reported further *FUT2* genotype-linked phylotype shifts, including the decrease of *Roseburia* and *Faecalibacterium* in endoscopic lavage samples from "nonsecretors"[41] as well as probiotic *Bifidobacterium* decrease in stool samples from "nonsecretors."[42] In contrast, stool sample analysis by two large studies failed to reveal any associations between *FUT2* genotype and gut microbiome shifts.[43,44] Still, it is well known that what is detected in stool may not be representative of what is occurring within the host.[35] For this reason, one can argue that samples obtained by mucosal biopsy or colonic lavage are preferable to stool for analyzing bacterial communities populating colonic mucus. In any case, it is evident that O-glycans associated with *MUC2* strongly influence the composition of the microbial population normally confined to the outer mucus layer in the colon. It was already noted that O-glycans can serve as a reserve nutrition resource for commensals in situations when the dietary supply of glycans is limited, but it is also important to stress that the same O-glycans can constitute scaffolds for host-derived antimicrobial factors. These functions were earlier reviewed in detail elsewhere.[36] One additional feature of mammalian gut mucus is a regiospecificity of the distribution of *MUC2* O-glycan patterns. In the mouse, sialylated and sulfated glycans prevailed in the small intestine, whereas the colon was dominated by highly charged fucosylated glycans.[45] This pattern correlated with the relative abundance of O-glycosyltransferases produced by the epithelial cells along the gut.[46] It is, however, believed that these differences develop in the postnatal life and are likely to be associated with the establishment of gut microbiota.[47] Indeed, experimental studies using mouse models have shown that commensal colonization of the gut promotes structural and physiological adaptations of the mucus barrier, thus contributing to intestinal homeostasis.[48,49] Also, it has recently been demonstrated that aging in mice causes a progressing decrease in protective mucus layer thickness that is accompanied by major changes in the fecal microbiota composition and considerably more frequent contacts of luminal bacteria with the epithelium.[50] A similar reduction of colonic mucus layer thickness was observed in aging rats.[51] Although age-related changes in gut mucus layer thickness have never been studied in humans, it is notable that that the composition of the intestinal microbiota in elderly subjects was reported to substantially differ from that in young adults, especially with regard to the lower proportion of phylum Firmicutes in the elderly.[52]

HOST CELL EXFOLIATION AND MIGRATION FROM THE EPITHELIAL SURFACE TO MUCUS LAYERS IN NORMAL PHYSIOLOGICAL CONDITIONS

The intestinal epithelium is the most actively renewing tissue of the human body. Before the discovery of colonic mucus structure and recognition of its importance, a simplistic view on epithelial cell renewal prevailed. It was traditionally presumed that terminally differentiated enterocytes or colonocytes undergo spontaneous apoptosis and are then "shed into the gut lumen,"[53] with millions of exfoliated cells potentially detectable in stool.[54] Our group, however, demonstrated that cell exfoliation in the normal human gut is by far less intense, with only rare single colonocytes present in mucus samples intrarectally collected from the surface of the rectal mucosa of healthy individuals.[30,31] This finding was later confirmed by analyzing colorectal mucus samples obtained noninvasively.[55] Likewise, the presence of small numbers of normal exfoliated colonocytes was earlier observed in mucus-containing washes from the surface of stool samples obtained from healthy volunteers.[56-58]

In view of the two-layer structure attributed to the colonic mucus **(Fig. 1)** and discussed above, an immediate question emerges: how exfoliated colonocytes manage to penetrate the dense inner mucus layer that is impenetrable for much smaller bacteria? Currently, there is no easy answer to this question, but upon colorectal mucus structure discovery, it was assumed that shed cells are "trapped in the mucus" and degraded there.[4] However, well-preserved colonocytes were observed in all studies that used mucus sampling.[30,31,55-58] While it could be argued that during intrarectal mucus collection[31] exfoliated colonocytes could be detached from the epithelium due to complete mucus removal by the mechanical contact of the collecting device with the rectal mucosa, this explanation is not valid when mucus samples were obtained noninvasively[55] or from the surface of freshly excreted stool.[56-58] It can be hypothesized that exfoliated cell migration through the inner colonic mucus layer can somehow be assisted by the rapid renewal of this layer[11] or that focal partial *MUC2* cleavage[5] may occur alongside colonocyte exfoliation, but mechanisms of this phenomenon currently remain obscure. In contrast, massive presence of both exfoliated colonocytes and migrating free cells of inflammation in colorectal mucus samples obtained from patients with IBD and CRC is easy to explain by severe deterioration of the colonic mucus barrier observed during these conditions and considered below. Despite the existing knowledge gaps regarding mechanisms involved in cell accumulation in colorectal mucus, it is indisputable that this easily accessible substance presents a highly informative material for diagnostic analysis.

GUT MUCUS CHANGES ASSOCIATED WITH INFLAMMATORY BOWEL DISEASE

Inflammatory bowel disease is a group of chronic relapsing inflammatory conditions, Crohn's disease (CD)[59] and ulcerative colitis (UC)[60] being its two main types. IBD has a complex etiopathogenesis that remains poorly understood, but certainly involves genetic components (that stronger influence CD) and impacts of environmental factors including gut microbiome shifts (dysbiosis). The disease is believed to be triggered by bacterial penetration through the intestinal protective barrier, which is followed by inadequate immune responses resulting in the development of chronic inflammation.[61-63] Gut mucus presents the first defensive line against the luminal microbiota, its inner layer making bacterial contact with the colonic epithelium impossible in the normal conditions.[4] Although loose mucus of the small intestine can be penetrated by bacteria, it is rich in antimicrobial substances, and its intense production by goblet cells in the normal conditions creates a permanent mucus flow preventing bacteria from entering intestinal crypts and reaching the epithelium.[2,64] Hence, only serious alterations of gut mucus layers can lead to exposing the surface of the epithelium to contacts with luminal microorganisms. The critical role of *MUC2*-rich mucus for gut protection was demonstrated by spontaneous colitis development in *MUC2*-knockout mice that are unable to produce *MUC2*.[65] Colonic mucus deterioration was similarly observed in patients with UC and CD by Swidsinski et al.,[66] and the authors concluded that the intestinal bacteria in these patients were usually confined to mucosa-adhering "biofilms" that can be defined as matrix-enclosed multispecies bacterial communities forming higher order structures.[37,67]

Gut mucus alterations occurring during CD and UC were shown to differ.[64] CD is very often initiated in the terminal ileum, where the protective effects of mucus primarily depend on the effective functioning of goblet cells and Paneth cells. These secretory functions become compromised in CD patients due to misfolding of proteins occurring during biosynthesis, especially in course of assembling complex secretory proteins in the endoplasmic reticulum (ER). Protein misfolding leads to ER stress that can trigger the unfolded protein response and induce inflammatory signaling.[68] It is remarkable that the *XBP1* locus known to be associated with CD risk was shown to control the development of ER stress in the intestinal epithelium.[61] Morphological manifestations of ER stress include reduced numbers of secretory granules combined with ER vacuolization, and these features associated with decreased production of both mucus by goblet cells and AMPs by Paneth cells are commonly observed in IBD.[68,69] It was, however, shown experimentally that anti-inflammatory cytokine interleukin-10 (IL-10) can prevent protein misfolding and ER stress by maintaining correct folding of *MUC2*, its transport from the ER, and its glycosylation and secretion.[70] In the small intestine, defects in the secretory activities of goblet cells and Paneth cells apparently result in the formation of functionally impaired mucus that fails to prevent bacteria from penetrating the crypts and initiating inflammation that leads to CD development.[69] It is not surprising that the total expression of mucin genes was found to be decreased in CD patients.[71]

In contrast, mucin gene total expression was reported to be increased in patients with UC,[72] albeit decreased numbers of colonic goblet cells[73-75] and both reduced thickness and disruption of colonic mucus layers were described in association with UC.[73,74,76] Importantly, colon mucus properties in UC patients were apparently changing as the inner mucus layer became highly penetrable for luminal bacteria.[76] It has recently been demonstrated that in active UC the secretory response of colonic goblet cells to microbes is impaired, with the number of sentinel goblet cells[21] considerably reduced in active UC.[77] Decreased sulfation of colonic mucins was also reported as an inflammation-related feature in patients with UC.[78] Although IBD in general is associated with apparent signs of intestinal barrier deterioration, differences between CD and UC patients were revealed in patterns of genetic and transcriptomic dysregulations.[79] Nevertheless, some genes encoding mucus barrier elements, including *MUC1*, *MUC4*, and *MUC22*, were identified as common candidates for the onset or perpetuation of chronic gastrointestinal inflammation in IBD.[79]

IBD-related gut mucus changes considered so far are defined by multiple functions of the gut epithelium, but mucus layer properties also strongly depend on gut microbiota.[1] Experiments in mice showed that the composition of intestinal microbiota is important for defining properties of the inner mucus layer,[48] and it was later demonstrated that dysbiosis in the mucus preceded experimental colitis development.[80] In humans, previously described mucus microbiota shifts caused by *FUT2* "nonsecretor" genotype are associated with a higher risk of developing CD,[40] and mucolytic bacteria presence was found to be increased in patients with both CD and UC.[81] Likewise, biofilm formation is a common feature of these diseases.[66] In addition, significant changes in the composition of colonic mucus microbiota were revealed in UC patients compared with healthy controls.[82] Details of host–microbiome interactions at the level of colonic mucus in the context of UC were previously reviewed by Lennon et al.[34]

Another important risk factor for IBD development is the modern Western diet characterized by decreased consumption of dietary fibers.[83,84] Indeed, it was previously demonstrated that dietary fiber deficiency can provoke gut microbiota switch to mucin *O*-glycan degradation that eventually causes mucus barrier disruption.[13,84] Conversely, fiber addition to the diet[85] and administration of probiotic microbiota, especially *Bifidobacterium* species,[85-87] restored gut mucus layer functionality and provided an anti-inflammatory effect in experimental models.[85-87] Likewise, tea polyphenols in vitro[88] and citrus flavonoids in vivo[89] were shown to protect colonic mucus integrity. However, further intense research is needed for achieving a clear understanding of complex interactions between dietary factors, gut microbiota, mucus layer preservation, and inflammation.

Concluding this section, it is necessary to highlight the often-forgotten dramatic changes in the host cell presence in colorectal mucus associated with IBD development. Although neutrophil- or eosinophil-derived biomarkers are commonly found in stool samples obtained from IBD patients, and stool calprotectin detection is widely used for diagnosing IBD,[90] the abundance of inflammatory cells in colorectal mucus collected from these patients was largely ignored. Our studies conducted since 2007 clearly demonstrated that numerous immune cells can always be seen in mucus samples collected from patients with active IBD either intrarectally[31,91] or noninvasively from the anal area following defecation.[55,92,93] Neutrophils are clearly the most frequent cell type **(Fig. 2)**, but macrophages, eosinophils (especially in UC cases), plasma cells, and lymphocytes were commonly found as well.[92] It is also remarkable that all these cells were extremely well preserved and appeared to be viable, because neutrophils and macrophages engaged in phagocytosis and erythrophagocytosis were clearly observed.[92] Moreover, it was suggested that

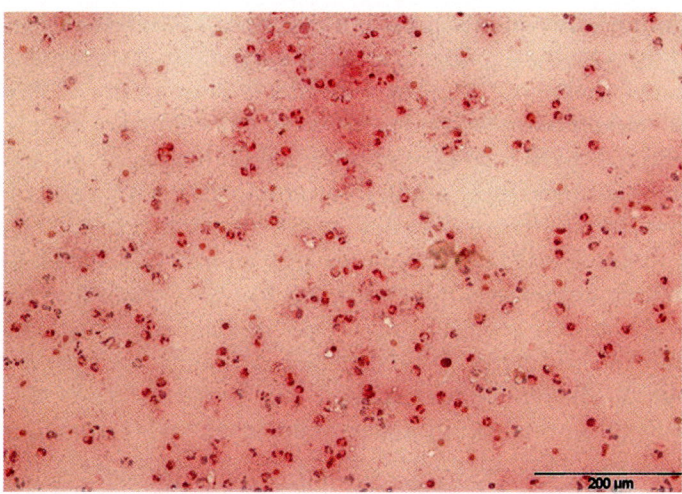

Fig. 2: Abundance of inflammatory cells (predominantly neutrophils) in colorectal mucus noninvasively collected from a patient with active ulcerative colitis.

neutrophils and probably eosinophils located in the mucus can frequently undergo ETosis (cell death associated with extracellular trap formation).[92,94]

Taken together, these observations allowed to assume that gut mucus in IBD may act as a unique supporting milieu for immune responses expanding from the mucosa.[94] Nevertheless, interactions of the migrating immune cells with mucus-dwelling bacteria on the one hand and with the epithelium on the other hand remain obscure; thus, this intriguing area needs further thorough investigation.

GUT MUCUS CHANGES ASSOCIATED WITH COLORECTAL CANCER

Sporadic CRC is a slowly developing malignancy, the early stages of which are confined exclusively to colorectal mucosa.[95] It was known for decades that genetic markers of CRC can be detected in the feces excreted by CRC patients,[96-98] and the presence of malignant cells on the stool surface was repeatedly demonstrated by several groups.[56-58,99,100] The importance of colonic mucus for the preservation of cells released from the tumor surface was highlighted for the first time by Ahlquist et al., who described the existence of a "mucocellular layer" covering the tumor and capturing all cells and cell fragments shed from its epithelium.[101] It was later demonstrated that this material can be collected intrarectally using a cytology brush[102] or a specially designed inflatable device.[31] Abundant malignant colonocytes and inflammatory cells were identifiable in the mucus from CRC patients, and cell numbers were much higher in the mucus overlaying tumor surface.[31,101] In addition, human DNA measurement in the mucus collected at equal distances proximally and distally from tumors (resected colon segments were examined) revealed significantly higher DNA levels in the samples collected distally, thus confirming distal movement of the mucus with all incorporated elements.[31] The latter finding led our group to developing a completely noninvasive technique for collecting colorectal mucus samples by swabbing the anal area immediately following defecation.[55] This technique was successfully applied for noninvasive CRC detection in our recent pilot study.[103] There is no doubt that colonic mucus can be regarded as a unique biological material possessing an enormous diagnostic potential due to abundant presence of different types of CRC-associated biomarkers comprising a range of proteins[103] and DNA[31] demonstrated in human studies and microRNAs, which have been detected in colonic mucus taken from rats during experimental induction of CRC.[104]

While the diagnostic significance of colonic mucus is gradually becoming recognized, this substance also emerges as an important pathogenetic factor in the development of CRC. Experimental studies have demonstrated that mice genetically deficient in the *MUC2* are predisposed to developing CRC.[105-107] Likewise, goblet cell depletion was demonstrated during 1,2-dimethylhydrazine-induced colon carcinogenesis in rats.[108] *MUC2* expression decrease in human colorectal tumors was shown to correlate with tumor progression from adenomas to advanced adenocarcinomas,[109] and reduced *MUC2* expression is usually associated with poor prognosis in CRC patients.[110,111] However, mucinous carcinomas demonstrating elevated levels of expression of several mucin-encoding genes constitute a notable exception[112-114] remaining to be explained. In addition, impaired colonic *O*-glycosylation was shown to stimulate colitis-associated carcinogenesis in genetically modified mice[115,116] and to contribute to CRC development in humans.[117] These observations suggest that CRC-associated compositional alterations of colonic mucus are likely to entail its structural changes, and recent advances in clarifying the impact of mucus-inhabiting microbiota in colorectal carcinogenesis are especially interesting in this context.

It is now well established that CRC development is accompanied by substantial changes in human gut microbiome composition.[118] Recent studies have also revealed that bacteria probably implicated in carcinogenesis can generate biofilms already mentioned in the context of IBD.[37,67] Biofilm formation in the colon of CRC patients is usually confined to the mucus overlaying tumor surface or margins, and the biofilms were shown to be located within the inner mucus layer,[67,119,120] which is sterile in the normal conditions, but apparently damaged in CRC patients. It was, however, unclear whether biofilm formation could be regarded as a carcinogenesis-triggering factor or a consequence of tumor growth.

Recent studies have demonstrated that biofilm presence was strongly associated with proximal tumors,[119,120] especially with mucinous CRC.[119,121] The main bacterial species identified in these biofilms were gut commensal *B. fragilis* that may generate enterotoxigenic strains[122] and oral pathogens including *Fusobacterium nucleatum*, *Parvimonas micra*, and *Peptostreptococcus stomatis*.[120] Further research of the same group revealed the presence of patchy bacterial biofilms composed predominantly of enterotoxigenic *B. fragilis* and colibactin-expressing *Escherichia coli* on the surface of the colonic mucosa of patients with familial adenomatous polyposis.[123] Importantly, the detected biofilms were not restricted to polyps and were not associated with proximal colon location.[123] Moreover, co-colonization of tumor-prone mice with these bacterial strains provoked DNA damage in colonic epithelium and accelerated experimental carcinogenesis.[123] The latter finding was later confirmed in three murine models, and bacterial biofilms obtained from both CRC patients and healthy individuals manifestly promoted colon carcinogenesis.[124] Interestingly, *F. nucleatum* was apparently not required for carcinogenesis in the latter case, being possibly involved in later stages of human CRC.[124] Taken together, these results indicate that polymicrobial bacterial biofilms may now be regarded as a potential additional colon carcinogen.

The described new developments related to the role of colonic mucus in CRC development reveal a previously unknown area of pathogenetically important interactions between gut mucus, luminal bacteria, epithelial cells (normal, malignant, and especially mucus-producing goblet cells), and immune cells actively migrating to colonic mucus through the epithelium. These interactions are schematically presented in **Figure 3**. It is evident that bacterial biofilm's direct contact with the epithelium can be damaging or carcinogenic *per se*, but the inevitably intervening immune response is another factor of great importance. The main antibacterial (and antibiofilm) roles of effector immune cells (especially neutrophils and eosinophils)

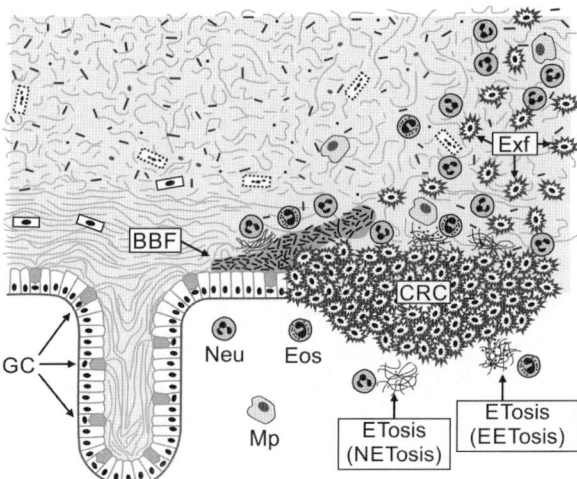

Fig. 3: Schematic of colorectal mucus-associated events involved in CRC development. (BBF: bacterial biofilm; Exf: exfoliated malignant cells of CRC; GC: goblet cells; Neu: neutrophils; Eos: eosinophils; Mp: macrophages; ETosis: extracellular DNA trap formation; NETosis: neutrophil-derived ETosis; EETosis: eosinophil-derived ETosis)

migrating to the colonic mucus include phagocytosis, release of cytotoxic proteins (during degranulation), and ETosis (formation of antibacterial extracellular DNA traps). However, in the loosened mucus overlaying tumor surface, both cytotoxic factors and ETosis can also harm host cells, damaging both malignant and healthy tissue elements. The significance of these impacts in the context of CRC remains obscure and requires further intense research. Elucidation of physiological mechanisms controlling biological and pathogenetic events occurring within colonic mucus is an obligatory prerequisite for possible development of new therapeutic approaches targeting CRC through the mucus of the gut.

CONCLUSION

The gut mucus layer is a highly dynamic and rapidly renewing barrier structure, the importance of which for gastrointestinal physiology and homeostasis maintenance was seriously underestimated until recently. The significance of colonic mucus impact in the pathogenesis of major colorectal diseases including IBD and CRC is only starting to emerge. Further progress in this field promises both devising more efficient noninvasive diagnostic approaches and creating new therapeutic strategies for these diseases.

REFERENCES

1. Hansson GC. Mucus and mucins in diseases of the intestinal and respiratory tracts. J Intern Med. 2019;285:479-90.
2. Pelaseyed T, Bergström JH, Gustafsson JK, Ermund A, Birchenough GM, Schütte A, et al. The mucus and mucins of the goblet cells and enterocytes provide the first defense line of the gastrointestinal tract and interact with the immune system. Immunol Rev. 2014;260:8-20.
3. Matsuo K, Ota H, Akamatsu T, Sugiyama A, Katsuyama T. Histochemistry of the surface mucous gel layer of the human colon. Gut. 1997;40:782-9.
4. Johansson ME, Phillipson M, Petersson J, Velcich A, Holm L, Hansson GC. The inner of the two *MUC2* mucin-dependent mucus layers in colon is devoid of bacteria. Proc Natl Acad Sci USA. 2008;105:15064-9.
5. Johansson ME, Holmén Larsson JM, Hansson GC. The two mucus layers of colon are organized by the *MUC2* mucin, whereas the outer layer is a legislator of host-microbial interactions. Proc Natl Acad Sci USA. 2011;108:4659-65.
6. Ermund A, Schütte A, Johansson ME, Gustafsson JK, Hansson GC. Studies of mucus in mouse stomach, small intestine, and colon. I. Gastrointestinal mucus layers have different properties depending on location as well as over the Peyer's patches. Am J Physiol Gastrointest Liver Physiol. 2013;305:G341-7.
7. Birchenough GM, Johansson ME, Gustaffson JK, Bergström JH, Hansson GC. New developments in goblet cell mucus secretion and function. Mucosal Immunol. 2015;8:712-9.
8. Johansson ME, Ambort E, Pelaseyed T, Schütte A, Gustafsson JK, Ermund A, et al. Composition and functional role of the mucus layers in the intestine. Cell Mol Life Sci. 2011;68:3635-41.

9. Johansson ME, Sjövall H, Hansson GC. The gastrointestinal mucus system in health and disease. Nat Rev Gastroenterol Hepatol. 2013;10:352-61.
10. Round AN, Rigby NM, Garcia de la Torre A, Macierzanka A, Mills EN, Mackie AR. Lamellar structures of *MUC2*-rich mucin: a potential role in governing the barrier and lubricating functions of intestinal mucus. Biomacromolecules. 2012;13:3253-61.
11. Johansson ME. Fast renewal of the distal colonic mucus layers by the surface goblet cells as measured by in vivo labelling of mucin glycoproteins. PLoS One. 2012;7:e41009.
12. Schütte A, Ermund A, Becker-Pauly C, Johansson ME, Rodríguez-Piñeiro AM, Bäckhed F, et al. Microbial-induced meprin β cleavage in *MUC2* mucin and a functional CFTR channel are required to release anchored small intestinal mucus. Proc Natl Acad Sci USA. 2014;111:12396-401.
13. Desai MS, Seekatz AM, Koropatkin NM, Kamada N, Hickey CA, Wolter M, et al. A dietary fiber-deprived gut microbiota degrades the colonic mucus barrier and enhances pathogen susceptibility. Cell. 2016;167:1339-53.
14. McGuckin MA, Eri R, Simms LA, Florin TH, Radford-Smith G. Intestinal barrier dysfunction in inflammatory bowel diseases. Inflamm Bowel Dis. 2009;15:100-13.
15. Mabbott NA, Donaldson DS, Ohno H, Williams IR, Mahajan A. Microfold (M) cells: important immunosurveillance posts in the intestinal epithelium. Mucosal Immunol. 2013;6:666-77.
16. Parikh K, Antanaviciute A, Fawkner-Corbett D, Jagielowicz M, Aulicino A, Lagerholm C, et al. Colonic epithelial cell diversity in health and inflammatory bowel disease. Nature. 2019;567:49-55.
17. Johansson ME, Hansson GC. Is the intestinal goblet cell a major immune cell? Cell Host Microbe. 2014;15:251-2.
18. McDole JR, Wheeler LW, McDonald KG, Wang B, Konjufca V, Knoop KA, et al. Goblet cells deliver luminal antigen to CD103+ dendritic cells in the small intestine. Nature. 2012;483:345-9.
19. Patel KK, Miyoshi H, Beatty WL, Head RD, Malvin NP, Cadwell K, et al. Autophagy proteins control goblet cell function by potentiating reactive oxygen species production. EMBO J. 2013;32:3130-44.
20. Wlodarska M, Thaiss CA, Nowarski R, Henao-Mejia J, Zhang JP, Brown EM, et al. NLRP6 inflammasome orchestrates the colonic host-microbial interface by regulating goblet cell mucus secretion. Cell. 2014;156:1045-59.
21. Birchenough GM, Nyström EE, Johansson ME, Hansson GC. A sentinel goblet cell guards the colonic crypt by triggering Nlrp6-dependent *MUC2* secretion. Science. 2016;352:1535-42.
22. Knoop KA, McDonald KG, McCrate S, McDole JR, Newberry RD. Microbial sensing by goblet cells controls immune surveillance of luminal antigens in the colon. Mucosal Immunol. 2015;8:198-210.
23. McGuckin MA, Hasnain SZ. Goblet cells as mucosal sentinels for immunity. Mucosal Immunol. 2017;10:1118-21.
24. Gassler N. Paneth cells in intestinal physiology and pathophysiology. World J Gastrointest Pathophysiol. 2017;8:150-60.
25. Renner M, Bergmann G, Krebs I, End C, Lyer S, Hilberg F, et al. *DMBT1* confers mucosal protection in vivo and a deletion variant is associated with Crohn's disease. Gastroenterology. 2007;133:1499-509.

26. Antoni L, Nuding S, Weller D, Gersemann M, Ott G, Wehkamp J, et al. Human colonic mucus is a reservoir for antimicrobial peptides. J Crohns Colitis. 2013;7:e652-64.
27. Johansen FE, Kaetzel CS. Regulation of the polymeric immunoglobulin receptor and IgA transport: new advances in environmental factors that stimulate pIgR expression and its role in mucosal immunology. Mucosal Immunol. 2011;4:598-602.
28. Rogier EW, Frantz AL, Bruno ME, Kaetzel CS. Secretory IgA is concentrated in the outer layer of colonic mucus along with gut bacteria. Pathogens. 2014;3:390-403.
29. Espey MG. Role of oxygen gradients in shaping redox relationships between the human intestine and its microbiota. Free Radic Biol Med. 2013;55:130-40.
30. Loktionov A. Cell exfoliation in the human colon: myth, reality and implications for colorectal cancer screening. Int J Cancer. 2007;120:2281-9.
31. Loktionov A, Bandaletova T, Llewelyn AH, Dion C, Lywood HG, Lywood RC, et al. Colorectal cancer detection by measuring DNA from exfoliated colonocytes obtained by direct contact with rectal mucosa. Int J Oncol. 2009;34:301-11.
32. Datta SS, Preska Steinberg A, Ismagilov RF. Polymers in the gut compress the colonic mucus hydrogel. Proc Natl Acad Sci USA. 2016;113:7041-6.
33. Kamphuis JBJ, Mercier-Bonin M, Eutamène H, Theodorou V. Mucus organisation is shaped by colonic content; a new view. Sci Rep. 2017;7:8527.
34. Lennon G, Balfe A, Earley G, et al. Influences of the colonic microbiome on the mucous gel layer in ulcerative colitis. Gut Microbes. 2014;5:277-85.
35. Tropini C, Earle KA, Huang KC, Devane LA, Lavelle A, Winter DC, et al. The gut microbiome: connecting spatial organization to function. Cell Host Microbe. 2017;21:433-42.
36. Bergstrom KS, Xia L. Mucin-type O-glycans and their roles in intestinal homeostasis. Glycobiology. 2013;23:1026-37.
37. Tytgat HLP, Nobrega FL, van der Oost J, de Vos WM. Bowel biofilms: tipping points between a healthy and compromised gut. Trends Microbiol. 2019;27:17-25.
38. Taylor SL, McGuckin MA, Wesselingh S, Rogrs GB. Infection's sweet tooth: how glycans mediate infection and disease susceptibility. Trends Microbiol. 2018;26:92-101.
39. Staubach F, Künzel S, Baines AC, Yee A, McGee BM, Bäckhed F, et al. Expression of the blood-group-related glycosyltransferase *B4GALNT2* influences the intestinal microbiota in mice. ISME J. 2012;6:1345-55.
40. Rausch P, Rehman A, Künzel S, Häsler R, Ott SJ, Schreiber S, et al. Colonic mucosa-associated microbiota is influenced by an interaction of Crohn disease and *FUT2* (Secretor) genotype. Proc Natl Acad Sci USA. 2011;108:19030-5.
41. Tong M, McHardy I, Ruegger P, Goudarzi M, Kashyap PC, Haritunians T, et al. Reprograming of gut microbiome energy metabolism by the *FUT2* Crohn's disease risk polymorphism. ISME J. 2014;8:2193-206.
42. Wacklin P, Mäkivuokko H, Alakulppi N, Nikkilä J, Tenkanen H, Räbinä J, et al. Secretor genotype (*FUT2* gene) is strongly associated with the composition of Bifidobacteria in the human intestine. PLoS One. 2011;6:e20113.
43. Davenport ER, Goodrich JK, Bell JT, Spector TD, Ley RE, Clark AG. ABO antigen and secretor statuses are not associated with gut microbiota composition in 1,500 twins. BMC Genomics. 2016;17:941.

44. Turpin W, Bedrani L, Espin-Garcia O, Xu W, Silverberg MS, Smith MI, et al. FUT2 genotype and secretory status are not associated with fecal microbial composition and inferred function in healthy subjects. Gut Microbes. 2018;9:357-68.
45. Holmén Larsson JM, Thomsson KA, Rodríguez-Piñeiro AM, Karlsson H, Hansson GC. Studies of mucus in mouse stomach, small intestine, and colon. III. Gastrointestinal *MUC5AC* and *MIC2* mucin O-glycan patterns reveal a regiospecific distribution. Am J Gastrointest Liver Physiol. 2013;305:G357-63.
46. Arike L, Holmén Larsson JM, Hansson GC. Intestinal *MUC2* mucin O-glycosylation is affected by microbiota and regulated by differential expression of glycosyltransferases. Glycobiology. 2017;27:318-28.
47. Rokhsefat S, Lin A, Comelli EM. Mucin-microbiota interaction during postnatal maturation of the intestinal ecosystem: Clinical implications. Dig Dis Sci. 2016;61:1473-86.
48. Jakobsson HE, Rodríguez-Piñeiro AM, Schütte A, Ermund A, Boysen P, Bemark M, et al. The composition of the gut microbiota shapes the colon mucus barrier. EMBO Rep. 2015;16:164-77.
49. Hayes CL, Dong J, Galipeau HJ, Jury J, McCarville J, Huang X, et al. Commensal microbiota induces colonic barrier structure and functions that contribute to homeostasis. Sci Rep. 2018;8:14184.
50. Sovran B, Hugenholtz F, Elderman M, Van Beek AA, Graversen K, Huijskes M, et al. Age-associated impairment of the mucus barrier function is associated with profound changes in microbiota and immunity. Sci Rep. 2019;9:1437.
51. Merchant HA, Rabbie SC, Varum FJ, Afonso-Pereira A, Basit AW. Influence of ageing on the gastrointestinal environment of the rat and its implications for drug delivery. Eur J Pharm Sci. 2014;62:76-85.
52. Claesson MJ, Cusack S, O'Sullivan O, Greene-Diniz R, de Weerd H, Flannery E, et al. Composition, variability, and temporal stability of the intestinal microbiota of the elderly. Proc Natl Acad Sci USA. 2011;108(Suppl 1):4586-91.
53. van der Flier LG, Clevers H. Stem cells, self-renewal, and differentiation in the intestinal epithelium. Annu Rev Physiol. 2009;71:241-60.
54. Nair P, Lagerholm S, Dutta S, Shami S, Davis K, Ma S, et al. Coprocytobiology: on the nature of cellular elements from stools in the pathophysiology of colonic disease. J Clin Gastroenterol. 2003;36(Suppl 5):S84-93.
55. Loktionov A, Chhaya V, Bandaletova T, Andrew P. Assessment of cytology and mucin 2 in colorectal mucus collected from patients with inflammatory bowel disease: results of a pilot trial. J Gastroenterol Hepatol. 2016;31:326-33.
56. Loktionov A, O'Neill IK, Silvester KR, Cummings JH, Middleton SJ, Miller R. Quantitation of DNA from exfoliated colonocytes isolated from human stool surface as a novel noninvasive screening test for colorectal cancer. Clin Cancer Res. 1998;4:337-42.
57. Bandaletova T, Bailey N, Bingham SA, Loktionov A. Isolation of exfoliated colonocytes from human stool as a new technique for colonic cytology. APMIS. 2002;110:239-46.
58. Davies RJ, Freeman A, Morris LS, Bingham S, Dilworth D, Scott I, et al. Analysis of minichromosome maintenance proteins as a novel method for detection of colorectal cancer in stool. Lancet. 2002;359:1917-9.

59. Torres J, Mehandru S, Colombel JF, Peyrin-Biroulet L. Crohn's disease. Lancet. 2017;389:1741-55.
60. Ungaro R, Mehandru S, Allen PB, Peyrin-Biroulet L, Colombel JF. Ulcerative colitis. Lancet. 2017;389:1756-70.
61. Kaser A, Zeissig S, Blumberg RS. Inflammatory bowel disease. Annu Rev Immunol. 2010;28:573-621.
62. Cader MZ, Kaser A. Recent advances in inflammatory bowel disease: mucosal immune cells in intestinal inflammation. Gut. 2013;62:1653-64.
63. de Souza HS, Fiocchi C. Immunopathogenesis of IBD: current state of the art. Nat Rev Gastroenterol Hepatol. 2016;13:13-27.
64. Johansson ME. Mucus layers in inflammatory bowel disease. Inflamm Bowel Dis. 2014;20:2124-31.
65. Van der Sluis M, De Koning BA, De Bruin AC, Velcich A, Meijerink JP, Van Goudoever JB, et al. *MUC2*-deficient mice spontaneously develop colitis, indicating that *MUC2* is critical for colonic protection. Gastroenterology. 2006;131:117-29.
66. Swidsinski A, Weber J, Loening-Baucke V, Hale LP, Lochs H, et al. Spatial organization and composition of the mucosal flora in patients with inflammatory bowel disease. J Clin Microbiol. 2005;43:3380-9.
67. Li S, Konstantinov SR, Smits R, Peppelenbosch MP. Bacterial biofilms in colorectal cancer initiation and progression. Trends Mol Med. 2017;23:18-30.
68. Hasnain SZ, Lourie R, Das I, Chen AC, Mcguckin MA. The interplay between endoplasmic reticulum stress and inflammation. Immunol Cell Biol. 2012;90:260-70.
69. Wehkamp J, Salzman NH, Porter E, Nuding S, Weichenthal M, Petras RE, et al. Reduced Paneth cell alpha-defensins in ileal Crohn's disease. Proc Natl Acad Sci USA. 2005;102:18129-34.
70. Hasnain SZ, Tauro S, Das I, Tong H, Chen AC, Jeffery PL, et al. IL-10 promotes production of intestinal mucus by suppressing protein misfolding and endoplasmic reticulum stress in goblet cells. Gastroenterology. 2013;144:357-68.
71. Niv Y. Mucin genes expression in the intestine of Crohn's disease patients: a systematic review and meta-analysis. J Gastrointestin Liver Dis. 2016;25:351-7.
72. Niv Y. Mucin genes expression in the intestine of ulcerative colitis patients: a systematic review and meta-analysis. Eur J Gastroenterol Hepatol. 2016;28:1241-5.
73. Swidsinski A, Loening-Baucke V, Theissig F, Engelhardt H, Bengmark S, Koch S, et al. Comparative study of the intestinal barrier in normal and inflamed colon. Gut. 2007;56:343-50.
74. Strugala V, Dettmar PW, Pearson JP. Thickness and continuity of the adherent colonic mucus barrier in active and quiescent ulcerative colitis and Crohn's disease. Int J Clin Pract. 2008;62:762-9.
75. Gersemann M, Becker S, Kübler I, Koslowski M, Wang G, Herrlinger KR, et al. Differences in goblet cell differentiation between Crohn's disease and ulcerative colitis. Differentiation. 2009;77:84-94.
76. Johansson ME, Gustafsson JK, Holmén-Larsson J, Jabbar KS, Xia L, Xu H, et al. Bacteria penetrate the normally impenetrable inner colon mucus layer in both murine colitis models and patients with ulcerative colitis. Gut. 2014;63:281-91.
77. van der Post S, Jabbar KS, Birchenough G, Arike L, Akhtar N, Sjovall H, et al. Structural weakening of the colonic mucus barrier is an early event in ulcerative colitis pathogenesis. Gut. 2019;68(12):2142-51.

78. Lennon G, Balfe Á, Bambury N, Lavelle A, Maguire N, Docherty J, et al. Correlations between colonic crypt mucin chemotype, inflammatory grade and Desulfovibrio species in ulcerative colitis. Colorectal Dis. 2014;16:O161-9.
79. Vancamelbeke M, Vanuytsel T, Farré R, Verstockt S, Ferrante M, Assche GV, et al. Genetic and transcriptomic bases of intestinal barrier dysfunction in inflammatory bowel disease. Inflamm Bowel Dis. 2017;23:1718-29.
80. Glymenaki M, Singh G, Brass A, Warhurst G, McBain AJ, Else KJ, et al. Compositional changes in the gut mucus microbiota precede the onset of colitis-induced inflammation. Inflamm Bowel Dis. 2017;23:912-22.
81. Png CW, Lindén SK, Gilshehan KS, Zoetendal EG, McSweeney CS, Sly LI, et al. Mucolytic bacteria with increased prevalence in IBD mucosa augment in vitro utilization of mucin by other bacteria. Am J Gastroenterol. 2010;105:2420-8.
82. Lavelle A, Lennon G, O'Sullivan O, Docherty N, Balfe A, Maguire A, et al. Spatial variation of the colonic microbiota in patients with ulcerative colitis and control volunteers. Gut. 2015;64:1553-61.
83. Kaplan GG, Ng SC. Understanding and preventing the global increase of inflammatory bowel disease. Gastroenterology. 2017;152:313-21.
84. Birchenough G, Schroeder BO, Bäckhed, Hansson GC. Dietary destabilisation of the balance between the microbiota and the colonic mucus barrier. Gut Microbes. 2019;10:246-50.
85. Schroeder BO, Birchenough GMH, Ståhlman M, Arike L, Johansson MEV, Hansson GC, et al. Bifidobacteria or fiber protects against diet-induced microbiota-mediated colonic mucus deterioration. Cell Host Microbe. 2018;23:27-40.
86. Kumar M, Kissoon-Singh V, Coria AL, Moreau F, Chade K. Probiotic mixture VSL#3 reduces colonic inflammation and improves intestinal barrier function in *MUC2* mucin-deficient mice. Am J Physiol Gastrointest Liver Physiol. 2017;312:G34-45.
87. Engevik MA, Luk B, Chang-Graham AL, Hall A, Herrmann B, Ruan W, et al. Bifidobacterium dentium fortifies the intestinal mucus layer via autophagy and calcium signalling pathways. MBio. 2019;10:e01087-19.
88. D'Agostino EM, Rossetti D, Atkins D, Ferdinando D, Yakubov GE. Interaction of tea polyphenols and food constituents with model gut epithelia: the protective role of the mucus gel layer. J Agric Food Chem. 2012;60:3318-28.
89. He W, Liu M, Li Y, Yu H, Wang D, Chen Q, et al. Flavonoids from Citrus aurantium ameliorate TNBS-induced ulcerative colitis through protecting colonic mucus layer integrity. Eur J Pharmacol. 2019;857:172456.
90. Sands BE. Biomarkers of inflammation in inflammatory bowel disease. Gastroenterology. 2015;149:1275-85.
91. Anderson N, Suliman I, Bandaletova T, Obichere A, Lywood R, Loktionov A, et al. Protein biomarkers in exfoliated cells collected from the human rectal mucosa: implications for colorectal disease detection and monitoring. Int J Colorectal Dis. 2011;26:1287-97.
92. Bandaletova T, Chhaya V, Poullis A, Loktionov A. Colorectal mucus non-invasively collected from patients with inflammatory bowel disease and its suitability for diagnostic cytology. APMIS. 2016;124:160-8.
93. Loktionov A, Chhaya V, Bandaletova T, Poullis A. Inflammatory bowel disease detection and monitoring by measuring biomarkers in non-invasively collected colorectal mucus. J Gastroenterol Hepatol. 2017;32:992-1002.

94. Loktionov A. Eosinophils in the gastrointestinal tract and their role in the pathogenesis of major colorectal disorders. World J Gastroent. 2019;25:3503-26.
95. Grady WM, Markowitz SD. The molecular pathogenesis of colorectal cancer and its potential application to colorectal cancer screening. Dig Dis Sci. 2015;60:762-72.
96. Sidransky D, Tokino T, Hamilton SR, Kinzler KW, Levin B, Frost P, et al. Identification of ras oncogene mutations in the stool of patients with curable colorectal tumors. Science. 1992;256:102-5.
97. Imperiale TF, Ransohoff DF, Itzkowitz SH, Turnbull BA, Ross ME. Fecal DNA versus fecal occult blood for colorectal-cancer screening in an average-risk population. N Engl J Med. 2004;351:2704-14.
98. Imperiale TF, Ransohoff DF, Itzkowitz SH, Levin TR, Lavin P, Lidgard, GP, et al. Multitarget stool DNA testing for colorectal-cancer screening. N Engl J Med. 2014;370:1287-97.
99. Matsushita H, Matsumura Y, Moriya Y, Akasu T, Fujita S, Yamamoto S, et al. A new method for isolating colonocytes from naturally evacuated feces and its clinical application to colorectal cancer diagnosis. Gastroenterology. 2005;129:1918-27.
100. White V, Scarpini C, Barbosa-Morais NL, Ikelle E, Carter S, Laskey RA, et al. Isolation of stool-derived mucus provides a high yield of colonocytes suitable for early detection of colorectal carcinoma. Cancer Epidemiol Biomarkers Prev. 2009;18:2006-13.
101. Ahlquist DA, Harrington JJ, Burgart LJ, Roche PC. Morphometric analysis of the "mucocellular layer" overlying colorectal cancer and normal mucosa: relevance to exfoliation and stool screening. Hum Pathol. 2000;31:51-7.
102. Hamer HM, Jonkers DM, Loof A, Vanhoutvin SA, Troost FJ, Venema K, et al. Analyses of human colonic mucus obtained by in vivo sampling technique. Dig Liver Dis. 2009;41:559-64.
103. Loktionov A, Soubieres A, Bandaletova T, Mathur J, Poullis A. Colorectal cancer detection by biomarker quantification in noninvasively collected colorectal mucus: preliminary comparison of 24 protein biomarkers. Eur J Gastroenterol Hepatol. 2019;31:1220-7.
104. Kunte DP, DelaCruz M, Wali RK, Menon A, Du M, Stypula Y, et al. Dysregulation of microRNAs in colonic field carcinogenesis: implications for screening. PLoS One. 2012;7:e45591.
105. Velcich A, Yang W, Heyer J, Fragale A, Nicholas C, Viani, S, et al. Colorectal cancer in mice genetically deficient in the mucin *MUC2*. Science. 2002;295:1726-9.
106. Yang K, Popova NV, Yang WC, Lozonschil, Tadesse S, Kent S, et al. Interaction of *MUC2* and *APC* on *WNT* signalling and in intestinal tumorigenesis: potential role of chronic inflammation. Cancer Res. 2008;68:7313-22.
107. Bao Y, Guo Y, Li Z, Fang W, Yang Y, Li X, et al. MicroRNA profiling in *MUC2* knockout mice of colitis-associated cancer model reveals epigenetic alterations during chronic colitis malignant transformation. PLoS One. 2014;9:e99132.
108. Novaes RD, Sequetto PL, Vilela Gonçalves R, Cupertino MC, Santos EC, Mello VJ, et al. Depletion of enteroendocrine and mucus-secreting cells is associated with colorectal carcinogenesis severity and impaired intestinal motility in rats. Microsc Res Tech. 2016;79:3-13.
109. Mizoshita T, Tsukamoto T, Inada KI, Naoki H, Masahiro T, Taketsune N, et al. Loss of *MUC2* expression correlates with progression along the adenoma-carcinoma

sequence pathway as well as de novo carcinogenesis in the colon. Histol Histopathol. 2007;22:251-60.
110. Betge J, Schneider NI, Harbaum L, Pollheimer MJ, Lindtner RA, Kornprat P, et al. *MUC1*, *MUC2*, *MUC5AC*, and *MUC6* in colorectal cancer: expression profiles and clinical significance. Virchows Arch. 2016;469:255-65.
111. Kasprzak A, Siodła E, Andrzejewska M, Szmeja J, Seraszek-Jaros A, Cofta S, et al. Differential expression of mucin 1 and mucin 2 in colorectal cancer. World J Gastroenterol. 2018;24:4164-77.
112. Tozawa E, Ajioka Y, Watanabe H, Nishikura K, Mukai G, Suda T, et al. Mucin expression, p53 overexpression, and peritumoral lymphocytic infiltration of advanced colorectal carcinoma with mucus component: is mucinous carcinoma a distinct histological entity? Pathol Res Pract. 2007;203:567-74.
113. Walsh MD, Clendenning M, Williamson E, Pearson SA, Walters JR, Nagler B, et al. Expression of *MUC2*, *MUC5AC*, *MUC5B*, and *MUC6* mucins in colorectal cancers and their association with the CpG island methylator phenotype. Mod Pathol. 2013;26:1642-56.
114. Li G, Yang S, Shen P, Wu B, Sun T, Sun H, et al. SCF/c-KIT signalling promotes mucus secretion of colonic goblet cells and development of mucinous colorectal adenocarcinoma. Am J Cancer Res. 2018;8:1064-73.
115. An G, Wei B, Xia B, Michael McDaniel J, Ju T, Cumming RD, et al. Increased susceptibility to colitis and colorectal tumors in mice lacking core 3-derived O-glycans. J Exp Med. 2007;204:1417-29.
116. Bergstrom K, Liu X, Zhao Y, Gao N, Wu Q, Song K, et al. Defective intestinal mucin-type O-glycosylation causes spontaneous colitis-associated cancer in mice. Gastroenterology. 2016;151:152-64.
117. Jiang Y, Liu Z, Xu F, Xichen D, Yurong C, Yizhang H, et al. Aberrant O-glycosylation contributes to tumorigenesis in human colorectal cancer. J Cell Mol Med. 2018;22:4875-85.
118. Wong SH, Yu J. Gut microbiota in colorectal cancer: mechanisms of action and clinical applications. Nat Rev Gastroenterol Hepatol. 2019;16:690-704.
119. Dejea CM, Wick EC, Hechenbleikner EM, White JR, Mark Wlech JL, Rosetti BJ, et al. Microbiota organization is a distinct feature of proximal colorectal cancers. Proc Natl Acad Sci USA. 2014;111:18321-6.
120. Drewes JL, White JR, Dejea CM, Paya, F, Thevambiga I, Januma V, et al. High-resolution bacterial 16S rRNA gene profile meta-analysis and biofilm status reveal common colorectal cancer consortia. NPJ Biofilms Microbiomes. 2017;3:34.
121. Li S, Peppelenbosch MP, Smits R. Bacterial biofilms as a potential contributor to mucinous colorectal cancer formation. Biochim Biophys Acta Rev Cancer. 2019;1872:74-9.
122. Sears CL. Enterotoxigenic Bacteroides fragilis: a rogue among symbiotes. Clin Microbiol Rev. 2009;22:349-69.
123. Dejea CM, Fathi P, Craig JM, Boleij A, Taddese R, Geis AL, et al. Patients with familial adenomatous polyposis harbour colonic biofilms containing tumorigenic bacteria. Science. 2018;359:592-7.
124. Tomkovich S, Dejea CM, Winglee K, Drewes JL, Chung L, Franck, H, et al. Human colon mucosal biofilms from healthy or colon cancer hosts are carcinogenic. J Clin Invest. 2019;130:1699-712.

CHAPTER

7

Ten Common Errors in the Treatment of *Helicobacter Pylori* Infection

Javier P Gisbert, Olga P Nyssen

INTRODUCTION

Helicobacter pylori infection affects billions of people worldwide. This infection is the main known cause of gastritis, peptic ulcer disease, and gastric cancer.[1] However, even after more than 30 years of experience in the treatment of *H. pylori*, the ideal regimen to treat this infection remains undefined. Antibiotic resistance has been identified as one of the major factors affecting our ability to cure *H. pylori* infection, and the rate of resistance—mainly to clarithromycin—seems to be increasing in many geographic areas.[2]

Constant decision-making is required in daily clinical practice, and each decision is open to possible errors. Misconceptions are very common in clinical practice, but can be prevented.[3-5] Since 1997, there has been a proliferation of literature, guidelines, and consensus conferences on *H. pylori* providing evidence-based recommendations that should be implemented in clinical practice. However, doubts have been raised in the field of implementation science on the delay and real penetration of guideline publications by themselves,[6,7] suggesting that in order to reach high levels of penetration and implementation, guidelines should comply with some basic attributes and must be assimilated by the practitioner.[8-10]

Our objective was to review 10 of the most common errors in the treatment of *H. pylori* infection **(Box 1)**. This chapter aims to state the commonly found

Box 1: Ten common errors in the treatment of *Helicobacter pylori* infection.

1. To consider sufficient an *H. pylori* cure rate of 80%
2. To use the standard triple therapy in areas where it is ineffective for *H. pylori* eradication
3. To prescribe *H. pylori* eradication therapy for only 7–10 days
4. To use a standard dose of proton-pump inhibitors in *H. pylori* eradication regimens
5. To underestimate the benefit of adding bismuth to antibiotic treatment to eradicate *H. pylori* infection
6. In patients allergic to penicillin, to prescribe always a triple therapy with clarithromycin and metronidazole
7. To systematically supplement *H. pylori* eradication treatment with probiotics
8. To repeat certain antibiotics, mainly after *H. pylori* eradication failure
9. To ignore the importance of compliance with treatment for *H. pylori* eradication
10. Not to check the success (or failure) of *H. pylori* eradication after treatment

errors in clinical practice, to review the related scientific evidence and, finally, to propose the adequate approach in each case.

COMMON ERRORS IN THE TREATMENT OF HELICOBACTER PYLORI INFECTION

Error 1: To Consider Sufficient a *Helicobacter Pylori* Cure Rate of 80%

The first and probably most frequent misconception is to consider a cure rate ≥80% as sufficient. In fact, in all previous European consensuses up to 2017, a threshold of 80% was agreed as an acceptable *H. pylori* eradication efficacy rate.[11-13] However, the usual cure rates of therapy for *H. pylori* infection are lower in spite of being considered acceptable for other serious, treatable bacterial infections. The expectation for most bacterial infections is that >95% of infections can be reliably cured with the first course of therapy.[14] Actually, patients' expectations of a minimal success rate of eradication therapy are higher than those of their physicians; in a study of real-world practice and expectations of Asia-Pacific physicians and patients, the expectation of minimal eradication rate among patients was 91% while that of physicians was only 86%.[15]

The approach to anti-*H. pylori* therapy differs from other common gastrointestinal conditions because, as an infectious disease, treatment success of more than 90–95% should be expected.[16] At present, an optimal anti-*H. pylori* regimen is therefore generally defined as one that reliably offers a cure rate of at least 90%, to meet the existing practice in the field of other common bacterial infectious diseases.[17,18] Therefore, *H. pylori* therapies have been suggested to be the best according to absolute outcome, since a cure rate of 90% or more is considered good, 95% excellent, and <90% unacceptable (bad).[16,17,19,20] Due to the lack of susceptibility data, an optimal therapy might be defined as one that consistently provides high cure rates (e.g., ≥90%) irrespective of the presence of antimicrobial resistance. Recently, in 2015, the Kyoto consensus report on *H. pylori* gastritis recommended, accordingly, that within any region, only regimens reliably producing eradication rates ≥90% in that population should be used for empirical treatment.[21]

Clearly, at the present time, most treatments' eradication rates cannot be considered "good," according to the aforementioned proposed report cards' grading system.[17] All treatments must be optimized in terms of duration, dose, and interval of administration of proton-pump inhibitors (PPIs) and antibiotics[22] in order to achieve this goal. Even so, although considerable emphasis has been placed on the need to cure >90% of infections, and on ruling out any treatment that does not reach this threshold, achieving very high cure rates is difficult and 100% cure rates are virtually impossible.[23] The most important reason for this statement is that the tests used to assess cure are not perfect—false-positive results range from 0 to 15% depending on the accuracy of the diagnostic method. Thus, even if a perfect "100% cure" treatment was tested, the cure rates observed would range between 85 and 95% and would only exceptionally reach 100%, with false-positive test results accounting for most of the "failures."[23]

In summary, an optimal *H. pylori* eradication therapy might be defined as one that consistently provides ≥90% cure rates irrespective of the presence of antimicrobial resistance; to achieve this goal, all treatments must be optimized in terms of duration, dose, and interval of administration of PPIs and antibiotics.

Error 2: To Use the Standard Triple Therapy in Areas Where It is Ineffective for *Helicobacter Pylori* Eradication

The traditionally most commonly used first-line triple therapies—a PPI plus two antibiotics—fail in approximately 20–40% of patients, as shown in large clinical trials and meta-analyses and in clinical practice where this rate might be even higher.[1,24] The primary cause of therapeutic failure in patients with infectious diseases, particularly *H. pylori* infection,[25] is probably antibiotic resistance. Thus, the success rate of standard triple therapies is declining due to the increased resistance to antibiotics, mainly clarithromycin—around the globe.[19,26,27] Consequently, the efficacy of standard triple therapy has been shown to be progressively declining to unacceptable levels.[28,29] Furthermore, the ethics of continued use of standard triple therapy has recently been questioned, and alternative approaches have been recommended.[30]

For example, already in the year 2000, a meta-analysis of studies combining a PPI plus clarithromycin and amoxicillin calculated a mean *H. pylori* eradication rate of only 81% by intention-to-treat (ITT) analysis.[28] In 2001, another meta-analysis revealed that the cure rate of triple therapy was <80%.[31] More recently, another meta-analysis of European abstracts presented at scientific meetings during 1997–2004 concluded that the eradication rate of PPI-based triple regimens was only 83% in 2004.[32] A recent chronological analysis performed between 1998 and 2010 of the results of all meta-analyses showed that first-line standard triple regimens achieved eradication rates (by ITT) of around 80% only.[33]

In 2011, the efficacy of standard triple therapy in the eradication of *H. pylori* was assessed through an epidemiological analysis of all published Spanish trials.[24] Overall, the analysis of the 32 studies (4,727 patients) showed, by ITT analysis, a mean *H. pylori* cure rate of 80%. Lately in 2013, the available evidence on the effectiveness of triple therapy in 3,147 Spanish patients over the previous years (2007–2012) was updated, and a mean cure rate of only 71% was calculated.[34] Similarly, in 2010, the Tokyo *H. pylori* study group revealed that in 14 hospitals over the Tokyo metropolitan area, the eradication rate of 7-day triple therapy was only 66% according to ITT analysis.[35]

All randomized, controlled trials conducted in the United States or Canada which had assessed the efficacy of this triple regimen since 2000 were identified and analyzed by the American College of Gastroenterology. Consistent with other meta-analyses, eradication rates in studies with 7 or 10 days of clarithromycin-based triple therapy were indeed <80%; eradication rates with 14 days of triple therapy were higher, but only two-arm studies with 195 subjects were included.[36]

In 2013, a systematic review and meta-analysis from the Cochrane Collaboration found that the standard triple therapy with a PPI, clarithromycin, and amoxicillin, even when prescribed for 14 days, was able to eradicate *H. pylori* infection in only 83% of the cases.[37]

Ideally, the choice of therapies for infectious disease is based on cultures and susceptibility testing for each patient; nonetheless, this strategy is hampered by the wide unavailability of these techniques, as well as the need for an invasive procedure (endoscopy), and the costs or time consumption.[38] The obvious alternative is to empirically choose a regimen based on the local pattern of resistance; in this instance, the best approach is to use regimens that have been proven to be reliably excellent in the targeted population.[18] Thus, currently, triple therapy with a PPI, clarithromycin, and amoxicillin is generally not recommended because of the variability of its efficacy, which in most cases does not reach 80%. Exceptionally, in the few privileged areas where resistances are still low, it could be maintained provided that monitoring of cure rates continues to show excellent results.[23] In summary, recommendations should be locally adapted.[23] For example, in some Nordic countries, the strict antibiotic policies applied may keep resistances low and the continued use of triple therapies may be allowed. As long as monitoring of cure rates confirms high effectiveness, there is no reason to change to more complicated schedules.

When the clarithromycin resistance rate in the region is >15%, PPI-clarithromycin-containing triple therapy without prior susceptibility testing should be abandoned as stated in the Maastricht V consensus report.[27] However, regarding the recommendation in consensus statements to adapt treatment to the local resistance pattern, these resistances are rarely (if ever) adequately known, because: (1) Resistances have been reported to vary from year to year and (2) they may change markedly from country to country (or even from area to area).[34] The decision to use triple therapies should then be based, ideally, not on published resistance data but according to the previous local experience. Furthermore, as stated, it is of the utmost importance to monitor cure rates in order to confirm that triple therapy continues to be effective.[23]

In order to produce descriptive studies of the management of *H. pylori* infection, the "European Registry on the management of *Helicobacter pylori* infection (Hp-EuReg)" aims to obtain a database registering systematically a large and representative sample of routine clinical practice of European gastroenterologists.[39] It is an international multicenter prospective non-interventionist registry promoted by the *European Helicobacter and Microbiota Study Group*. At present, over 30,000 patients have been included from 27 European countries. Recently, an interim analysis of more than 21,000 patients treated with a first-line regimen showed that triple therapy with amoxicillin and clarithromycin was the most commonly prescribed (40%), achieving, overall, a 68% ITT eradication rate.[40] Therefore, it was concluded that the management of *H. pylori* infection by European gastroenterologists is heterogeneous, suboptimal, and frequently discrepant with current recommendations. Only quadruple therapies lasting at least 10 days were shown to be able to achieve >90% eradication rates.[40] Similarly, a questionnaire from Asia-Pacific countries showed that the most commonly used regimen was clarithromycin-based standard triple therapy (81%), which suggested that physicians have ignored the newer and more efficacious anti-*H. pylori* regimens recommended by the Kyoto consensus report.[15]

In this respect, the impact of time of consensus, prescription choices, and efficacy trends on clinical practice has not been studied in depth. Thus, in the previously mentioned European Registry, first-line treatment use and efficacy trends in 2013–2018 were evaluated.[41] Although, overall, the most commonly prescribed treatments in the 2013–2018 period were triple therapies, a shift in antibiotic regimens was identified: Triple therapies decreased from >50% of prescriptions in 2013/14 to <25% in 2017/18 while, e.g., Pylera® (bismuth, metronidazole, and tetracycline) increased from 1% (2014/15) to 25% (2018). Regarding the time trend of *H. pylori* treatment efficacy, approximately a 10% overall improvement in first-line efficacy has been reported. Therefore, it can be concluded that European gastroenterological practice is constantly adapting to the newest published evidence and recommendations, and although this shift is delayed and slow, it improves clinical practice outcomes.

On the other hand, we recently performed an open online survey in order to evaluate adherence of Spanish primary care physicians to recommendations, where a total of 1,445 responses were analyzed.[42] Even at present, the most common first-line treatment in primary care in Spain is still triple therapy with clarithromycin and amoxicillin (by 56% of doctors, a figure similar to that reported by European gastroenterologists; see above). Likewise, >70% of primary care doctors in the United States prescribed treatments with efficacies <80%, although these data correspond to more than a decade ago.[43]

In the search for better cure rates, several new treatments (different from the standard triple therapy) have been evaluated.[23] Of all of them, quadruple therapies have been the most successful alternatives. In the overall literature,[23] three main groups of quadruple therapies have been assessed: (1) Adding metronidazole to classical clarithromycin-containing triple therapy, (2) classical PPI–bismuth–metronidazole–tetracycline quadruple therapy, and (3) adding bismuth to triple therapy, as it will be briefly reviewed below.

1. *Adding metronidazole to triple therapy*: Therapies using a PPI, amoxicillin, clarithromycin, and metronidazole have been extensively evaluated. A total of three main therapies have been assessed, all containing a PPI, clarithromycin, metronidazole, and amoxicillin. "Concomitant" therapy

uses all four drugs for 10–14 days; hybrid therapy consists of a PPI plus amoxicillin for 10–14 days, adding clarithromycin and metronidazole for the last 5–7 days; and sequential treatment gives a PPI for 10–14 days, administering amoxicillin in the first 5–7 days and clarithromycin and metronidazole for the remaining half of the treatment. Meta-analyses have found these quadruple therapies to be superior to 14-day triple therapy, except for sequential treatment.[44,45] Cure rates were better with concomitant than with sequential therapy as reported in an updated meta-analysis specifically performed by the Toronto Consensus.[46] Cure rates of around 90% with concomitant therapy have consistently been reported in most published studies.[47] For all these reasons, concomitant therapy may be a first-line treatment of choice.[27]

2. *Combination of a PPI, bismuth, metronidazole, and tetracycline*: Usually named "classical" or "bismuth" quadruple therapy, this therapy has long been used for *H. pylori* treatments. In most recent meta-analyses,[48-50] it has been shown to be superior to triple therapy. Even in the presence of in vitro resistance to metronidazole,[50] the combination seems to work acceptably. In many western countries a 3-in-1 pill is available, combining metronidazole, tetracycline, and bismuth. This presentation simplifies dosing for patients and allows the use of this quadruple therapy in countries where tetracycline or bismuth is not available. In most published studies, this combination has also been shown to achieve cure rates >90%.[51,52] A very recent meta-analysis evaluated the efficacy and safety of single capsule Pylera® (bismuth, metronidazole, and tetracycline) plus a PPI, including 30 studies and 6,482 patients, and the ITT efficacy was 90%.[52]

3. *Adding bismuth to triple therapy*: This combination will be reviewed in detail in the corresponding section (see below).

In summary, in most geographical areas, the efficacy of the standard triple therapy—a combination of a PPI plus two antibiotics—is clearly suboptimal and therefore should be abandoned. Quadruple regimens—including bismuth and non-bismuth regimens—should be prescribed instead.

Error 3: To Prescribe *Helicobacter pylori* Eradication Therapy for Only 7–10 Days

Overwhelming evidence is available supporting the use of longer—14 days—treatments for most of the eradication regimens,[22] as will be reviewed here.

Triple Therapy

Four meta-analyses have been carried out and yielded very similar results, that is, a 10-day treatment improves the eradication rate by 4% and a 14-day treatment improves the eradication rate by 5–6%, in comparison to a 7-day treatment.[53-56] However, there was no difference regarding the rate of side effects. The benefit of prolonging the length of triple therapy has also been disclosed in more recent articles,[57-59] whereas only a few could not demonstrate the advantage of this strategy.[60,61] Accordingly, the Maastricht V Consensus Report stated that "the treatment duration of PPI–clarithromycin-based triple therapy should be extended to 14 days, unless shorter therapies are proven effective locally."[27] Similarly, the Toronto Consensus pointed that "in patients with *H. pylori* infection, we recommend a treatment duration of 14 days."[46]

A recent meta-analysis from the Cochrane Collaboration aimed to assess the relative effectiveness of different durations (7, 10, or 14 days) of a variety of regimens for eradicating *H. pylori*.[37] Only parallel group randomized controlled trials (RCTs) assessing the efficacy of 1–2 weeks' duration of first-line *H. pylori* eradication regimens in adults were eligible. The overall conclusion was that increasing the duration of PPI-based triple therapy increases *H. pylori* eradication rates. Specifically for the PPI–clarithromycin–amoxicillin regimen, prolonging the treatment duration from 7 to 10 days or from 10 to 14 days was associated with a significantly higher eradication rate, and therefore it was concluded that for this therapy (and also for PPI–amoxicillin–nitroimidazole) the optimal duration is at least 14 days. However, more data are needed to confirm if there is any benefit in increasing the duration of therapy for PPI–clarithromycin–metronidazole therapy.[37]

It is well known that the main limitation of the PPI–clarithromycin–amoxicillin regimen is clarithromycin resistance, with success depending on the resistance rate to this antibiotic and, as previously stated, the duration of therapy.[18] With 14-day therapy, the combination remains effective until clarithromycin resistance exceeds approximately 15%, whereas 7-day therapy is compromised by clarithromycin resistance exceeding 5%. There are few regions in the world where clarithromycin resistance is currently <15% (i.e., the 14-day regimen is still useful in such areas as Northern Europe and Thailand).[18,26]

On the other hand, when prescribing a triple therapy with a PPI, amoxicillin, and metronidazole, it has been shown that prolonging the treatment duration can overcome the negative effect of metronidazole resistance.[58,62,63] Thus, for patients with resistant strains, prolongation of treatment results in statistically significant improvements in eradication success.[58] Moreover, a 2-week metronidazole-containing second-line triple therapy provides high efficacy after failure of the standard PPI–clarithromycin–amoxicillin regimen.[64] It can therefore be concluded that the major advantage of 14-day metronidazole regimens is related to overcoming the influence of overall bacterial resistance on eradication success.[58]

Sequential Therapy

The sequential treatment comprises a simple dual regimen including a PPI plus amoxicillin followed by a triple regimen with PPI, clarithromycin, and nitroimidazole.[44,45] Some studies have suggested that prolonging the duration of sequential treatment (from 10 days onward) may be beneficial. In an RCT published by Lee et al., the treatment efficacy of 15-day and 10-day sequential therapies was compared:[65] The eradication rates by ITT analysis were 80% and 72%, respectively. Even though statistical significance was not reached in the ITT analysis, the efficacy of 15-day sequential therapy was statistically higher in the per-protocol (PP) analysis. The difference appeared to be originated from the patients with resistant *H. pylori* isolates. That is, in nine patients with single clarithromycin or metronidazole resistance isolates, the eradication rate was higher with the 15-day sequential therapy than with the 10-day sequential therapy.[65] In this same line, recent meta-analyses have confirmed that sequential therapy given for 14 days, but not for 10 days, was more effective than 14-day triple therapy as first-line treatment.[44,66]

Nevertheless, although a 14-day sequential therapy may achieve relatively high eradication rates, its efficacy in patients with clarithromycin-resistant strains was only 75%; this is not consistent with the hypothesis that extending sequential therapy to 14 days would lead to further improve the eradication rate for clarithromycin-resistant infections.[67] Furthermore, patients with clarithromycin and metronidazole dual resistance showed poor eradication results, which might suggest that 14-day sequential therapy is not capable of overcoming dual antibiotic resistance.[65]

Concomitant Therapy

Traditional standard triple therapy (PPI–clarithromycin–amoxicillin) can easily be converted to concomitant therapy by the addition of metronidazole or tinidazole twice daily.[47,68] In the latest consensus conferences, this regimen has been recommended as first-line treatment, especially in areas with high clarithromycin resistance.[27,46] Concomitant therapy was originally developed in an attempt to decrease the duration of treatment for *H. pylori* infection. In studies performed in the late 1990s, data from Europe and Japan suggested that a short course of 3–5 days with three antibiotics and a PPI could achieve reasonable eradication rates.[69]

Despite the very short duration of some of the trials, Essa et al.[70] showed in their meta-analysis (nine studies) that concomitant therapy yielded excellent results but the duration of therapy became a significant variable, with longer duration tending to produce higher eradication rates. More recently, Gisbert and Calvet showed in their systematic review that, for different durations of treatment, mean *H. pylori* eradication rates were 3 days (85%), 4 days (88%), 5 days (89%), 7 days (93%), and 10 days (92%). Therefore, a trend toward better results was also observed with longer treatments.[47]

Very recently, Gisbert and McNicholl, in a large meta-analysis involving 55 studies ($n = 6,906$), were unable to find clear evidence for higher eradication results with longer treatments.[68] However, several RCTs have compared, in the same study and with the same protocol, two different durations of concomitant therapy and demonstrated that the longer duration was more effective.[71-74] Moreover, suboptimal ITT results have been observed with a 5-day treatment duration in Latin America (73%)[75] and South Korea (59%)[76] and in two studies of 14-day treatment from Turkey (75%)[77] and South Korea (81%).[78] These poorer results have been attributed to the high prevalence of *H. pylori* strains resistant to clarithromycin and metronidazole, and consequently dual resistances in these populations.[18,79]

The efficacy and tolerability of the standard and the so-called optimized concomitant regimen (new generation PPIs at high doses and longer treatment duration) has been compared in a recent prospective multicenter study in over 800 patients, achieving a 5% advantage with the optimized regimen and reaching over 90% ITT eradication rate.[80] The authors concluded that an optimized (14-day and high-dose esomeprazole) nonbismuth quadruple concomitant regimen is more effective than the standard treatment for the eradication of *H. pylori*; they also concluded that although the incidence of adverse events is higher with the optimized treatment, these are mostly mild and do not negatively impact on compliance. However, this study does not allow drawing conclusions regarding which percentage of improvement is due to the longer treatment duration or to the potency of high acid inhibition.

In the OPTRICON trial, another multicenter study performed in Spain, the authors compared the effectiveness and safety of two "optimized" therapies—triple and concomitant.[81] The first 402 patients received an optimized triple therapy—esomeprazole (40 mg/12 h), amoxicillin (1 g/12 h), and clarithromycin (500 mg/12 h) for 14 days; and the last 375 patients received an optimized concomitant treatment—optimized triple therapy plus metronidazole (500 mg/12 h). The optimized concomitant therapy achieved significantly higher eradication rates in the ITT analysis (81% vs. 90%; $p < 0.001$). Therefore, the authors concluded that empiric optimized concomitant therapy achieves significantly higher cure rates (>90%) than optimized triple therapy.[81]

Accordingly, the Maastricht V Consensus Report stated that "the recommended treatment duration of nonbismuth quadruple therapy (concomitant) is 14 days, unless 10-day therapies are proven effective locally."[27] Similarly, the Toronto Consensus pointed out that "in patients with *H. pylori* infection, we recommend treatment duration of 14 days."[46]

Hybrid, Sequential, and Concomitant Regimen

Hybrid therapy is generally prescribed for 2 weeks.[82] However, a recent study showed that excellent cure rates (>95%) for hybrid therapy could be maintained despite shortening the duration of therapy from 14 to 10 days.[83] Patients were randomized to 10-day, 12-day, or 14-day hybrid therapy consisting of esomeprazole 40 mg and amoxicillin 1 g/12 h for 10, 12, or 14 days plus clarithromycin 500 mg, and metronidazole 500 mg/12 h for the final 7 days. The PP eradication rates were similar—95% for 10-day, 95% for 12-day, and

93% for 14-day hybrid therapies. Nonetheless, the aforementioned study was conducted in a relatively low-resistance area and it may not be transferable to an area with high-resistance levels.[83] Therefore, these results suggest that in regions of moderate-to-low clarithromycin and/or metronidazole resistance it may be feasible to shorten hybrid therapy to 10 or 12 days. In regions with moderate-to-high clarithromycin and/or metronidazole resistance, further studies are needed to evaluate hybrid therapy.

Bismuth Quadruple Therapy

Bismuth quadruple therapy has been recommended as one of the treatments of choice for both first-line and rescue therapies.[27,46] In the latter scenario, the eradication rates of bismuth quadruple therapy have been reported to range from 57 to 95%, with a mean value of only 77%.[84] Therefore, it is clear that, for this combination, there is still room for improvement. When the traditional bismuth quadruple therapy is prescribed,[85] treatment duration is a critical determinant of outcome.

In a meta-analysis performed by Fischbach et al.,[86] the efficacy, adverse events, and adherence related to first-line *H. pylori* quadruple eradication therapies were evaluated. Bismuth quadruple therapy for 1–3, 4, or 7 days was less effective than for 10–14 days. Even in areas with a high prevalence of metronidazole resistance, the combination of PPI, bismuth, metronidazole, and tetracycline lasting 10–14 days achieved ≥85% eradication rate. In this respect, the efficacy and safety of single-capsule Pylera® plus a PPI were evaluated in a very recent meta-analysis including 30 studies and 6,482 patients; the ITT efficacy was 90%, while for metronidazole-resistant infection, the ITT efficacy as first-line therapy was as high as 93%.[52]

A Cochrane Collaboration systematic review involving 75 studies evaluated the optimum duration for *H. pylori* eradication regimens,[37] and only six studies (1,157 patients) provided data for PPI–bismuth plus two antibiotics quadruple therapy. The combined antibiotics included tetracycline and metronidazole, furazolidone and amoxicillin, and clarithromycin and amoxicillin. *H. pylori* eradication was compared for 14 versus 7 days, 10 versus 7 days, and 14 versus 10 days. None of the comparisons suggested that increased duration significantly improved the treatment effect for bismuth-based PPI quadruple therapy. However, the small number and heterogeneity of the studies included prevented solid conclusions to be drawn on the optimum duration for bismuth quadruple therapy.

Recent studies have shown that, in different regions of the world, 14-day bismuth quadruple therapy has achieved ≥85% eradication.[85,87,88] Asian studies also suggest some benefit with longer treatments.[89-92] In a randomized study,[91] 227 patients were assigned to receive 1- or 2-week bismuth quadruple therapy, the eradication rates being higher for the longer treatment (83% vs. 64% by ITT). Lee et al. treated patients with a bismuth-containing quadruple regimen for 7 and 14 days in a nonrandomized study;[89] the 14-day regimen showed a higher eradication rate than the 7-day regimen, although this difference was not statistically significant (53% vs. 73% by ITT; however, a *beta* error cannot be excluded due to the low statistical power). Finally, a 2-week quadruple therapy was somewhat more effective than 1-week treatment in another retrospective study (88% vs. 77%), although, again, probably due to insufficient statistical power, no statistically significant differences were demonstrated.[90]

In non-naïve patients to *H. pylori* eradication treatment, it was generally considered that a 7-day treatment duration seemed to be sufficient when the bismuth quadruple therapy was used after a failed first-line regimen, as quite similar eradication rates with 7, 10, and 14 days were reported.[84,93] These results are in agreement with those previously reported more than 20 years ago with quadruple therapy as first-line treatment, when 1-week therapy appeared sufficient, and prolonging treatment did not increase efficacy.[93] The metronidazole resistance rate is 20–40% in the United States and Europe, but in developing countries the prevalence is higher, from 50 to 80%.[94] Therefore, it may be expected that the increased duration of bismuth-containing quadruple therapy would be more effective, mainly in high metronidazole-resistant areas or in those patients with a previous failure with a metronidazole-containing treatment.[95] However, a recent RCT showed that a 7-day bismuth quadruple regimen, when administered as a second-line rescue therapy, was not statistically inferior to the 14-day regimen.[96] However, the authors concluded that it would be better to extend the duration of treatment to 2 weeks for *H. pylori* second-line treatment.[96] Similarly, Yoon et al. prospectively investigated patients with a persistent *H. pylori* infection after first-line triple therapy. Patients were randomized to receive either 1- or 2-week bismuth quadruple therapy. The 1-week group achieved 83% and the 2-week group achieved 88% eradication rate (ITT analyses), not reaching statistically significant differences. Therefore, it is clear that more comparative studies evaluating efficacy, safety, and cost are warranted to precisely define the ideal duration of the bismuth quadruple therapy, both in first-line and in rescue regimens.

In summary, it is known that bacterial resistance to metronidazole has a negative impact on the effectiveness of bismuth-containing quadruple therapy, but it may be possible to overcome this drawback by increasing the duration of treatment.[94] A critical determinant of outcome is the antimicrobial duration, e.g., in areas where metronidazole resistance is 40% or greater,[85] 7-day bismuth quadruple regimens typically produce unacceptably low-cure rates. Therefore, bismuth quadruple therapy should achieve acceptable results provided the doses are sufficient and the duration is at least 10 but preferably 14 days, especially where metronidazole resistance is likely.[87,97,98] Accordingly, recent consensus conferences recommended generally extending the duration of bismuth quadruple therapy to 14 days (unless 10-day therapies are proven locally effective).[27,46]

Quinolone-based Treatments

The duration of quinolone therapy, more than the dosage, seems to be the crucial factor affecting the eradication rate.[99] Three meta-analyses[100-102] found higher cure rates with 10- to 14-day than with 7-day levofloxacin-containing regimens, as did three recent RCTs.[100,103,104] Furthermore, the efficacy of 14- and 10-day levofloxacin-containing triple therapy as rescue regimen was compared in a very recent study, and a higher eradication rate was demonstrated with the longest regimen.[105] On the other hand, triple therapy with moxifloxacin for 10 days was reported to be more effective than the same treatment for 5 or 7 days in two recent studies.[106,107] Increasing the duration of therapy was expected to increase the eradication rate in another study, but the expected increase did not materialize, most likely because of a coincident marked increase in the prevalence of resistance to moxifloxacin.[108] Finally, in a recent RCT, 14 days of moxifloxacin treatment significantly increased eradication compared with a 7-day regimen.[109]

In the European Registry, the efficacy (by ITT) of the PPI–clarithromycin–amoxicillin triple therapy for 7, 10, and 14 days was 63, 74, and 82%, respectively.[40] Similarly, the efficacy of the concomitant therapy for 10 and 14 days was 85 and 91%, respectively.[40] Fortunately, in Europe, the prescription of 14-day treatments increased markedly from <20% in 2013 to almost 50% in 2018 while the prescription of 7-day treatments almost disappeared, which is in line with the current recommendations.[41] The primary care practice is also adapting to the newest recommendations, although this shift is still delayed: in an open online survey to evaluate adherence of Spanish primary care physicians to recommendations, treatments (mainly the standard triple therapy) were prescribed for 10 days in 43% of the cases.[42]

In summary, for most *H. pylori* eradication regimens, a higher effectiveness has been demonstrated for longer treatments. Therefore, the treatment duration should be extended to 14 days for all treatments, unless shorter therapies are proven effective locally.

Error 4: To Use a Standard Dose of Proton-pump Inhibitors in *Helicobacter Pylori* Eradication Regimens

Acid inhibition is a key component of *H. pylori* treatment. Acid inhibition increases luminal concentrations of antibiotics by decreasing their acid-related degradation, in addition to a possible antibacterial effect of the PPIs. Abundant evidence is available supporting the use of high-dose PPIs,[22] as will be reviewed in the following section.

Triple Therapy

There is indirect and direct evidence that high-dose PPI can improve the cure rates of *H. pylori* eradication treatment.[13] Indirect evidence comes from multiple old studies showing that high-dose PPI was necessary for the efficacy of dual therapies and a meta-analysis showing that in triple therapy, twice-a-day PPI was better than a single daily dose.[110]

In addition, standard triple therapy cure rates depend on the availability of PPI, which depends on polymorphisms on the *CYP2C19* and multidrug-resistant (*MDR*) transporter genes. A meta-analysis showed that extensive PPI metabolizers had lower eradication rates, although this difference was only seen with omeprazole.[111] A lower eradication rate was also obtained when the MDR T/T genotype was present compared with the T/C and C/C genotypes.[112] As for the different PPI molecules available, a recent meta-analysis disclosed that at the standard doses, the efficacy of omeprazole- and lansoprazole-based first-line triple therapies was dependent on the *CYP2C19* genotype status, which appeared to lack an effect on the efficacy of the regimens including rabeprazole.[113] In line with this finding, two other recent meta-analyses have demonstrated that better overall *H. pylori* eradication rates were reported with esomeprazole and rabeprazole, especially in *CYP2C19* extensive metabolizers.[114,115]

Direct evidence comes from a meta-analysis showing that high-dose PPI increases cure rates by around 6–10% in comparison with standard doses.[116,117] A subanalysis of these data showed that the maximal effect was seen when high doses of the more potent second-generation PPIs—namely, 40 mg of esomeprazole twice a day—was compared with a standard dose of a first-generation PPI also twice a day.[117] Based on this subanalysis, increasing the dose of PPI from, for e.g., 20 mg omeprazole twice daily to 40 mg of esomeprazole or rabeprazole twice daily may increase cure rates by 8–12%. Furthermore, in a recent meta-analysis, esomeprazole (and rabeprazole) has shown better *H. pylori* eradication rates than first-generation PPIs;[114] again, this clinical benefit was more pronounced in esomeprazole 40 mg/12 h regimens.[114] Accordingly, in the Maastricht V consensus report, it was stated that "the use of high-dose PPI twice daily increases the efficacy of triple therapy."[27]

A combined strategy, increasing duration of treatment, prescribing adequate antibiotic dose and frequency, and using high-dose potent PPIs would be the ideal one. Puig et al. performed a systematic review and meta-analysis to evaluate the efficacy of triple therapy including a PPI, amoxicillin, and metronidazole.[118] A total of 94 studies (7,974 patients) were included. Overall, the mean cure rate was only 76%; however, eradication rates increased when PPIs were administered at high doses and twice a day and when antibiotics were administered three times a day, with 14-day treatment schedules. Thus, in high-dose 14-day schedules (4 studies, 233 patients), the PP eradication rate was as high as 90%. Regarding efficacy in resistant bacteria, in patients harboring metronidazole-susceptible strains, the eradication rate was 89% versus 60% in resistant strains, with a risk difference of 30%. However, in 14-day schedules, this difference decreased to 20%. Although this regimen is, overall, 30% less effective in metronidazole-resistant strains, high-dose 14-day schedules partially overcome the resistance effect.[118]

Concomitant Therapy

In a noncomparative subanalysis performed in a recent meta-analysis, the effect of using single- or double-dose PPI (bioequivalent to omeprazole 40 mg twice daily) was evaluated. The results showed superior ITT and PP eradication rates (91 and 94%, respectively) in studies using double-dose PPI, as compared to those obtained in single-dose studies (86 and 89%), suggesting that double-dose PPI may be able to increase the efficacy of concomitant treatment up to 5%.[68]

Rifabutin Therapy

In a recent study, *H. pylori*-infected patients with two previous eradication failures were randomly assigned to receive either lansoprazole 30 mg/12 h or lansoprazole 60 mg/12 h, together with amoxicillin (1 g/8 h) and rifabutin (150 mg/12 h) during 7 days.[119] In the high-dose PPI group, eradication rates were higher (96% vs. 78%). Therefore, increasing doses of PPI might be the key to successful rescue therapy with rifabutin–amoxicillin–PPI regimen.

In the European Registry, the multivariate analysis showed that, in general, most treatments benefit from the use of double-dose PPI.[40] Fortunately, the daily PPI dose in Europe has increased from a dose equivalent to 60 mg of omeprazole in 2013 to 80 mg in 2018.[41]

In summary, the use of high-dose PPI twice daily increases the efficacy of most eradication therapy regimens and is therefore recommended.

Error 5: To Underestimate the Benefit of Adding Bismuth to Antibiotic Treatment to Eradicate *Helicobacter Pylori* Infection

Bismuth is one of the few antimicrobials to which resistance is not developed.[120] In addition, bismuth has an additive effect with antibiotics, overcomes clarithromycin and levofloxacin resistance, and its efficacy is not affected by metronidazole resistance.[120,121] Thus, combining bismuth and several antibiotics in the same regimen may be a promising option, as it will be summarized below.

Addition of Bismuth to Triple Therapy

Several studies have evaluated the effectiveness of adding bismuth to a standard triple therapy **(Table 1)**.[122-139] In a recent study, *H. pylori*-positive patients were randomized to receive the PPI–clarithromycin–amoxicillin regimen or this standard triple therapy plus bismuth for 7 days.[134] The

Table 1: Efficacy of standard triple therapy (proton-pump inhibitor, clarithromycin, and amoxicillin) plus bismuth as a first-line treatment for *Helicobacter pylori* infection.

Author	Year	Country	Treatment	Duration (days)	Eradication n/N (ITT %)
Ergúl[122]	2013	Turkey	L 30 mg/ 12 h A 1 g/ 12 h C 500 mg/ 12 h Bi 300 mg/ 12 h	14	88/97 (91%)
Fakheri[123]	2001	Iran	O 20 mg/ 12 h A 1 g/ 12 h C 500 mg/ 12 h Bi 240 mg/ 12 h	14	47/55 (85%)
Gao[124]	2012	China	E A C Bi	7	178/220 (81%)
Guo[125]	2019	China	E 20 mg/ 12 h A 1 g/ 12 h C 500 mg/ 12 h Bi 220 mg/ 12 h	14	90/102 (88%)
Leow[126]	2018	Malaysia	R 20 mg/ 12 h A 1 g/ 12 h C 500 mg/ 12 h Bi 240 mg/ 12 h	7	98/120 (82%)
Liang[127]	2012	China	O 20 mg/ 12 h A 1 g/ 12 h C 500 mg/ 12 h Bi 110 mg/ 12 h	10	106/156 (68%)
Lu[139]	2019	China	O 20 mg/ 12 h A 1 g/ 12 h C 250–500 mg/ 12 h Bi 600 mg/ 12 h	14	187/212 (87%)
McNicholl[128]	2019	Spain	O, P, R or E 20–40/ 12 h A 1 g/ 12 h C 500 mg/ 12 h Bi 120/6h or 240 mg/ 12 h	10-14	1002/1141 (88%)
Mu[129]	2007	China	L 30 mg/ 12 h A 1 g/ 12 h C 250 mg/ 12 h Bi 220 mg/ 12 h	7	26/30 (86%)
Shavakhi[130]	2013	Iran	O 20 mg/ 12 h A 1 g/ 12 h C 500 mg/ 12 h Bi 240 mg/ 12 h	14	70/86 (81%)

Contd...

Contd...

Author	Year	Country	Treatment	Duration (days)	Eradication n/N (ITT %)
Srinarong[131]	2014	Thailand	L 30 mg/ 12 h A 1 g/ 12 h C (long-acting) 1 g/ 12 h Bi 1,048 mg/ 12 h	7	23/25 (92%)
Srinarong[131]	2014	Thailand	L 30 mg/ 12 h A 1 g/ 12 h C (long-acting) 1 g/ 12 h Bi 1,048 mg/ 12 h	14	24/25 (96%)
Sun[132]	2010	China	O 20 mg/ 12 h A 1 g/ 12 h C 500 mg/ 12 h Bi 220 mg/ 12 h	7	64/80 (80%)
Sun[132]	2010	China	O 20 mg/ 12 h A 1 g/ 12 h C 500 mg/ 12 h Bi 220 mg/ 12 h	14	75/80 (94%)
Xie[133]	2018	China	O 20 mg/ 12 h A 1 g/ 12 h C 500 mg/ 12 h Bi 600 mg/ 12 h	10	169/192 (88%)
Xu[134]	2011	China	E 20 mg/ 12 h A 1 g/ 12 h C 500 mg/ 12 h Bi 220 mg/ 12 h	7	55/67 (82%)
Yagbasan[135]	2018	Turkey	L 30 mg/ 12 h A 1 g/ 12 h C 500 mg/ 12 h Bi 600 mg/ 12 h	7	28/35 (80%)
Yagbasan[135]	2018	Turkey	L 30 mg/ 12 h A 1 g/ 12 h C 500 mg/ 12 h Bi 600 mg/ 12 h	14	29/35 (83%)
Yi[136]	2019	China	E 20 mg/ 12 h A 1 g/ 12 h C 500 mg/ 12 h Bi 220 mg/ 12 h	14	79/92 (86%)
Zhang[137]	2015	China	L 30 mg/ 12 h A 1 g/ 12 h C 500 mg/ 12 h Bi 220 mg/ 12 h	14	95/107 (89%)
Zhou[138]	2014	China	E 20 mg/ 12 h A 1 g/ 12 h C 500 mg/ 12 h Bi 220 mg/ 12 h	10	271/350 (77%)

(A: amoxicillin; Bi: bismuth; C: clarithromycin; E: esomeprazole; ITT: intention-to-treat; L: lansoprazole; N: number of patients; O: omeprazole; P: pantoprazole; R: rabeprazole.)

eradication rate of the quadruple therapy group (82%) was higher than that of the triple therapy group (67%). Thus, the bismuth-containing quadruple therapy, regimen compared to the standard triple therapy regimen, has a higher eradication rate and thus has even been recommended as a first-line treatment for *H. pylori* infection.[134] In areas with low clarithromycin resistance such as Thailand, another randomized study confirmed that a 7-day standard triple therapy plus bismuth and probiotic can provide an excellent cure rate of *H. pylori* (100%).[131] Also, in the randomized study by Sun et al., the duration of treatments using bismuth optimization was evaluated, showing higher eradication rates with 14 than with 7 days (94% vs. 80%), an improvement related to the higher efficacy of the longer treatment under clarithromycin resistance.[120] These results suggest that addition of bismuth and prolonging treatment duration can overcome *H. pylori* resistance to clarithromycin. Finally, in the more extensive study so far, including more than 1,000 patients treated with bismuth plus standard triple regimen, an 88% eradication rate was achieved (by ITT), which increased up to 93% when 14-day treatment was prescribed.[128]

Addition of Bismuth to Levofloxacin Therapy

Some authors have evaluated a combination of a triple therapy with PPI–amoxicillin–levofloxacin but adding bismuth and thus converting this triple regimen into a quadruple one, with encouraging results **(Table 2)**.[121,140-151] Some of these levofloxacin–bismuth studies were specifically focused on

Table 2: Studies evaluating the efficacy of a combination of a proton-pump inhibitor, amoxicillin, levofloxacin, and bismuth for the eradication of *H. pylori* infection.

Author	Year	Country	Treatment order	Duration (days)	Eradication n/N (ITT %)
Bago[140]	2007	Croatia	First	7	57/66 (86%)
Cao[141]	2015	China	Frist	14	117/141 (83%)
Fu[142]	2017	China	First	14	167/200 (84%)
Gao[143]	2010	China	First	10	60/72 (83%)
Gisbert[144]	2015	Spain	Second	14	180/200 (90%)
Gan[145]	2018	China	First	14	314/400 (79%)
Hsu[146]	2008	Taiwan	Third	10	31/37 (84%)
Kahramanoglu[147]	2017	Turkey	First	14	93/111 (84%)
Liao[121]	2013	China	First	14	70/80 (87.5%)
Song[148]	2016	China	Second	14	97/132 (74%)
Su[149]	2017	China	First	7	78/90 (87%)
Wu[150]	2017	China	Second	10	28/33 (85%)
Yee[151]	2007	China	≥Second	7	37/51 (73%)

patients with one previous *H. pylori* eradication failure, achieving high eradication rates, which may be considered encouraging, particularly considering that the rescue regimen was prescribed empirically. With levofloxacin–bismuth-based quadruple therapy, only few studies reported cure rates <80%, which might be explained by inclusion of patients with one or more failures of eradication therapies, of whom some had previously received levofloxacin.[151]

With respect to the additive or synergistic effect of the bismuth compound, two RCTs have shown that adding bismuth to a triple therapy that included a PPI, amoxicillin and levofloxacin or moxifloxacin for first-line treatment of *H. pylori* infection increased the eradication rate of the same therapy without bismuth.[121,152] The mechanism of action of bismuth appears to be more antiseptic than antibiotic, and no resistance has been described for it.[153,154] Bismuth exerts its antibacterial action by decreasing mucin viscosity, by binding toxins produced by *H. pylori*, and by preventing bacterial colonization and adherence to gastric epithelium.[155] In addition, bismuth reduces the bacterial load and has a synergistic effect with antibiotics.[120] In this respect, the combination of bismuth subcitrate with the older quinolone, oxolinic acid, produced synergistic activity against *H. pylori*.[156]

Resistance of *H. pylori* to fluoroquinolones is increasing worldwide, mainly in countries with a high consumption of these drugs.[2,157,158] In a recent study, the efficacy and effect of fluoroquinolone resistance on levofloxacin-containing triple therapy with or without the addition of bismuth was assessed.[121] Patients were randomized to receive a PPI, amoxicillin, and levofloxacin with or without bismuth for 14 days. The eradication rate was slightly higher with the bismuth-based regimen (87% vs. 83%); however, the most remarkable finding was that, for levofloxacin-resistant strains, the bismuth combination was still relatively effective (71%) while the nonbismuth regimen achieved *H. pylori* eradication in only 37% of the patients.[121] The cutoff level of resistance at which success would fall below 90% has been calculated:[97] When fluoroquinolone resistance rates exceed approximately 12%, treatment success will fall below this efficacy threshold with a 14-day fluoroquinolone triple therapy, whereas in areas with a fluoroquinolone resistance of up to approximately 25%, 14-day bismuth-containing fluoroquinolone quadruple therapy could be used.[121] Thus, in regions where fluoroquinolone resistance is increasing but is still not very high, 14-day fluoroquinolone plus bismuth quadruple therapy may be especially useful.

Nonbismuth quadruple sequential and concomitant regimens, including a PPI, amoxicillin, clarithromycin, and nitroimidazole, are increasingly used as first-line treatments for *H. pylori* infection as their effectiveness is considerably high.[47,68] However, these patients have limited options for further (rescue) therapy because they already have received three different relevant antibiotics—amoxicillin, clarithromycin, and metronidazole; the best rescue therapy following the failure of these regimens remains unknown.

There is only one study evaluating the levofloxacin–bismuth quadruple rescue regimen after these therapies.[144] Cure rates were similar when compared depending on the previous treatment (standard triple therapy 88%, sequential 94%, and concomitant 92%). Therefore, the levofloxacin–bismuth-containing quadruple therapy constitutes an encouraging second-line strategy not only in patients with previous standard triple therapy but also in those with nonbismuth quadruple sequential or concomitant treatment failure, even improving the results previously obtained with a levofloxacin triple therapy.[159-163] Thus, in a recent meta-analysis, after the failure of concomitant and sequential treatment the eradication rates of a 10-day levofloxacin–amoxicillin-PPI therapy were 78% and 81%, respectively,[164] while optimization of the regimen through addition of bismuth (plus high-dose PPI and lengthening the treatment duration) increased eradication rates by 10%, reaching the 90% threshold.[144]

Adverse events associated with the bismuth–levofloxacin–amoxicillin treatment have been relatively frequent but only in a very low proportion of the cases; these adverse events were classified as intense, and none of them was classified as a serious adverse event. Accordingly, treatment withdrawal due to levofloxacin-related adverse events has been exceptional.[121,140-151] Regarding bismuth safety, in the context of *H. pylori* eradication, the drug doses currently used in the quadruple regimen are relatively low and are administered for a short period of time, leading to safe blood levels.[165] Correspondingly, there was no significant difference in the incidence of side effects when comparing a levofloxacin-containing triple therapy with or without the addition of bismuth.[121]

Addition of Bismuth to Rifabutin Therapy

To evaluate the therapeutic gain of the addition of bismuth to a rifabutin-containing triple therapy with amoxicillin and a PPI for the treatment of third-line *H. pylori* infection, a recent study compared two treatment groups: (1) rifabutin 150 mg/12 h, pantoprazole 20 mg/12 h, and amoxicillin 1 g/12 h for 10 days and (2) the same treatment plus bismuth subcitrate 240 mg/12 h for 10 days.[166] Cure rates were 67% and 97%, respectively. Both treatments were well tolerated with no reported relevant side effects. Therefore, the authors concluded that the addition of bismuth to a triple therapy that includes a PPI, amoxicillin, and rifabutin resulted in a 30% therapeutic gain.

In summary, bismuth coadministered with antibiotics against *H. pylori* can hinder the emergence of antibiotic resistance, inhibit the growth of *H. pylori*, have an additive effect on antibiotics and, consequently, improve the efficacy of eradication treatment.[132,167-170] To date, no resistance to bismuth has been reported. Furthermore, to assess the safety of bismuth, a meta-analysis including 35 RCTs and 4,763 patients was published, where it was found that no serious adverse events occurred with bismuth therapy, which was safe and well tolerated.[171]

Error 6: In Patients Allergic to Penicillin, to Prescribe always a Triple Therapy with Clarithromycin and Metronidazole

Amoxicillin is one of the most effective antimicrobial agents against *H. pylori*, and therefore most eradication regimens include this antibiotic. In some countries, triple therapy including a PPI and two antibiotics, mainly amoxicillin and clarithromycin, still constitutes the standard treatment for *H. pylori* infection. However, when penicillin allergy is present—a relatively frequent scenario—replacing amoxicillin with metronidazole has been recommended in PPI-based triple combinations.[13,172]

Gisbert et al. prescribed this triple regimen (PPI–clarithromycin–metronidazole, for 7 days) to 12 patients allergic to penicillin in a prospective single center study, and in only 58% of the cases was *H. pylori* eradication (by ITT analysis) achieved.[173] In a more recent prospective study including 50 consecutive patients allergic to penicillin, a relatively low efficacy of a combination of a PPI, clarithromycin, and metronidazole (for 7 days), with an ITT eradication rate of only 55%, was confirmed.[28] In a meta-analysis conducted in 2000, the PPI–clarithromycin–nitroimidazole regimen was considered quite effective to treat *H. pylori* infection, with mean eradication rates >80%.[28] The disappointing cure rates (<60%) in recent aforementioned studies in some countries might be related, at least in part, to increasing resistance rates to both clarithromycin and metronidazole.[2,34,174]

On the other hand, an 80–85% ITT eradication rate was reported by two other research groups prescribing a 10-day regimen of PPI, tetracycline, and metronidazole to 5 and 17 patients with documented allergy to penicillin.[175,176] These encouraging results suggest that this triple combination (or even better, with the addition of bismuth, resulting in a quadruple regimen) may be a better alternative for first-line treatment in the presence of penicillin allergy (mainly in areas with high metronidazole and/or clarithromycin resistance), probably because the negative effect of metronidazole resistance is mostly overcome by the coadministration of bismuth[86] and because the efficacy of this regimen is not influenced by clarithromycin resistance.[177]

In this respect, a first-line treatment comprising 7-day omeprazole–clarithromycin–metronidazole and 10-day omeprazole–bismuth–tetracycline–metronidazole was given to 267 patients allergic to penicillin in a recent prospective multicenter study.[178] The ITT eradication rate was 57% for the triple therapy, while it was higher (74%) for the quadruple regimen. Compliance with treatment was 94% and 98%, respectively. Adverse events were reported in 14% of the cases with both regimens (all mild).

In the study by Liang et al.,[98] 109 patients allergic to penicillin (most of them having failed with PPI–clarithromycin–metronidazole) were randomized to receive a 2-week eradication regimen with a classical bismuth quadruple therapy (PPI–bismuth–tetracycline–metronidazole) or a modified bismuth quadruple regimen with PPI–bismuth–tetracycline–furazolidone.

The ITT eradication rates were 88% and 92%, respectively, supporting the effectiveness of bismuth-containing regimens in penicillin-allergic patients.

Finally, Gao et al.[179] prescribed the classical bismuth quadruple therapy (PPI–bismuth–tetracycline–metronidazole) to 120 penicillin-allergic patients in a study performed in China, and achieved *H. pylori* eradication in 87% and 94% of the patients by ITT and PP, respectively.

In summary, and in accordance with Maastricht consensus recommendations,[27] in patients with penicillin allergy, in areas of low-clarithromycin resistance, for a first-line treatment, a PPI–clarithromycin–metronidazole combination may be prescribed, but in areas of high-clarithromycin resistance, the bismuth quadruple therapy should be preferred.

Error 7: To Systematically Supplement *Helicobacter Pylori* Eradication Treatment with Probiotics

A probiotic is defined as a living microbial species that may have a positive effect on the bowel microecology and improve health.[180] Probiotics, besides preventing antibiotic side effects, may modulate the human microbiota, stimulate the immune response, and directly compete with pathogenic bacteria.[181] Indeed, probiotics have exhibited inhibitory activity against *H. pylori* in vitro and in vivo.[182,183] Theoretically, probiotics may inhibit *H. pylori* through several mechanisms, including the release of antimicrobial products or the competition with *H. pylori* for colonization and survival. Currently, the most studied probiotics are lactic acid-producing bacteria, particularly *Lactobacillus* species.[184]

At present, the role of probiotics as an adjuvant to the antibiotic treatment with the aim of increasing *H. pylori* cure rates remains unclear. A number of meta-analyses of RCTs have assessed the capacity of probiotics to increase the efficacy of *H. pylori* eradication therapies (mainly triple therapies), with controversial results.[185-203] In meta-analyses in which subgroup analysis was performed, only certain strains maintained significance, including different *Lactobacillus* strains, *Bifidobacterium* strains, and *Saccharomyces boulardii*.[27] These data highlight the impropriety of pooling the data from studies investigating different probiotic species, strains, and concentrations.[204]

Currently, data on the usefulness of probiotics for *H. pylori* eradication with quadruple therapies are exceptional.[205] Recent studies have shown a reduction of side effects with probiotics combined with bismuth quadruple or sequential regimens, but no increase in cure rates.[130,159,206] However, a more recent study concluded that adding *B. infantis* as an adjuvant to sequential therapy significantly improved cure rates.[207] A recent meta-analysis included RCTs examining effects of probiotics supplementation on the eradication rate and found that it was only useful in less effective (<80% eradication rate) antibiotic therapies.[185] Thus, these results suggest that supplementation with specific strains of probiotics may be considered an option for increasing eradication rates, particularly when antibiotic therapies are relatively ineffective, but in effective regimens, such as the concomitant treatment, probiotic supplementation may not be needed. On the other hand, the impact of probiotics on side effects associated with the concomitant therapy remains unclear and more trials are thus needed.

Finally, it should be taken into account that probiotics add complexity as they mean adding a fourth or fifth capsule, in the case of triple and quadruple therapies respectively, which may increase the risk of poor compliance with therapy. Furthermore, probiotics are "over-the-counter" medications and the cost of eradication therapy may rise notably.

In summary, before a general recommendation in clinical practice can be made, further studies refining the most effective probiotic and the profile of the patient most likely to benefit from probiotic supplementation are needed.

Error 8: To Repeat Certain Antibiotics, Mainly after *Helicobacter Pylori* Eradication Failure

In the absence of local or even regional *H. pylori* antibiotic-resistance data, it is very important to ask patients about previous exposure to antibiotics for any reason, particularly macrolides and fluoroquinolones, as this provides a proxy for underlying *H. pylori* antibiotic resistance.[2,208] Accordingly, the Maastricht V consensus report stated that "for an individual patient a history of any prior use of one of the key antibiotics proposed will identify likely antibiotic resistance despite low resistance rates in the population."[27] Similarly, it was pointed out by the American College of Gastroenterology that "patients should be asked about any previous antibiotic exposure(s) and this information should be taken into consideration when choosing an *H. pylori* treatment regimen. In regions where *H. pylori* clarithromycin resistance is known to be <15% and in patients with no previous history of macrolide exposure for any reason, clarithromycin triple therapy consisting of a PPI, clarithromycin, and amoxicillin or metronidazole for 14 days remains a recommended treatment option."[36]

On the other hand, as Calvet has accurately stated, one of the "rules of thumb" to correctly treat *H. pylori* infection is "do not repeat antibiotics after treatment failure."[23] After a failed first treatment, the remaining *H. pylori* will show very high resistances to some (though not all) of the antibiotics administered. Due to the specific characteristics of the bacteria, resistance to amoxicillin, tetracycline, and rifabutin is extremely rare, even after treatment failure including those antibiotics. By contrast, after treatment failure, resistances to clarithromycin, quinolones, and metronidazole approach virtually 100%. As the efficacy of clarithromycin- and quinolone-containing regimens is strongly affected by clarithromycin and quinolone resistance, repeating these drugs in rescue treatments is discouraged; so, these antibiotics should not be repeated after treatment failure.

With regard to metronidazole, some articles suggest that in vitro metronidazole resistance has a limited impact in the efficacy of *H. pylori* treatments when using sufficiently long treatments and high doses.[209] However, a recent multicenter study has shown that cure rates of a 14-day, high-dose, rescue triple metronidazole–amoxicillin–PPI therapy were as low as 37% in patients with previous metronidazole administration.[210] Therefore, it is suggested to repeat this antibiotic only when it is indispensable and in the setting of 14-day quadruple therapies.[211]

Finally, the acquisition of resistance to amoxicillin and tetracycline is remarkably rare and these antibiotics can be used more than once in the same patients without a significant reduction in efficacy. The same applies to bismuth, although its antibacterial activity mechanism remains uncertain, no in vitro resistance to this drug has been described.[212] Therefore, bismuth, amoxicillin, and tetracycline can be used more than once in the same patients, as they remain active despite previous treatment failure.

Although it may seem illogical, some studies have demonstrated that the repetition, even of exactly the same antibiotic regimen after *H. pylori* eradication failure, is not exceptional in clinical practice.[213] Thus, Li et al. found that, to eradicate *H. pylori* infection in Shanghai, the clarithromycin-containing regimens were repeatedly used in 178 patients (61%) and the levofloxacin-containing regimens were repeated in 88 patients (30%).[214]

In summary, in order to increase the success of *H. pylori* eradication therapy, the effect of prior therapies needs to be given more consideration. Clearly, doctors and patients should be educated about the important effect of prior antibiotic use on adversely affecting the outcome of *H. pylori* therapy. Antibiotics (mainly clarithromycin and quinolones) should not be repeated, especially after *H. pylori* eradication failure.

Error 9: To Ignore the Importance of Compliance with Treatment for *Helicobacter Pylori* Eradication

Together with antibiotic resistance, compliance with therapy is the most important factor in *H. pylori* eradication. Unfortunately, the problem of compliance is quite frequent. Thus, it has been proven that 10% of patients prescribed *H. pylori* eradication therapy will fail to take even 60% of medications.[215] In another study, only 88% of the patients consumed >85% of doses and were considered as "good compliers."[216] Forgetfulness has been demonstrated to be the reason for missing dose in a majority (80%) of the nonadherent patients.[217] However, estimates of compliance with *H. pylori* eradication treatment may not accurately reflect normal clinical practice, as they are derived mostly from clinical trials with highly filtered patient populations. In addition, as compliance in these studies is usually measured by interview or pill count only, and both measures tend to overestimate compliance, the compliance rates for eradication therapy may be lower than reported.

Poorer levels of compliance with therapy are associated with significantly lower levels of *H. pylori* eradication. The most common causes for reliably good or excellent regimens to fail are the presence of organisms resistant to one or more of the antimicrobials used and poor compliance. Compliance was the most important factor predicting success in the pioneer study by Graham et al.: The success rate was 96% for patients who took >60% of the prescribed medications and 69% for patients who took less.[218] Similarly, in another study, successful eradication was achieved for 89% of patients who received at least 90% of the prescribed drugs, whereas the eradication rate for nonadherent patients was only 37%.[219]

Some authors have evaluated and recommended medication counseling as it has been shown to improve the outcome and compliance in *H. pylori* therapy.[220] In a study prescribing bismuth, metronidazole, and tetracycline triple therapy for 14 days, patients were randomized to a control group or to a group receiving medication counseling (written and oral) from a pharmacist, along with a medication calendar and a minipill box, as well as a follow-up phone call after initiation of therapy, while compliance was assessed by a pill count.[215] There was a statistically significant difference in the number of patients taking >90% of the medications—67% of the control group versus 89% of the medication counseling group. In another study, patients received a 1-week triple therapy comprising a PPI, amoxicillin, and clarithromycin all twice daily, and compliance was assessed using MEMS(R) containers (Medication Event Monitoring System) which recorded the time of medicine consumption. On multivariate analysis, *H. pylori* eradication was inversely associated with poor compliance.[216] In a different study, *H. pylori*-positive patients were prospectively randomized to receive either PPI–amoxicillin–metronidazole twice daily for 10 days or this same regimen plus compliance-enhancing measures (medication in a dose-dispensing unit, medication chart, an information sheet about *H. pylori* treatment, and phone call 2 days after starting therapy), and, unsuspectedly, *H. pylori* was eradicated in 89% of patients in both groups, while compliance was also similar (97%) in the two groups.[221] Finally, a study carried out in Northern Ireland compared an approach including informing the patient of the risks of *H. pylori* infection, structured counseling, and follow-up with a "prescription and discharge" strategy; this revealed significantly increased levels of both compliance and eradication in the cohort who had been provided with greater knowledge of their illness and the importance of compliance.[220]

Compliance is a multifactorial process in *H. pylori* eradication regimens.[222] Complex and prolonged eradication regimens are recommended by current evidence and published guidelines. This complexity provides challenges for both the physician and the patient. The motivated physician can offer information to the patient which will lead to his/her empowerment to play an active role in his/her treatment by complying with therapy.[222]

The impact of motivated physicians on ensuring compliance may reflect the setting in which the prescription is issued. The opportunity to educate the patient on the importance of compliance is surely greater in a physician's office setting than in the case of prescribing eradication therapy for a patient possibly still under the effect of sedation in an endoscopy unit where a positive rapid urease test has been recorded.[222]

It has been shown that treatment failure and decreased compliance are significantly associated with side effects.[221] Although the side effects of standard therapies are common, they rarely result in severe adverse events mandating discontinuation of therapy.[18,214,223] However, the most common adverse events recorded are bothersome symptoms such as diarrhea, nausea, and vomiting which have significant physical and social impacts. Again, the central themes of physician motivation and patient information assume an importance here. The patient is more likely to tolerate "minor" adverse events if the goals of therapy are clear in his/her mind.[222]

Compliance with therapy is finally about much more than swallowing pills at regular intervals; it involves a partnership between the physician and the patient with a plan for eradication. As such, the importance of structured aftercare and follow-up of patients is of critical significance. The time spent by the physician in explaining the rationale behind complex treatments is of inestimable value for good compliance.[224]

In the European Registry, compliance was defined as having taken at least 90% of the prescribed drugs and was evaluated through patient interrogation with both open-ended questions and a predefined questionnaire. Compliance with treatment was the most relevant factor in all multivariate models for achieving successful eradication (with odds ratios ranging from 6 to 40 in the logistic regression), regardless of the treatment chosen or the clinical context.[40,41]

In summary, poor compliance remains a clinically relevant and potentially modifiable source of *H. pylori* treatment failure. The fact that *H. pylori* therapy often involves multiple drugs and multiple dosing intervals makes patient education extremely important. In this context, the doctor–patient relationship is of paramount importance. It is worthwhile to consider direct counseling regarding the regimen and the need to be compliant as well as to give handouts regarding the objectives and the details of the regimen. As a final point, doctors need to do a better job in explaining to the patient that side effects might occur but that these are temporary and most often harmless.

Error 10: Not to Check the Success (or Failure) of *Helicobacter Pylori* Eradication after Treatment

The decision to perform a diagnostic test to establish cure of an infection depends on several factors, including effectiveness of therapy, clinical ramifications of persistent infection, patient desire to confirm cure, test accuracy, and cost.[225] Recommendations on whether or not to determine the cure of *H. pylori* infection have varied from some doctors performing systematic control to others being more lax, indicating that eradication should be checked only in serious diseases [peptic ulcer and complicated ulcer, early gastric cancer, and MALT (mucosa-associated lymphoid tissue) lymphoma] and that, on the other hand, control after eradication is optional in cases of dyspepsia.[226]

In all treated peptic ulcer disease patients, routine *H. pylori* confirmatory testing is supported by the morbidity and costs associated with the increased risk of ulcer recurrence (and its potential complications such as bleeding or perforation) in patients who remain infected after an attempt of eradication. Moreover, there are also arguments in favor of systematically checking eradication after the treatment in all patients, as summarized here.

- With increasing antibiotic resistance and declining success rates for *H. pylori* eradication therapy, many patients will be persistently infected after treatment and will therefore remain at risk for the complications of *H. pylori*-related disease, such as peptic ulceration and gastric malignancy. The effectiveness of *H. pylori* treatment in clinical practice is much less than optimum, as previously reviewed, being even lower than 80% in many settings. Thus, after a first *H. pylori* eradication attempt, at least 20% of the patients will remain infected.

- There is an imperfect correlation between the success/failure of *H. pylori* eradication and the persistence/disappearance of the digestive symptoms. Although the disappearance of dyspeptic symptoms correlates well with the cure of infection, as shown in some cohort studies,[227,228] this has not been confirmed in many others; in fact, in the case of functional dyspepsia, symptoms usually persist after successful *H. pylori* eradication.[229] Post-treatment testing would facilitate the direction of any further management on an individual basis, either as re-treatment in the case of treatment failure or switch to symptomatic therapy.

- Fortunately, there is widespread availability of relatively inexpensive, nonendoscopic diagnostic tests, including the ^{13}C-urea breath test[230] and the stool antigen test,[231] which allow ease of monitoring for treatment success. These noninvasive tests should be employed for confirmation of eradication except, for instance, in cases where repeat endoscopy is indicated, as in patients with gastric ulcer.

- The arguments supporting routine post-treatment testing are intuitively obvious when there is already a clear indication for *H. pylori* treatment. However, the scientific evidence to support such a strategy from a cost-effectiveness viewpoint is not so clear.[36] In fact, in patients with uncomplicated duodenal ulcers, the arguments in favor of not carrying out treatment systematically are based on cost-effectiveness.[232] However, for bleeding peptic ulcers associated with *H. pylori*, modeling studies do support the cost-effectiveness of routinely testing to confirm *H. pylori* eradication.[233,234]

- Patients' own desires on the need to confirm eradication should also be taken into consideration, as their wish to get rid of what is a potentially carcinogenic bacterium may ultimately drive shared decision-making in favor of retesting.[36] In patients with peptic ulcer disease, in order to estimate patients' desire for confirmatory testing in the absence of symptoms, Fendrick et al. used a willingness-to-pay methodology.[225] Most of the patients (90%) responded that they would prefer to undergo confirmatory testing if asymptomatic, as opposed to delaying testing until symptoms recurred. The authors concluded that patients' desire for confirmation of cure, coupled with a frequent need for confirmatory testing as a result of recurrent symptoms after therapy, may justify routine confirmatory testing after *H. pylori* treatment.

- An additional argument in favor of post-treatment testing is to provide data on which to make rational community-based decisions. Without retesting, it is impossible to obtain information on a practitioner's or community's eradication success and on the need to modify antibiotic regimens.[36]
- Finally, both the Maastricht Consensus report[11,12] and the American College of Gastroenterology[36] recommend that successful eradication should always be confirmed after *H. pylori* treatment.

In the European Registry, confirmation of eradication was performed in >90% of the cases by the participant gastroenterologists.[40] However, as summarized in **Table 3**, including the surveys evaluating the percentage

Table 3: Surveys evaluating the percentage of patients in whom *Helicobacter pylori* eradication was confirmed in different countries and settings.

Author	Setting	Country	Publication year	% of patients with confirmed eradication
Ahmed[235]	Primary care	Pakistan	2009	57
Boekema[236]	Gastroenterology	The Netherlands	1997	42
Boltin[237]	Primary care	Israel	2016	44
Cano-Contreras[238]	Primary care	Peru	2018	92
Gene[239]	Primary care	Spain	2002	48
Gene[240]	Primary care	Spain	2008	42
Lim[241]	Primary care	United Kingdom	1997	57
Luman[242]	Primary care	Singapore	2001	8
Markus[243]	Primary care and internal medicine	Hungary	2019	88
McNicholl[42]	Primary care	Spain	2019	68
Milne[244]	Gastroenterology	United Kingdom	1995	22
Murakami[245]	Gastroenterology	United States	2017	58
Shirin[246]	Primary care, internal medicine, and gastroenterology	Israel	2004	24

> **Box 2:** Ten "rules of thumb" to correctly treat *Helicobacter pylori* infection and avoid common errors.
>
> 1. *H. pylori* eradication treatments must achieve ≥90% eradication rates; to achieve this goal, all treatments must be optimized in terms of duration, dose, and interval of administration of proton-pump inhibitors (PPIs) and antibiotics.
> 2. The efficacy of the standard triple therapy is clearly suboptimal and therefore should be abandoned in most geographical areas. Quadruple regimens—including bismuth and nonbismuth regimens—should be prescribed instead.
> 3. Eradication treatments should be generally prescribed for 14 days, unless shorter therapies are proven effective locally.
> 4. The use of high-dose PPI twice daily increases the efficacy of most eradication therapy regimens and is therefore recommended.
> 5. The efficacy of triple therapies can be significantly improved by the addition of bismuth salts, which offer an additive effect in combination with antibiotics.
> 6. In patients with penicillin allergy, the bismuth quadruple therapy should be preferred in areas of high clarithromycin resistance.
> 7. Probiotics cannot be generally recommended for clinical practice.
> 8. Antibiotics (mainly clarithromycin and quinolones) should not be repeated, especially after *H. pylori* eradication failure.
> 9. Compliance with therapy is, together with antibiotic resistance, the most important factor in *H. pylori* eradication. In this context, the importance of the doctor–patient relationship is paramount.
> 10. Cure of *H. pylori* infection should be systematically checked after eradication treatment in all patients.

of patients in whom *H. pylori* eradication was confirmed in different countries and settings (primary care and gastroenterology), figures ranged widely from 8 to 92%, with a mean value of 50%.[42,235-246] As an example, in the aforementioned survey of Spanish primary care, 33% of the physicians did not systematically refer to an eradication confirmation test.[42] Restricted use of retesting probably reflects, at least in part, the limited availability of noninvasive diagnostic tests, such as the urea breath test.[247] Thus, in this last study, 16% reported no direct access to any validated diagnostic method and only 44% to urea breath test.[42]

In summary, considering the pros and cons of confirmation of the cure of *H. pylori* infection after treatment, it is recommended to check this in all cases.

CONCLUSION

In this chapter, 10 of the most common errors in the treatment of *H. pylori* infection **(Box 1)** and the related scientific evidence have been reviewed. This has allowed drawing specific take-home messages that should be taken into consideration when deciding how to prescribe the best eradication treatment. These 10 "rules of thumb" to correctly treat *H. pylori* infection are summarized in **Box 2**.

We should never lose sight that *H. pylori* is an infectious organism when treating it and clinicians should expect, and in fact demand, that recommended treatments provide cure rates ≥90%. Should the treatment score lower, it may be either tailored to the resistance pattern (patient or population based, which is not available in most centers), discarded or optimized. In most geographical areas, the efficacy of the standard triple therapy is clearly suboptimal and therefore should be abandoned. Quadruple regimens, including bismuth and nonbismuth regimens, should be prescribed instead. In order to reach the desired threshold, different strategies may be applied to different treatments. The most direct way to optimize a treatment is by prescribing it for 14 days, unless a shorter scheme has been shown locally to be equally effective. For most eradication therapy regimens, high-dose PPI therapy is also recommended. Also, the addition of bismuth salts offers an additive effect in combination with antibiotics and therefore the efficacy of triple therapies can be significantly improved. For a first-line treatment, in patients with penicillin allergy, in areas of low-clarithromycin resistance, a PPI–clarithromycin–metronidazole combination may be prescribed; but in areas of high-clarithromycin resistance, the bismuth quadruple therapy should be preferred. Overall, probiotics seem to reduce antibiotic side effects, but they cannot be generally recommended for clinical practice yet, given that the increase on eradication rates is not so evident. In order to increase the success of *H. pylori* eradication therapy, more consideration needs to be given to the effect of prior therapies, and certain antibiotics (mainly clarithromycin and quinolones) should not be repeated. Poor compliance remains a clinically relevant and potentially modifiable source of *H. pylori* treatment failure, thus emphasizing the paramount importance of the doctor–patient relationship. Finally, considering the pros and cons of confirmation of eradication of *H. pylori* infection, cure of the infection should be systematically checked after treatment in all patients.

The level of penetration of recommendations is still poor and delayed even though some improvements from guidelines have been partially incorporated. The barriers for implementation, access to diagnostic tests and treatments and to continuous medical education, should be removed in order to provide optimal care. One of the main reasons for poor adherence is lack of or scarce dissemination, and this is a shared responsibility between medical societies, health systems/providers, and individual professionals.

CONFLICT OF INTEREST

Dr Gisbert has served as a speaker, a consultant, and advisory member for or has received research funding from Casen Recordati, Mayoly, Allergan, Advia, Diasorin.

Dr P Nyssen has received research funding from Allergan.

REFERENCES

1. Graham DY, Fischbach L. *Helicobacter pylori* infection. N Engl J Med. 2010;363:595-6.
2. Megraud F, Coenen S, Versporten A, Kist M, Lopez-Brea M, Hirschl AM, et al. *Helicobacter pylori* resistance to antibiotics in Europe and its relationship to antibiotic consumption. Gut. 2013;62:34-42.
3. Helmreich RL. On error management: Lessons from aviation. BMJ. 2000;320:781-5.
4. Reason J. Human error: Models and management. BMJ. 2000;320:768-70.
5. Studdert DM, Mello MM, Gawande AA, Gandhi TK, Kachalia A, Yoon C, et al. Claims, errors, and compensation payments in medical malpractice litigation. N Engl J Med. 2006;354:2024-33.
6. Grimshaw JM, Russell IT. Effect of clinical guidelines on medical practice: A systematic review of rigorous evaluations. Lancet. 1993;342:1317-22.
7. Damschroder LJ, Aron DC, Keith RE, Kirsh SR, Alexander JA, Lowery JC. Fostering implementation of health services research findings into practice: A consolidated framework for advancing implementation science. Implement Sci, 2009;4:50.
8. Grimshaw JM, Russell IT. Achieving health gain through clinical guidelines II: Ensuring guidelines change medical practice. Qual Health Care. 1994;3:45-52.
9. Pronovost PJ. Enhancing physicians' use of clinical guidelines. J Am Med Assoc. 2013;310:2501-02.
10. Grol R, Dalhuijsen J, Thomas S, Veld C, Rutten G, Mokkink H. Attributes of clinical guidelines that influence use of guidelines in general practice: Observational study. BMJ. 1998;317:858-61.
11. Malfertheiner P, Megraud F, O'Morain C, Hungin AP, Jones R, Axon A, et al. Current concepts in the management of *Helicobacter pylori* infection: The Maastricht 2-2000 Consensus Report. Aliment Pharmacol Ther. 2002;16:167-80.
12. Malfertheiner P, Megraud F, O'Morain C, Bazzoli F, El-Omar E, Graham D, et al. Current concepts in the management of *Helicobacter pylori* infection: The Maastricht III Consensus Report. Gut. 2007;56:772-81.
13. Malfertheiner P, Megraud F, O'Morain CA, Atherton J, Axon AT, Bazzoli F, et al. Management of *Helicobacter pylori* infection: The Maastricht IV/Florence Consensus Report. Gut. 2012;61:646-64.
14. Graham DY, Shiotani A. New concepts of resistance in the treatment of *Helicobacter pylori* infections. Nat Clin Pract Gastroenterol Hepatol. 2008;5:321-31.
15. Chuah YY, Wu DC, Chuah SK, Yang JC, Lee TH, Yeh HZ, et al. Real-world practice and expectation of Asia-Pacific physicians and patients in *Helicobacter Pylori* eradication (REAP-HP Survey). Helicobacter. 2017;22(3).
16. Graham DY. *Helicobacter pylori* eradication therapy research: Ethical issues and description of results. Clin Gastroenterol Hepatol. 2010;8:1032-6.
17. Graham DY, Lu H, Yamaoka Y. A report card to grade *Helicobacter pylori* therapy. Helicobacter. 2007;12:275-8.
18. Graham DY, Lee YC, Wu MS. Rational *Helicobacter pylori* therapy: Evidence-based medicine rather than medicine-based evidence. Clin Gastroenterol Hepatol. 2014;12:177-86.e3.

19. Graham DY, Fischbach L. *Helicobacter pylori* treatment in the era of increasing antibiotic resistance. Gut. 2010;59:1143-53.
20. Graham DY. Efficient identification and evaluation of effective *Helicobacter pylori* therapies. Clin Gastroenterol Hepatol. 2009;7:145-8.
21. Sugano K, Tack J, Kuipers EJ, Graham DY, El-Omar EM, Miura S, et al. Kyoto global consensus report on *Helicobacter pylori* gastritis. Gut. 2015;64:1353-67.
22. Gisbert JP, McNicholl AG. Optimization strategies aimed to increase the efficacy of H. pylori eradication therapies. *Helicobacter*. 2017;22.
23. Calvet X. Dealing with uncertainty in the treatment of *Helicobacter pylori*. Ther Adv Chronic Dis. 2018;9:93-102.
24. Gisbert JP, Calvet X. Review article: The effectiveness of standard triple therapy for *Helicobacter pylori* has not changed over the last decade, but it is not good enough. Aliment Pharmacol Ther. 2011;34:1255-68.
25. Megraud F. *H. pylori* antibiotic resistance: Prevalence, importance, and advances in testing. Gut. 2004;53:1374-84.
26. Thung I, Aramin H, Vavinskaya V, Gupta S, Park JY, Crowe SE, et al. Review article: The global emergence of *Helicobacter pylori* antibiotic resistance. Aliment Pharmacol Ther. 2016;43:514-33.
27. Malfertheiner P, Megraud F, O'Morain CA, Gisbert JP, Kuipers EJ, Axon AT, et al. Management of *Helicobacter pylori* infection-the Maastricht V/Florence Consensus Report. Gut. 2017;66:6-30.
28. Gisbert JP, Gonzalez L, Calvet X, García N, López T, Roqué M, et al. Proton pump inhibitor, clarithromycin and either amoxycillin or nitroimidazole: A meta-analysis of eradication of *Helicobacter pylori*. Aliment Pharmacol Ther. 2000;14:1319-28.
29. Gisbert JP, Pajares R, Pajares JM. Evolution of *Helicobacter pylori* therapy from a meta-analytical perspective. *Helicobacter*. 2007;12 Suppl 2:50-8.
30. Graham DY, Lu H, Yamaoka Y. Therapy for *Helicobacter pylori* infection can be improved: Sequential therapy and beyond. Drugs. 2008;68:725-36.
31. Janssen MJ, Van Oijen AH, Verbeek AL, Jansen JB, De Boer WA. A systematic comparison of triple therapies for treatment of *Helicobacter pylori* infection with proton pump inhibitor/ranitidine bismuth citrate plus clarithromycin and either amoxicillin or a nitroimidazole. Aliment Pharmacol Ther. 2001;15:613-24.
32. Buzas GM, Jozan J. First-line eradication of H. pylori infection in Europe: A meta-analysis based on congress abstracts, 1997-2004. World J Gastroenterol. 2006;12:5311-9.
33. Buzas GM. First-line eradication of *Helicobacter pylori*: are the standard triple therapies obsolete? A different perspective. World J Gastroenterol. 2010;16:3865-70.
34. Molina-Infante J, Gisbert JP. [Update on the efficacy of triple therapy for *Helicobacter pylori* infection and clarithromycin resistance rates in Spain (2007-2012)]. Gastroenterol Hepatol. 2013;36:375-81.
35. Kawai T, Takahashi S, Suzuki H, Sasaki H, Nagahara A, Asaoka D, et al. Changes in the first line *Helicobacter pylori* eradication rates using the triple therapy-a multicenter study in the Tokyo metropolitan area (Tokyo *Helicobacter pylori* study group). J Gastroenterol Hepatol. 2014;29 Suppl 4:29-32.
36. Chey WD, Leontiadis GI, Howden CW, Moss SF. ACG Clinical Guideline: Treatment of *Helicobacter pylori* infection. Am J Gastroenterol. 2017;112:212-39.

37. Yuan Y, Ford AC, Khan KJ, Gisbert JP, Forman D, Leontiadis GI, et al. Optimum duration of regimens for *Helicobacter pylori* eradication. Cochrane Database Syst Rev. 2013;12:CD008337.
38. Gisbert JP. "Rescue" regimens after *Helicobacter pylori* treatment failure. World J Gastroenterol. 2008;14:5385-402.
39. McNicholl AG, O'Morain CA, Megraud F, Gisbert JP. Protocol of the European Registry on the management of *Helicobacter pylori* infection (Hp-EuReg). *Helicobacter*. 2019;24(5):e12630.
40. McNicholl A, Nyssen OP, Bordin DS, Tepes B, Perez-Aisa A, Vaira D, et al. First-line *H. pylori* eradication therapy in Europe: Results from 21,487 cases of the European Registry on *H. pylori* Management (Hp-EuReg). United European Gastroenterol J. 2019;in press.
41. McNicholl A, Nyssen OP, Bordin DS, Tepes B, Perez-Aisa A, Vaira D, et al. Pan-European Registry on *H. pylori* Management (Hp-EuReg): First-line treatment use and efficacy trends in 2013-2018. United European Gastroenterol J. 2019;in press.
42. McNicholl AG, Amador J, Ricote M, Cañones-Garzón PJ, Gene E, Calvet X, et al. Spanish primary care survey on the management of *Helicobacter pylori* infection and dyspepsia: Information, attitudes, and decisions. *Helicobacter*. 2019;24(4):e12593.
43. Breuer T, Goodman KJ, Malaty HM, Sudhop T, Graham DY. How do clinicians practicing in the U.S. manage *Helicobacter pylori*-related gastrointestinal diseases? A comparison of primary care and specialist physicians. Am J Gastroenterol. 1998;93:553-61.
44. Nyssen OP, McNicholl AG, Megraud F, Savarino V, Oderda G, Fallone CA, et al. Sequential versus standard triple first-line therapy for *Helicobacter pylori* eradication. Cochrane Database Syst Rev. 2016:CD009034.
45. Gisbert JP, Calvet X, O'Connor A, Megraud F, O'Morain CA. Sequential therapy for *Helicobacter pylori* eradication: A critical review. J Clin Gastroenterol. 2010;44:313-25.
46. Fallone CA, Chiba N, van Zanten SV, Fischbach L, Gisbert JP, Hunt RH, et al. The Toronto consensus for the treatment of *Helicobacter pylori* infection in adults. Gastroenterology. 2016;151:51-69.e14.
47. Gisbert JP, Calvet X. Review article: non-bismuth quadruple (concomitant) therapy for eradication of *Helicobater pylori*. Aliment Pharmacol Ther. 2011;34:604-17.
48. Gene E, Calvet X, Azagra R, Gisbert JP. Triple vs. quadruple therapy for treating *Helicobacter pylori* infection: A meta-analysis. Aliment Pharmacol Ther. 2003;17:1137-43.
49. Luther J, Higgins PD, Schoenfeld PS, Moayyedi P, Vakil N, Chey WD. Empiric quadruple vs. triple therapy for primary treatment of *Helicobacter pylori* infection: Systematic review and meta-analysis of efficacy and tolerability. Am J Gastroenterol. 2010;105:65-73.
50. Venerito M, Krieger T, Ecker T, Leandro G, Malfertheiner P. Meta-analysis of bismuth quadruple therapy versus clarithromycin triple therapy for empiric primary treatment of *Helicobacter pylori* infection. Digestion 2013;88:33-45.
51. Gisbert JP. *Helicobacter pylori* eradication: A new, single-capsule bismuth-containing quadruple therapy. Nat Rev Gastroenterol Hepatol. 2011;8:307-9.
52. Nyssen OP, McNicholl AG, Gisbert JP. Meta-analysis of three-in-one single capsule bismuth-containing quadruple therapy for the eradication of *Helicobacter pylori*. *Helicobacter*. 2019;24:e12570.

53. Calvet X, Garcia N, Lopez T, Gisbert JP, Gene E, Roque M. A meta-analysis of short versus long therapy with a proton pump inhibitor, clarithromycin and either metronidazole or amoxycillin for treating *Helicobacter pylori* infection. Aliment Pharmacol Ther. 2000;14:603-9.
54. Ford A, Moayyedi P. How can the current strategies for *Helicobacter pylori* eradication therapy be improved? Can J Gastroenterol. 2003;17 Suppl B:36B-40B.
55. Fuccio L, Minardi ME, Zagari RM, Grilli D, Magrini N, Bazzoli F. Meta-analysis: Duration of first-line proton-pump inhibitor based triple therapy for *Helicobacter pylori* eradication. Ann Intern Med. 2007;147:553-62.
56. Flores HB, Salvana A, Ang ELR, Estanislao NI, Velasquez ME, Ong J, et al. Duration of proton-pump inhibitor-based triple therapy for *Helicobacter pylori* eradication: A meta-analysis. Gastroenterology. 2010;138(suppl.1):S-340.
57. Karatapanis S, Georgopoulos SD, Papastergiou V, Skorda L, Papantoniou N, Lisgos P, et al. 7, 10 and 14-days rabeprazole-based standard triple therapies for *H. pylori* eradication: Are they still effective? A randomized trial. Acta Gastroenterol Belg. 2011;74:407-12.
58. Filipec Kanizaj T, Katicic M, Skurla B, Ticak M, Plecko V, Kalenic S. *Helicobacter pylori* eradication therapy success regarding different treatment period based on clarithromycin or metronidazole triple-therapy regimens. Helicobacter. 2009;14:29-35.
59. Arama SS, Tiliscan C, Negoita C, Croitoru A, Arama V, Mihai CM, et al. Efficacy of 7-day and 14-day triple therapy regimens for the eradication of *Helicobacter pylori*: A comparative study in a cohort of romanian patients. Gastroenterol Res Pract. 2016;2016:5061640.
60. Choi HS, Chun HJ, Park SH, Keum B, Seo YS, Kim YS, et al. Comparison of sequential and 7-, 10-, 14-d triple therapy for *Helicobacter pylori* infection. World J Gastroenterol. 2012;18:2377-82.
61. Usta Y, Saltik-Temizel IN, Demir H, Uslu N, Ozen H, Gurakan F, et al. Comparison of short- and long-term treatment protocols and the results of second-line quadruple therapy in children with *Helicobacter pylori* infection. J Gastroenterol. 2008;43:429-33.
62. van der Hulst RW, van der Ende A, Homan A, Roorda P, Dankert J, Tytgat GN. Influence of metronidazole resistance on efficacy of quadruple therapy for *Helicobacter pylori* eradication. Gut. 1998;42:166-9.
63. Graham DY, Osato MS, Hoffman J, Opekun AR, Anderson SY, Kwon DH, et al. Metronidazole containing quadruple therapy for infection with metronidazole resistant *Helicobacter pylori*: A prospective study. Aliment Pharmacol Ther. 2000;14:745-750.
64. Hori K, Miwa H, Matsumoto T. Efficacy of 2-week, second-line *Helicobacter pylori* eradication therapy using rabeprazole, amoxicillin, and metronidazole for the Japanese population. Helicobacter. 2011;16:234-40.
65. Lee JW, Kim N, Kim JM, Nam RH, Kim JY, Lee JY, et al. A comparison between 15-day sequential, 10-day sequential and proton pump inhibitor-based triple therapy for *Helicobacter pylori* infection in Korea. Scand J Gastroenterol. 2014;49:917-24.
66. Liou JM, Chen CC, Lee YC, Chang CY, Wu JY, Bair MJ, et al. Systematic review with meta-analysis: 10- or 14-day sequential therapy vs. 14-day triple therapy in the first line treatment of *Helicobacter pylori* infection. Aliment Pharmacol Ther. 2016;43:470-81.

67. Hsu PI, Wu DC, Wu JY, Graham DY. Is there a benefit to extending the duration of *Helicobacter pylori* sequential therapy to 14 days? *Helicobacter*. 2011;16:146-52.
68. Gisbert JP, McNicholl AG. Eradication of *Helicobacter pylori* infection with non-bismuth quadruple concomitant therapy. In: Atta-ur-Rahman, Choudhary MI (Eds). Frontiers in Anti-infective Drug Discovery, Vol 8. Sarjah, UAE: Bentham Science Publishers; 2019.
69. Vakil N. *H. pylori* treatment: New wine in old bottles? *Am J Gastroenterol*. 2009;104: 26-30.
70. Essa AS, Kramer JR, Graham DY, Treiber G. Meta-analysis: Four-drug, three-antibiotic, non-bismuth-containing "concomitant therapy" versus triple therapy for *Helicobacter pylori* eradication. *Helicobacter*. 2009;14:109-18.
71. De Francesco V, Hassan C, Ridola L, Giorgio F, Ierardi E, Zullo A. Sequential, concomitant and hybrid first-line therapies for *Helicobacter pylori* eradication: A prospective randomized study. *J Med Microbiol*. 2014;63:748-52.
72. Treiber G, Wittig J, Ammon S, Walker S, van Doorn LJ, Klotz U. Clinical outcome and influencing factors of a new short-term quadruple therapy for *Helicobacter pylori* eradication: A randomized controlled trial (MACLOR study). *Arch Intern Med*. 2002;162:153-60.
73. Kongchayanun C, Vilaichone RK, Pornthisarn B, Amornsawadwattana S, Mahachai V. Pilot studies to identify the optimum duration of concomitant *Helicobacter pylori* eradication therapy in Thailand. *Helicobacter*. 2012;17:282-5.
74. Mahachai V, Thong-Ngam D, Noophun P, Tumwasorn S, Kullavanijaya P. Efficacy of clarithromycin-based triple therapy for treating *Helicobacter pylori* in Thai non-ulcer dyspeptic patients with clarithromycin-resistant strains. *J Med Assoc Thai*. 2006;89 Suppl 3:S74-8.
75. Greenberg ER, Anderson GL, Morgan DR, Torres J, Chey WD, Bravo LE, et al. 14-day triple, 5-day concomitant, and 10-day sequential therapies for *Helicobacter pylori* infection in seven Latin American sites: A randomised trial. *Lancet*. 2011;378:507-14.
76. Kim SY, Lee SW, Hyun JJ, Jung SW, Koo JS, Yim HJ, et al. Comparative study of *Helicobacter pylori* eradication rates with 5-day quadruple "concomitant" therapy and 7-day standard triple therapy. *J Clin Gastroenterol*. 2013;47:21-4.
77. Toros AB, Ince AT, Kesici B, Saglam M, Polat Z, Uygun A. A new modified concomitant therapy for *Helicobacter pylori* eradication in Turkey. *Helicobacter*. 2011;16:225-8.
78. Lim JH, Lee DH, Choi C, Lee ST, Kim N, Jeong SH, et al. Clinical outcomes of two-week sequential and concomitant therapies for *Helicobacter pylori* eradication: A randomized pilot study. *Helicobacter*. 2013;18:180-6.
79. Molina-Infante J, Gisbert JP. Optimizing clarithromycin-containing therapy for *Helicobacter pylori* in the era of antibiotic resistance. *World J Gastroenterol*. 2014;20:10338-47.
80. McNicholl A, Molina-Infante J, Bermejo F, Harb Y. Non-bismuth quadruple concomitant therapies in the eradication of *Helicobacter pylori*: Standard vs. optimized (14 days, high-dose PPI) regimens in clinical practice. *Helicobacter*. 2014;19(Suppl. 1):11.
81. Molina-Infante J, Lucendo AJ, Angueira T, Rodriguez-Tellez M, Perez-Aisa A, Balboa A, et al. Optimised empiric triple and concomitant therapy for *Helicobacter pylori* eradication in clinical practice: The OPTRICON study. *Aliment Pharmacol Ther*. 2015;41:581-9.

82. Molina-Infante J, Romano M, Fernandez-Bermejo M, Federico A, Gravina AG, Pozzati L, et al. Optimized nonbismuth quadruple therapies cure most patients with *Helicobacter pylori* infection in populations with high rates of antibiotic resistance. Gastroenterology. 2013;145:121-8.e121.

83. Wu JY, Hsu PI, Wu DC, Graham DY, Wang WM. Feasibility of shortening 14-day hybrid therapy while maintaining an excellent *Helicobacter pylori* eradication rate. Helicobacter. 2014;19:207-13.

84. Gisbert JP, Pajares JM. Review article: *Helicobacter pylori* "rescue" regimen when proton pump inhibitor-based triple therapies fail. Aliment Pharmacol Ther. 2002;16:1047-57.

85. Lu H, Zhang W, Graham DY. Bismuth-containing quadruple therapy for *Helicobacter pylori*: Lessons from China. Eur J Gastroenterol Hepatol. 2013;25:1134-40.

86. Fischbach L, Evans EL. Meta-analysis: The effect of antibiotic resistance status on the efficacy of triple and quadruple first-line therapies for *Helicobacter pylori*. Aliment Pharmacol Ther. 2007;26:343-57.

87. Salazar CO, Cardenas VM, Reddy RK, Dominguez DC, Snyder LK, Graham DY. Greater than 95% success with 14-day bismuth quadruple anti-*Helicobacter pylori* therapy: A pilot study in US Hispanics. Helicobacter. 2012;17:382-90.

88. Rimbara E, Fischbach LA, Graham DY. Optimal therapy for *Helicobacter pylori* infections. Nat Rev Gastroenterol Hepatol. 2011;8:79-88.

89. Lee ST, Lee DH, Lim JH, Kim N, Park YS, Shin CM, et al. Efficacy of 7-day and 14-day bismuth-containing quadruple therapy and 7-day and 14-day moxifloxacin-based triple therapy as second-line eradication for *Helicobacter pylori* infection. Gut Liver. 2015;9:478-85.

90. Choung RS, Lee SW, Jung SW, Han WS, Kim MJ, Jeen YT, et al. [Comparison of the effectiveness of quadruple salvage regimen for *Helicobacter pylori* infection according to the duration of treatment]. Korean J Gastroenterol. 2006;47:131-5.

91. Lee BH, Kim N, Hwang TJ, Lee SH, Park YS, Hwang JH, et al. Bismuth-containing quadruple therapy as second-line treatment for *Helicobacter pylori* infection: Effect of treatment duration and antibiotic resistance on the eradication rate in Korea. Helicobacter. 2010;15:38-45.

92. Park SC, Chun HJ, Jung SW, Keum B, Han WS, Choung RS, et al. [Efficacy of 14 day OBMT therapy as a second-line treatment for *Helicobacter pylori* infection]. Korean J Gastroenterol. 2004;44:136-41.

93. de Boer WA, Driessen WM, Potters VP, Tytgat GN. Randomized study comparing 1 with 2 weeks of quadruple therapy for eradicating *Helicobacter pylori*. Am J Gastroenterol. 1994;89:1993-7.

94. Megraud F, Lamouliatte H. Review article: The treatment of refractory *Helicobacter pylori* infection. Aliment Pharmacol Ther. 2003;17:1333-43.

95. de Boer WA. Bismuth triple therapy: Still a very important drug regimen for curing *Helicobacter pylori* infection. Eur J Gastroenterol Hepatol. 1999;11:697-700.

96. Chung JW, Lee JH, Jung HY, Yun SC, Oh TH, Choi KD, et al. Second-line *Helicobacter pylori* eradication: A randomized comparison of 1-week or 2-week bismuth-containing quadruple therapy. Helicobacter. 2011;16:289-94.

97. Graham DY, Shiotani A. Which Therapy for *Helicobacter pylori* Infection? Gastroenterology. 2012;143:10-12.

98. Liang X, Xu X, Zheng Q, Zhang W, Sun Q, Liu W, et al. Efficacy of bismuth-containing quadruple therapies for clarithromycin-, metronidazole-, and fluoroquinolone-resistant *Helicobacter pylori* infections in a prospective study. Clin Gastroenterol Hepatol. 2013;11:802-7.e1.
99. Di Caro S, Franceschi F, Mariani A, Thompson F, Raimondo D, Masci E, et al. Second-line levofloxacin-based triple schemes for *Helicobacter pylori* eradication. Dig Liver Dis. 2009;41:480-5.
100. Gisbert JP, Morena F. Systematic review and meta-analysis: Levofloxacin-based rescue regimens after *Helicobacter pylori* treatment failure. Aliment Pharmacol Ther. 2006;23:35-44.
101. Saad RJ, Schoenfeld P, Kim HM, Chey WD. Levofloxacin-based triple therapy versus bismuth-based quadruple therapy for persistent *Helicobacter pylori* infection: A meta-analysis. Am J Gastroenterol. 2006;101:488-96.
102. Li Y, Huang X, Yao L, Shi R, Zhang G. Advantages of moxifloxacin and levofloxacin-based triple therapy for second-line treatments of persistent *Helicobacter pylori* infection: A meta-analysis. Wien Klin Wochenschr. 2010;122:413-22.
103. Ercin CN, Uygun A, Toros AB, Kantarcioğlu M, Kilciler G, Polat Z, et al. Comparison of 7- and 14-day first-line therapies including levofloxacin in patients with *Helicobacter pylori* positive non-ulcer dyspepsia. Turk J Gastroenterol. 2010;21:12-6.
104. Telaku S, Manxhuka-Kerliu S, Kraja B, Qirjako G, Prifti S, Fejza H. The efficacy of levofloxacin-based triple therapy for first-line *Helicobacter pylori* eradication. Med Arch. 2013;67:348-50.
105. Tai WC, Chuah SK, Wu KL. The efficacy of second-line anti-*Helicobacter pylori* eradication using 10-day and 14-day levofloxacin-containing triple therapy. United Eur Gastroenterol J. 2013;1(1S):A5.
106. Sacco F, Spezzaferro M, Amitrano M, Grossi L, Manzoli L, Marzio L. Efficacy of four different moxifloxacin-based triple therapies for first-line *H. pylori* treatment. Dig Liver Dis. 2010;42:110-4.
107. Bago J, Majstorovic K, Belosic-Halle Z, Kućisec N, Bakula V, Tomić M, et al. Antimicrobial resistance of *H. pylori* to the outcome of 10-days vs. 7-days Moxifloxacin-based therapy for the eradication: A randomized controlled trial. Ann Clin Microbiol Antimicrob. 2010;9:13.
108. Yoon H, Kim N, Lee BH, Hwang TJ, Lee DH, Park YS, et al. Moxifloxacin-containing triple therapy as second-line treatment for *Helicobacter pylori* infection: Effect of treatment duration and antibiotic resistance on the eradication rate. Helicobacter. 2009;14:77-85.
109. Miehlke S, Krasz S, Schneider-Brachert W, Kuhlisch E, Berning M, Madisch A, et al. Randomized trial on 14 versus 7 days of esomeprazole, moxifloxacin, and amoxicillin for second-line or rescue treatment of *Helicobacter pylori* infection. Helicobacter. 2011;16:420-6.
110. Vallve M, Vergara M, Gisbert JP, Calvet X. Single vs. double dose of a proton pump inhibitor in triple therapy for *Helicobacter pylori* eradication: A meta-analysis. Aliment Pharmacol Ther. 2002;16:1149-56.
111. Padol S, Yuan Y, Thabane M, Padol IT, Hunt RH. The effect of *CYP2C19* polymorphisms on *H. pylori* eradication rate in dual and triple first-line PPI therapies: A meta-analysis. Am J Gastroenterol. 2006;101:1467-75.

112. Furuta T, Sugimoto M, Shirai N, Matsushita F, Nakajima H, Kumagai J, et al. Effect of *MDR1 C3435T* polymorphism on cure rates of *Helicobacter pylori* infection by triple therapy with lansoprazole, amoxicillin and clarithromycin in relation to *CYP2C19* genotypes and 23S rRNA genotypes of *H. pylori*. Aliment Pharmacol Ther. 2007;26:693-703.

113. Zhao F, Wang J, Yang Y, Wang X, Shi R, Xu Z, et al. Effect of *CYP2C19* genetic polymorphisms on the efficacy of proton pump inhibitor-based triple therapy for *Helicobacter pylori* eradication: A meta-analysis. *Helicobacter*. 2008;13:532-41.

114. McNicholl AG, Linares PM, Nyssen OP, Calvet X, Gisbert JP. Meta-analysis: Esomeprazole or rabeprazole vs. first-generation pump inhibitors in the treatment of *Helicobacter pylori* infection. Aliment Pharmacol Ther. 2012;36:414-25.

115. Tang HL, Li Y, Hu YF, Xie HG, Zhai SD. Effects of *CYP2C19* loss-of-function variants on the eradication of *H. pylori* infection in patients treated with proton pump inhibitor-based triple therapy regimens: A meta-analysis of randomized clinical trials. PLoS One. 2013;8:e62162.

116. Villoria A. [Acid-related diseases: Are higher doses of proton pump inhibitors more effective in the treatment of *Helicobacter pylori* infection?]. Gastroenterol Hepatol. 2008;31:546-7.

117. Villoria A, Garcia P, Calvet X, Gisbert JP, Vergara M. Meta-analysis: High-dose proton pump inhibitors vs. standard dose in triple therapy for *Helicobacter pylori* eradication. Aliment Pharmacol Ther. 2008;28:868-77.

118. Puig I, Baylina M, Sanchez-Delgado J, López-Gongora S, Suarez D, García-Iglesias P, et al. Systematic review and meta-analysis: Triple therapy combining a proton-pump inhibitor, amoxicillin and metronidazole for *Helicobacter pylori* first-line treatment. J Antimicrob Chemother. 2016;71(10):2740-53.

119. Lim HC, Lee YJ, An B, Lee SW, Lee YC, Moon BS. Rifabutin-based high-dose proton-pump inhibitor and amoxicillin triple regimen as the rescue treatment for *Helicobacter pylori*. *Helicobacter*. 2014;19:455-61.

120. Malfertheiner P. Infection: Bismuth improves PPI-based triple therapy for *H. pylori* eradication. Nat Rev Gastroenterol Hepatol. 2010;7:538-9.

121. Liao J, Zheng Q, Liang X, Zhang W, Sun Q, Liu W, et al. Effect of fluoroquinolone resistance on 14-day levofloxacin triple and triple plus bismuth quadruple therapy. *Helicobacter*. 2013;18:373-7.

122. Ergul B, Dogan Z, Sarikaya M, Filik L. The efficacy of two-week quadruple first-line therapy with bismuth, lansoprazole, amoxicillin, clarithromycin on *Helicobacter pylori* eradication: A prospective study. *Helicobacter*. 2013;18:454-8.

123. Fakheri H, Malekzadeh R, Merat S, Khatibian M, Fazel A, Alizadeh BZ, et al. Clarithromycin vs. furazolidone in quadruple therapy regimens for the treatment of *Helicobacter pylori* in a population with a high metronidazole resistance rate. Aliment Pharmacol Ther. 2001;15:411-6.

124. Gao W, Cheng H, Hu FL, Lü NH, Xie Y, Sheng JQ, et al. [Ilaprazole based bismuth-containing quadruple regimen for the first-line treatment of *Helicobacter pylori* infection: a multicenter, randomized, controlled clinical study]. Zhonghua Yi Xue Za Zhi. 2012;92:2108-12.

125. Guo T, Wang Q, Wu X, Li XQ, Li Y, Fei GJ, et al. [Amoxicillin-clarithromycin-containing bismuth quadruple therapy for primary eradication of *Helicobacter pylori*]. Zhongguo Yi Xue Ke Xue Yuan Xue Bao. 2019;41:75-9.

126. Leow AH, Azmi AN, Loke MF, Vadivelu J, Graham DY, Goh KL. Optimizing first line 7-day standard triple therapy for *Helicobacter pylori* eradication: Prolonging treatment or adding bismuth: Which is better? J Dig Dis. 2018;19:674-7.
127. Liang J, Li J, Han Y, Xia J, Yang Y, Li W, et al. *Helicobacter pylori* eradication with ecabet sodium, omeprazole, amoxicillin, and clarithromycin versus bismuth, omeprazole, amoxicillin, and clarithromycin quadruple therapy: A randomized, open-label, phase IV trial. *Helicobacter*. 2012;17:458-65.
128. McNicholl AG, Bordin DS, Lucendo A, Fadeenko G, Fernandez MC, Voynovan I, et al. Combination of bismuth and standard triple therapy eradicates *Helicobacter pylori* infection in more than 90% of patients. Clin Gastroenterol Hepatol. 2020;18(1):89-98.
129. Mu F, Hu FL, Yang GB, Cheng HA. Clinical study of proton pump inhibitor containig quadruple regimen as first-line therapy for *Helicobacter pylori* eradication. Clin J Gastroenterol. 2007;12:531-4.
130. Shavakhi A, Tabesh E, Yaghoutkar A, Hashemi H, Tabesh F, Khodadoostan M, et al. The effects of multistrain probiotic compound on bismuth-containing quadruple therapy for *Helicobacter pylori* infection: A randomized placebo-controlled triple-blind study. *Helicobacter*. 2013;18:280-4.
131. Srinarong C, Siramolpiwat S, Wongcha-Um A, Mahachai V, Vilaichone RK. Improved eradication rate of standard triple therapy by adding bismuth and probiotic supplement for *Helicobacter pylori* treatment in Thailand. Asian Pac J Cancer Prev. 2014;15:9909-13.
132. Sun Q, Liang X, Zheng Q, Liu W, Xiao S, Gu W, et al. High efficacy of 14-day triple therapy-based, bismuth-containing quadruple therapy for initial *Helicobacter pylori* eradication. *Helicobacter*. 2010;15:233-8.
133. Xie Y, Pan X, Li Y, Wang H, Du Y, Xu J, et al. New single capsule of bismuth, metronidazole and tetracycline given with omeprazole versus quadruple therapy consisting of bismuth, omeprazole, amoxicillin and clarithromycin for eradication of *Helicobacter pylori* in duodenal ulcer patients: A Chinese prospective, randomized, multicentre trial. J Antimicrob Chemother. 2018;73:1681-7.
134. Xu MH, Zhang GY, Li CJ. [Efficacy of bismuth-based quadruple therapy as first-line treatment for *Helicobacter pylori* infection]. Zhejiang Da Xue Xue Bao Yi Xue Ban. 2011;40:327-31.
135. Yagbasan A, Coskun DO, Ozbakir O, Deniz K, Gursoy S, Yucesoy M. A prospective, randomized study comparing 7-day and 14-day quadruple therapies as first-line treatments for *Helicobacter pylori* infection in patients with functional dyspepsia. Niger J Clin Pract. 2018;21:54-8.
136. Yi DM, Yang TT, Chao SH, Li YX, Zhou YL, Zhang HH, et al. Comparison the cost-efficacy of furazolidone-based versus clarithromycin-based quadruple therapy in initial treatment of *Helicobacter pylori* infection in a variable clarithromycin drug-resistant region, a single-center, prospective, randomized, open-label study. Medicine (Baltimore). 2019;98:e14408.
137. Zhang W, Chen Q, Liang X, Liu W, Xiao S, Graham DY, et al. Bismuth, lansoprazole, amoxicillin and metronidazole or clarithromycin as first-line *Helicobacter pylori* therapy. Gut. 2015;64:1715-20.
138. Zhou L, Song Z, Zhang J, He L, Li Y, Qian J, et al. Tailored versus bismuth quadruple versus concomitant therapy for the first-line treatment of *helicobacter pylori* in chinese patients: A multicentre, open-label, randomized control trial. *Helicobacter*. 2014;19 (Suppl.1):80.

139. Lu B, Wang J, Li J, Liu L, Chen Y. Half-dose clarithromycin-containing bismuth quadruple therapy is effective and economical in treating *Helicobacter pylori* infection: A single-center, open-label, randomized trial. *Helicobacter*. 2019;24:e12566.

140. Bago P, Vcev A, Tomic M, Rozankovic M, Marusic M, Bago J. High eradication rate of *H. pylori* with moxifloxacin-based treatment: A randomized controlled trial. Wien Klin Wochenschr. 2007;119:372-8.

141. Cao Z, Chen Q, Zhang W, Liang X, Liao J, Liu W, et al. Fourteen-day optimized levofloxacin-based therapy versus classical quadruple therapy for *Helicobacter pylori* treatment failures: A randomized clinical trial. Scand J Gastroenterol. 2015;50: 1185-90.

142. Fu W, Song Z, Zhou L, Xue Y, Ding Y, Suo B, et al. Randomized clinical trial: Esomeprazole, bismuth, levofloxacin, and amoxicillin or cefuroxime as first-line eradication regimens for *Helicobacter pylori* infection. Dig Dis Sci. 2017;62:1580-9.

143. Gao XZ, Qiao XL, Song WC, Wang XF, Liu F. Standard triple, bismuth pectin quadruple and sequential therapies for *Helicobacter pylori* eradication. World J Gastroenterol. 2010;16:4357-62.

144. Gisbert JP, Romano M, Gravina AG, Solís-Muñoz P, Bermejo F, Molina-Infante J, et al. *Helicobacter pylori* second-line rescue therapy with levofloxacin- and bismuth-containing quadruple therapy, after failure of standard triple or non-bismuth quadruple treatments. Aliment Pharmacol Ther. 2015;41:768-75.

145. Gan HY, Peng TL, Huang YM, Su KH, Zhao LL, Yao LY, et al. Efficacy of two different dosages of levofloxacin in curing *Helicobacter pylori* infection: A prospective, single-center, randomized clinical trial. Sci Rep. 2018;8:9045.

146. Hsu PI, Wu DC, Chen A, Peng NJ, Tseng HH, Tsay FW, et al. Quadruple rescue therapy for *Helicobacter pylori* infection after two treatment failures. Eur J Clin Invest. 2008;38:404-9.

147. Kahramanoglu Aksoy E, Pirincci Sapmaz F, Goktas Z, Uzman M, Nazligul Y. Comparison of *Helicobacter pylori* eradication rates of 2-week levofloxacin-containing triple therapy, levofloxacin-containing bismuth quadruple therapy, and standard bismuth quadruple therapy as a first-line regimen. Med Princ Pract. 2017;26:523-9.

148. Song Z, Zhou L, Zhang J, He L, Bai P, Xue Y. Levofloxacin, bismuth, amoxicillin and esomeprazole as second-line *Helicobacter pylori* therapy after failure of non-bismuth quadruple therapy. Dig Liver Dis. 2016;48:506-11.

149. Su J, Zhou X, Chen H, Hao B, Zhang W, Zhang G. Efficacy of 1st-line bismuth-containing quadruple therapies with levofloxacin or clarithromycin for the eradication of *Helicobacter pylori* infection: A 1-week, open-label, randomized trial. Medicine (Baltimore). 2017;96:e5859.

150. Wu TS, Hsu PI, Kuo CH, Hu HM, Wu IC, Wang SSW, et al. Comparison of 10-day levofloxacin bismuth-based quadruple therapy and levofloxacin-based triple therapy for *Helicobacter pylori*. J Dig Dis. 2017;18:537-42.

151. Yee YK, Cheung TK, Chu KM, Chan CK, Fung J, Chan P, et al. Clinical trial: Levofloxacin-based quadruple therapy was inferior to traditional quadruple therapy in the treatment of resistant *Helicobacter pylori* infection. Aliment Pharmacol Ther. 2007;26:1063-7.

152. Ciccaglione AF, Cellini L, Grossi L, Marzio L. Quadruple therapy with moxifloxacin and bismuth for first-line treatment of *Helicobacter pylori*. World J Gastroenterol. 2012;18:4386-90.

153. Goodwin CS, Marshall BJ, Blincow ED, Wilson DH, Blackbourn S, Phillips M. Prevention of nitroimidazole resistance in Campylobacter pylori by coadministration of colloidal bismuth subcitrate: Clinical and in vitro studies. J Clin Pathol. 1988;41:207-10.

154. Megraud F. The challenge of *Helicobacter pylori* resistance to antibiotics: The comeback of bismuth-based quadruple therapy. Therap Adv Gastroenterol. 2012;5:103-9.

155. Wagstaff AJ, Benfield P, Monk JP. Colloidal bismuth subcitrate. A review of its pharmacodynamic and pharmacokinetic properties, and its therapeutic use in peptic ulcer disease. Drugs. 1988;36:132-57.

156. Van Caekenberghe DL, Breyssens J. In vitro synergistic activity between bismuth subcitrate and various antimicrobial agents against Campylobacter pyloridis (C. pylori). Antimicrob Agents Chemother. 1987;31:1429-30.

157. Gao W, Cheng H, Hu F, Li J, Wang L, Yang G, et al. The evolution of *Helicobacter pylori* antibiotics resistance over 10 years in Beijing, China. Helicobacter. 2010;15:460-6.

158. De Francesco V, Giorgio F, Hassan C, Manes G, Vannella L, Panella C, et al. Worldwide H. pylori antibiotic resistance: A systematic review. J Gastrointestin Liver Dis. 2010;19:409-14.

159. Manfredi M, Bizzarri B, De'angelis GL. *Helicobacter pylori* infection: Sequential therapy followed by levofloxacin-containing triple therapy provides a good cumulative eradication rate. Helicobacter. 2012;17:246-53.

160. Perna F, Zullo A, Ricci C, Hassan C, Morini S, Vaira D. Levofloxacin-based triple therapy for *Helicobacter pylori* re-treatment: role of bacterial resistance. Dig Liver Dis. 2007;39:1001-5.

161. Pontone S, Standoli M, Angelini R, Pontone P. Efficacy of *H. pylori* eradication with a sequential regimen followed by rescue therapy in clinical practice. Dig Liver Dis. 2010;42:541-3.

162. Zullo A, De Francesco V, Hassan C. Second-line treatment for *Helicobacter pylori* eradication after sequential therapy failure: A pilot study. Therapy. 2006;3:251-4.

163. Gisbert JP, Perez-Aisa A, Bermejo F, Castro-Fernández M, Almela P, Barrio J, et al. Second-line therapy with levofloxacin after failure of treatment to eradicate *helicobacter pylori* infection: Time trends in a Spanish multicenter study of 1000 patients. J Clin Gastroenterol. 2013;47:130-5.

164. Marín AC, McNicholl AG, Gisbert JP. Efficacy of a second-line levofloxacin-containing triple therapy after the failure of the non-bismuth sequential or concomitant treatments: Systematic review and meta-analysis. Helicobacter. 2014;19(Suppl.1):139.

165. Hillemand P, Palliere M, Laquais B, Bouvet P. [Bismuth treatment and blood bismuth levels]. Sem Hop. 1977;53:1663-9.

166. Ciccaglione AF, Tavani R, Grossi L, Cellini L, Manzoli L, Marzio L. Rifabutin containing triple therapy and rifabutin with bismuth containing quadruple therapy for third-line treatment of *Helicobacter pylori* infection: Two pilot studies. Helicobacter. 2016;21:375-81.

167. Carvalho AF, Fiorelli LA, Jorge VN, Da Silva CM, De Nucci G, Ferraz JG, et al. Addition of bismuth subnitrate to omeprazole plus amoxycillin improves eradication of *Helicobacter pylori*. Aliment Pharmacol Ther. 1998;12:557-61.

168. Bland MV, Ismail S, Heinemann JA, Keenan JI. The action of bismuth against *Helicobacter pylori* mimics but is not caused by intracellular iron deprivation. Antimicrob Agents Chemother. 2004;48:1983-8.
169. Meyer JM, Ryu S, Pendland SL, Danziger LH. In vitro synergy testing of clarithromycin and 14-hydroxyclarithromycin with amoxicillin or bismuth subsalicylate against *Helicobacter pylori*. Antimicrob Agents Chemother. 1997;41:1607-8.
170. Chiba N. Effects of in vitro antibiotic resistance on treatment: Bismuth-containing regimens [In Process Citation]. Can J Gastroenterol. 2000;14:885-9.
171. Ford AC, Malfertheiner P, Giguere M, Santana J, Khan M, Moayyedi P. Adverse events with bismuth salts for *Helicobacter pylori* eradication: Systematic review and meta-analysis. World J Gastroenterol. 2008;14:7361-70.
172. Gisbert JP, Calvet X, Bermejo F, Boixeda D, Bory F, Bujanda L, et al. [III Spanish Consensus Conference on *Helicobacter pylori* infection]. Gastroenterol Hepatol. 2013;36:340-74.
173. Gisbert JP, Gisbert JL, Marcos S, Olivares D, Pajares JM. *Helicobacter pylori* first-line treatment and rescue options in patients allergic to penicillin. Aliment Pharmacol Ther. 2005;22:1041-6.
174. Gisbert JP, Maria Pajares J. *Helicobacter pylori* resistance to metronidazole and to clarithromycin in Spain. A systematic review. Med Clin (Barc). 2001;116:111-6.
175. Rodriguez-Torres M, Salgado-Mercado R, Rios-Bedoya CF, Aponte-Rivera E, Marxuach-Cuétara AM, Rodríguez-Orengo JF, et al. High eradication rates of *Helicobacter pylori* infection with first- and second-line combination of esomeprazole, tetracycline, and metronidazole in patients allergic to penicillin. Dig Dis Sci. 2005;50:634-9.
176. Matsushima M, Suzuki T, Kurumada T, Watanabe S, Watanabe K, Kobayashi K, et al. Tetracycline, metronidazole and amoxicillin-metronidazole combinations in proton pump inhibitor-based triple therapies are equally effective as alternative therapies against *Helicobacter pylori* infection. J Gastroenterol Hepatol. 2006;21:232-6.
177. Malfertheiner P, Bazzoli F, Delchier JC, Celiñski K, Giguère M, Rivière M, et al. *Helicobacter pylori* eradication with a capsule containing bismuth subcitrate potassium, metronidazole, and tetracycline given with omeprazole versus clarithromycin-based triple therapy: A randomised, open-label, non-inferiority, phase 3 trial. Lancet. 2011;377:905-13.
178. Gisbert JP, Barrio J, Modolell I, Molina-Infante J, Aisa AP, Castro-Fernández M, et al. *Helicobacter pylori* first-line and rescue treatments in the presence of penicillin allergy. Dig Dis Sci. 2015;60:458-64.
179. Gao W, Zheng SH, Cheng H, Wang C, Li YX, Xu Y, et al. [Tetracycline and metronidazole based quadruple regimen as first line treatment for penicillin allergic patients with *Helicobacter pylori* infection]. Zhonghua Yi Xue Za Zhi. 2019;99:1536-40.
180. Fuller R. Probiotics in human medicine. Gut. 1991;32:439-42.
181. Vitor JM, Vale FF. Alternative therapies for *Helicobacter pylori*: Probiotics and phytomedicine. FEMS Immunol Med Microbiol. 2011;63:153-64.
182. Aiba Y, Suzuki N, Kabir AM, Takagi A, Koga Y. Lactic acid-mediated suppression of *Helicobacter pylori* by the oral administration of *Lactobacillus* salivarius as a probiotic in a gnotobiotic murine model. Am J Gastroenterol. 1998;93:2097-101.
183. Pinchuk IV, Bressollier P, Verneuil B, Fenet B, Sorokulova IB, Mégraud F, et al. In vitro anti-*Helicobacter pylori* activity of the probiotic strain *Bacillus* subtilis 3 is due to secretion of antibiotics. Antimicrob Agents Chemother. 2001;45:3156-61.

184. Rolfe RD. The role of probiotic cultures in the control of gastrointestinal health. J Nutr. 2000;130:396S-402S.
185. Dang Y, Reinhardt JD, Zhou X, Zhang G. The effect of probiotics supplementation on *Helicobacter pylori* eradication rates and side effects during eradication therapy: A meta-analysis. PLoS One. 2014;9:e111030.
186. Lv Z, Wang B, Zhou X, Wang F, Xie Y, Zheng H, et al. Efficacy and safety of probiotics as adjuvant agents for *Helicobacter pylori* infection: A meta-analysis. Exp Ther Med. 2015;9:707-16.
187. Tong JL, Ran ZH, Shen J, Zhang CX, Xiao SD. Meta-analysis: The effect of supplementation with probiotics on eradication rates and adverse events during *Helicobacter pylori* eradication therapy. Aliment Pharmacol Ther. 2007;25:155-68.
188. Wang ZH, Gao QY, Fang JY. Meta-analysis of the efficacy and safety of *Lactobacillus*-containing and Bifidobacterium-containing probiotic compound preparation in *Helicobacter pylori* eradication therapy. J Clin Gastroenterol. 2013;47:25-32.
189. Zhang MM, Qian W, Qin YY, He J, Zhou YH. Probiotics in *Helicobacter pylori* eradication therapy: A systematic review and meta-analysis. World J Gastroenterol. 2015;21:4345-57.
190. Zheng X, Lyu L, Mei Z. *Lactobacillus*-containing probiotic supplementation increases *Helicobacter pylori* eradication rate: evidence from a meta-analysis. Rev Esp Enferm Dig. 2013;105:445-53.
191. Zhu R, Chen K, Zheng YY, Zhang HW, Wang JS, Xia YJ, et al. Meta-analysis of the efficacy of probiotics in *Helicobacter pylori* eradication therapy. World J Gastroenterol. 2014;20:18013-21.
192. Zou J, Dong J, Yu X. Meta-analysis: Lactobacillus containing quadruple therapy versus standard triple first-line therapy for *Helicobacter pylori* eradication. Helicobacter 2009;14:97-107.
193. Li S, Huang XL, Sui JZ, Chen SY, Xie YT, Deng Y, et al. Meta-analysis of randomized controlled trials on the efficacy of probiotics in *Helicobacter pylori* eradication therapy in children. Eur J Pediatr. 2014;173:153-61.
194. Sachdeva A, Nagpal J. Effect of fermented milk-based probiotic preparations on *Helicobacter pylori* eradication: A systematic review and meta-analysis of randomized-controlled trials. Eur J Gastroenterol Hepatol. 2009;21:45-53.
195. Szajewska H, Horvath A, Piwowarczyk A. Meta-analysis: The effects of *Saccharomyces boulardii* supplementation on *Helicobacter pylori* eradication rates and side effects during treatment. Aliment Pharmacol Ther. 2010;32:1069-79.
196. Gong Y, Li Y, Sun Q. Probiotics improve efficacy and tolerability of triple therapy to eradicate *Helicobacter pylori*: A meta-analysis of randomized controlled trials. Int J Clin Exp Med. 2015;8:6530-43.
197. Lu C, Sang J, He H, Wan X, Lin Y, Li L, et al. Probiotic supplementation does not improve eradication rate of *Helicobacter pylori* infection compared to placebo based on standard therapy: A meta-analysis. Sci Rep. 2016;6:23522.
198. McFarland LV, Huang Y, Wang L, Malfertheiner P. Systematic review and meta-analysis: Multi-strain probiotics as adjunct therapy for *Helicobacter pylori* eradication and prevention of adverse events. United Eur Gastroenterol J. 2016;4:546-61.
199. Lu M, Yu S, Deng J, Yan Q, Yang C, Xia G, et al. Efficacy of probiotic supplementation therapy for *Helicobacter pylori* eradication: A meta-analysis of randomized controlled trials. PLoS One. 2016;11:e0163743.

200. Wang F, Feng J, Chen P, Liu X, Ma M, Zhou R, et al. Probiotics in *Helicobacter pylori* eradication therapy: Systematic review and network meta-analysis. Clin Res Hepatol Gastroenterol. 2017;41:466-75.
201. Feng JR, Wang F, Qiu X, McFarland LV, Chen PF, Zhou R, et al. Efficacy and safety of probiotic-supplemented triple therapy for eradication of *Helicobacter pylori* in children: A systematic review and network meta-analysis. Eur J Clin Pharmacol. 2017;73:1199-208.
202. Wen J, Peng P, Chen P, Zeng L, Pan Q, Wei W, et al. Probiotics in 14-day triple therapy for Asian pediatric patients with *Helicobacter pylori* infection: A network meta-analysis. Oncotarget. 2017;8:96409-18.
203. Shi X, Zhang J, Mo L, Shi J, Qin M, Huang X. Efficacy and safety of probiotics in eradicating *Helicobacter pylori*: A network meta-analysis. Medicine (Baltimore). 2019;98:e15180.
204. Molina-Infante J, Gisbert JP. Probiotics for *Helicobacter pylori* eradication therapy: Not ready for prime time. Rev Esp Enferm Dig. 2013;105:441-4.
205. McNicholl AG, Molina-Infante J, Lucendo AJ, Calleja JL, Pérez-Aisa Á, Modolell I, et al. Probiotic supplementation with *Lactobacillus plantarum* and *Pediococcus acidilactici* for *Helicobacter pylori* therapy: A randomized, double-blind, placebo-controlled trial. Helicobacter. 2018;23:e12529.
206. Efrati C, Nicolini G, Cannaviello C, O'Sed NP, Valabrega S. *Helicobacter pylori* eradication: Sequential therapy and *Lactobacillus reuteri* supplementation. World J Gastroenterol. 2012;18:6250-4.
207. Dajani AI, Abu Hammour AM, Yang DH, Chung PC, Nounou MA, Yuan KY, et al. Do probiotics improve eradication response to *Helicobacter pylori* on standard triple or sequential therapy? Saudi J Gastroenterol. 2013;19:113-20.
208. McMahon BJ, Hennessy TW, Bensler JM, Bruden DL, Parkinson AJ, Morris JM, et al. The relationship among previous antimicrobial use, antimicrobial resistance, and treatment outcomes for *Helicobacter pylori* infections. Ann Intern Med. 2003;139:463-9.
209. Laine L, Hunt R, El-Zimaity H, Nguyen B, Osato M, Spenard J. Bismuth-based quadruple therapy using a single capsule of bismuth biskalcitrate, metronidazole, and tetracycline given with omeprazole versus omeprazole, amoxicillin, and clarithromycin for eradication of *Helicobacter pylori* in duodenal ulcer patients: A prospective, randomized, multicenter, North American trial. Am J Gastroenterol. 2003;98:562-7.
210. Puig I, Gonzalez-Santiago JM, Molina-Infante J, Barrio J, Herranz MT, Algaba A, et al. Fourteen-day high-dose esomeprazole, amoxicillin and metronidazole as third-line treatment for *Helicobacter pylori* infection. Int J Clin Pract. 2017;71.
211. Muller N, Amiot A, Le Thuaut A, Bastuji-Garin S, Deforges L, Delchier JC. Rescue therapy with bismuth-containing quadruple therapy in patients infected with metronidazole-resistant *Helicobacter pylori* strains. Clin Res Hepatol Gastroenterol. 2016;40:517-24.
212. Dore MP, Lu H, Graham DY. Role of bismuth in improving *Helicobacter pylori* eradication with triple therapy. Gut. 2016;65:870-8.
213. Ribaldone DG, Astegiano M, Pellicano R. *Helicobacter pylori* eradication: Poor medical compliance from East to West of the world. Scand J Gastroenterol. 2018;53:265.

214. Li H, Liang X, Chen Q, Zhang W, Lu H. Inappropriate treatment in *Helicobacter pylori* eradication failure: A retrospective study. Scand J Gastroenterol. 2018;53:130-3.
215. Lee M, Kemp JA, Canning A, Egan C, Tataronis G, Farraye FA. A randomized controlled trial of an enhanced patient compliance program for *Helicobacter pylori* therapy. Arch Intern Med. 1999;159:2312-6.
216. Wermeille J, Cunningham M, Dederding JP, Girard L, Baumann R, Zelger G, et al. Failure of *Helicobacter pylori* eradication: Is poor compliance the main cause? Gastroenterol Clin Biol. 2002;26:216-9.
217. Shakya Shrestha S, Bhandari M, Thapa SR, Shrestha R, Poudyal R, Purbey B, et al. Medication adherence pattern and factors affecting adherence in *Helicobacter Pylori* eradication therapy. Kathmandu Univ Med J (KUMJ). 2016;14:58-64.
218. Graham DY, Lew GM, Malaty HM, Evans DG, Evans DJ Jr, Klein PD, et al. Factors influencing the eradication of *Helicobacter pylori* with triple therapy. Gastroenterology. 1992;102:493-6.
219. Kotilea K, Mekhael J, Salame A, Mahler T, Miendje-Deyi VY, Cadranel S, et al. Eradication rate of *Helicobacter pylori* infection is directly influenced by adherence to therapy in children. *Helicobacter*. 2017;22.
220. Al-Eidan FA, McElnay JC, Scott MG, McConnell JB. Management of *Helicobacter pylori* eradication: The influence of structured counselling and follow-up. Br J Clin Pharmacol. 2002;53:163-71.
221. Henry A, Batey RG. Enhancing compliance not a prerequisite for effective eradication of *Helicobacter pylori*: The HelP Study. Am J Gastroenterol. 1999;94:811-5.
222. O'Connor JP, Taneike I, O'Morain C. Improving compliance with *Helicobacter pylori* eradication therapy: When and how? Therap Adv Gastroenterol. 2009;2:273-9.
223. Li BZ, Threapleton DE, Wang JY, Xu JM, Yuan JQ, Zhang C, et al. Comparative effectiveness and tolerance of treatments for *Helicobacter pylori*: Systematic review and network meta-analysis. BMJ. 2015;351:h4052.
224. Malfertheiner P. Compliance, adverse events and antibiotic resistance in *Helicobacter pylori* treatment. Scand J Gastroenterol Suppl. 1993;196:34-7.
225. Fendrick AM, Chey WD, Margaret N, Palaniappan J, Fennerty MB. Symptom status and the desire for *Helicobacter pylori* confirmatory testing after eradication therapy in patients with peptic ulcer disease. Am J Med 1999;107:133-6.
226. Bytzer P, Dahlerup JF, Eriksen JR, Jarbøl DE, Rosenstock S, Wildt S, et al. Diagnosis and treatment of *Helicobacter pylori* infection. Dan Med Bull. 2011;58:C4271.
227. Phull PS, Halliday D, Price AB, Jacyna MR. Absence of dyspeptic symptoms as a test of *Helicobacter pylori* eradication. BMJ. 1996;312:349-50.
228. McColl KE, el-Nujumi A, Murray LS, el-Omar EM, Dickson A, Kelman AW, et al. Assessment of symptomatic response as predictor of *Helicobacter pylori* status following eradication therapy in patients with ulcer. Gut. 1998;42:618-22.
229. Delaney B, Ford AC, Forman D, Moayyedi P, Qume M. Initial management strategies for dyspepsia. Cochrane Database Syst Rev. 2005:CD001961.
230. Gisbert JP, Pajares JM. Review article: 13C-urea breath test in the diagnosis of *Helicobacter pylori* infection: A critical review. Aliment Pharmacol Ther. 2004;20:1001-17.
231. Gisbert JP, Pajares JM. Stool antigen test for the diagnosis of *Helicobacter pylori* infection: A systematic review. *Helicobacter*. 2004;9:347-68.

232. Gene E, Calvet X, Azagra R. Diagnosis of *Helicobacter pylori* after triple therapy in uncomplicated duodenal ulcers: A cost-effectiveness analysis. Aliment Pharmacol Ther. 2000;14:433-42.
233. Ofman J, Wallace J, Badamgarav E, Chiou CF, Henning J, Laine L. The cost-effectiveness of competing strategies for the prevention of recurrent peptic ulcer hemorrhage. Am J Gastroenterol. 2002;97:1941-50.
234. 234. Pohl H, Finlayson SR, Sonnenberg A, Robertson DJ. *Helicobacter pylori*-associated ulcer bleeding: Should we test for eradication after treatment? Aliment Pharmacol Ther. 2005;22:529-37.
235. Ahmed S, Salih M, Jafri W, Ali Shah H, Hamid S. *Helicobacter pylori* infection: Approach of primary care physicians in a developing country. BMC Gastroenterol. 2009;9:23.
236. Boekema PJ, Veenendaal RA, van Berge-Henegouwen GP. After a decade of *Helicobacter pylori* in The Netherlands. A survey of the practice of the members of the Dutch Society of Gastroenterology. Neth J Med. 1997;51:129-33.
237. Boltin D, Kimchi N, Dickman R, Gingold-Belfer R, Niv Y, Birkenfeld S. Attitudes and practice related to *Helicobacter pylori* infection among primary care physicians. Eur J Gastroenterol Hepatol. 2016;28:1035-40.
238. Cano-Contreras AD, Rascon O, Amieva-Balmori M, Ríos-Gálvez S, Maza YJ, Meixueiro-Daza A, et al. Approach, attitudes, and knowledge of general practitioners in relation to *Helicobacter pylori* is inadequate. There is much room for improvement! Rev Gastroenterol Mex. 2018;83:16-24.
239. Gene E, Calvet X, Azagra R, Lopez T, Cubells MJ. [Management of dyspepsia, gastroduodenal ulcer and *Helicobacter pylori* infection in primary care]. Aten Primaria. 2002;29:486-94.
240. Gene E, Sanchez-Delgado J, Calvet X, Azagra R. [Management of *Helicobacter pylori* infection in primary care in Spain]. Gastroenterol Hepatol. 2008;31:327-34.
241. Lim AG, Martin RM, Montileone M, Walker AC, Gould SR. *Helicobacter pylori* serology and the management of young dyspeptics: A UK survey of gastroenterologists and general practitioners with an interest in gastroenterology. Aliment Pharmacol Ther. 1997;11:299-303.
242. Luman W, Ng HS. Survey of dyspepsia management in community. Singapore Med J. 2001;42:26-9.
243. Markus B, Herszenyi L, Matyasovszky M, Vörös K, Torzsa P, Rurik I, et al. The diagnosis and therapy of *Helicobacter pylori* infection in Hungary: Comparison of strategies applied by family physicians and internists. Dig Dis. 2019:1-10.
244. Milne R, Logan RP, Harwood D, Misiewicz JJ, Forman D. *Helicobacter pylori* and upper gastrointestinal disease: A survey of gastroenterologists in the United Kingdom. Gut. 1995;37:314-8.
245. Murakami TT, Scranton RA, Brown HE, Harris RB, Chen Z, Musuku S, et al. Management of *Helicobacter pylori* in the United States: Results from a national survey of gastroenterology physicians. Prev Med. 2017;100:216-22.
246. Shirin H, Birkenfeld S, Shevah O, Levine A, Epstein J, Boaz M, et al. Application of Maastricht 2-2000 guidelines for the management of *Helicobacter pylori* among specialists and primary care physicians in Israel: Are we missing the malignant potential of *Helicobacter pylori*? J Clin Gastroenterol. 2004;38:322-5.
247. Rubin G, Stevens R. Laboratory tests for *Helicobacter pylori* should be more widely available. BMJ. 1996;313:172-3.

CHAPTER

8

Artificial Intelligence in Gastroenterology

Corinna Hauff, Her Hsin Tsai

INTRODUCTION

Artificial intelligence (AI) is already in use in various forms, whether we are aware of it or not. Face recognition AI software is widely used in immigration and passport controls. The vast amount of data collected by online retailers to build up a picture of your buying habits in order to more accurately target sales is another example. In the field of medicine, the first areas in which AI will impact will be the image-based specialties such as dermatology, radiology, and diagnostic endoscopy. The latter will doubtless impact on gastrointestinal (GI) physicians in the not too distant future, and modern GI specialists will have to have an understanding of AI in order to harness the available and evolving tools effectively and know their limitations.

Artificial intelligence is defined loosely as the use of machines to mimic human thought and brain processing. It thus mimics human "cognitive" functions in order to harness both learning and problem-solving functions. McCarthy is often accredited with the first proposal in 1957 at the Dartmouth conference.[1] They proposed a supercomplex computer with characteristics similar to human intelligence, e.g., AI that thinks like human beings with human senses and thinking power. With the rapid advances in computing power in the latter half of the 20th century, this aspiration has finally become a reality.

Moore's law predicts a doubling of transistors into integrated circuits every year and this is leading to an exponential increase in computing power. The story of AI can be illustrated by the example of the use of computers to play chess and to try to beat the best chess grandmasters. Until 1997, the best chess players would triumph over machine. Then the IBM Deep Blue supercomputer competed against the then world champion Gary Kasparov over two series of six matches. Their first match was in 1996 when Kasparov defeated Deep Blue.[2-4] However, improvement to its algorithms and the ability to learn meant that on the return matches in 1998, Deep Blue beat Kasparov 3½–2½.[3] This is an example of "machine learning (ML)".

By 2010, chess playing "engines" would readily beat even the very best human players such that rival programs would play each other in their own computer versus computer matches. These engines are based on algorithms and calculations of possible future moves and their relative merits. Then in 2018 an AI company DeepMind (a Google subsidiary) used neural network program and with no advance knowledge of chess theory, but simply the rules of the game, and made it play against itself and learning what works. After 4 hours of self-play, it reached a level above most human players and after 9 hours it could beat the then champion chess computer program Stockfish 8 in a time-controlled 100-game tournament (28 wins, 0 losses, and 72 draws).[4] AlphaZero thus successfully demonstrated the power of "deep learning (DL)."

Many terms used in AI can seem a little confusing. More generally, AI refers to a field of computer science that creates systems for performing tasks that usually require human intelligence. There are two nonmutually exclusive methods to achieve this. Machine learning is a term introduced by Arthur Samuel in 1959 to describe a subfield of AI that includes all those approaches that allow computers to learn from data without being explicitly programmed.[5] ML has been extensively applied to medical imaging. Among the techniques that fall under the ML umbrella is DL and it has emerged as one of the most promising. It is best to think of DL as a subset of ML and both under the umbrella term of AI **(Fig. 1)**.

Artificial intelligence terminology:

Artificial intelligence	Machine intelligence that has cognitive functions similar to those of humans such as "learning" and "problem solving."
Machine learning	Mathematical algorithms which are automatically built from given data (known as input training data) and predict or make decisions in uncertain conditions without being explicitly programmed
Support vector machines	Discriminative classifier formally defined by an optimizing hyperplane with the largest functional margin
Artificial neural networks	Multilayered interconnected network which consists of an input, hidden connection (between the input and output layers), and output layer
Deep learning	Subset of machine learning technique that is composed of multiple-layered neural network algorithms
Convolutional neural networks	Specific class of artificial neural networks that consists of: (1) Convolutional and pooling layers, which are the two main components to extract distinct features; (2) Fully connected layers to make an overall classification
Overfitting	Modelling error which occurs when a certain learning model tailors itself too much on the training dataset and predictions are not well generalized to new datasets
Spectrum bias	Systematic error occurs when the dataset used for model development does not adequately represent or reflect the range of patients who will be applied in clinical practice (target population)

Depending on the task required, computer programs can apply the many tools they possess to achieve AI. These tools include search algorithms which search for the most appropriate path. Other tools include statistical

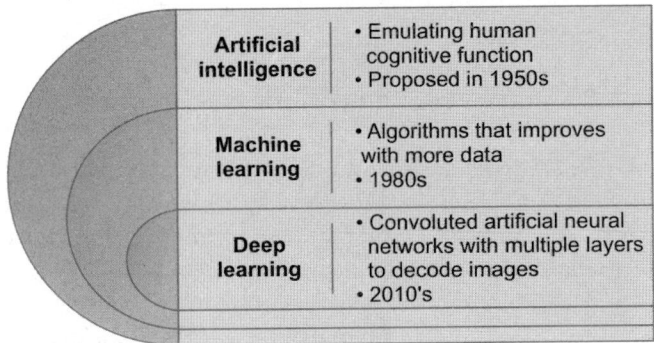

Fig. 1: Artificial intelligence can be seen as an umbrella term that includes machine learning (ML) and deep leaning a subset of ML.

models such as Bayesian models which use probability models to find the best solution. In medical imaging and endoscopy, the main concern is image recognition. Here, the most important tool is the use of artificial neural networks (ANNs). Hinton and LeCun are widely regarded as the two major pioneers of multilayered neural networks as the basis of AI.[6] The rapid advancement in recent years has been the catalyst to AI development in medical imaging and endoscopy.

Machine learning is a subfield of computer science that enables computers to learn without being explicitly programmed to do so. The technology of ML incorporates computational models and algorithms that are similar to the structure and function of our own brain's biologic neural networks. These computational models are often referred to as ANNs. When these ANNs process information (i.e., digital data) from numerous input flows, they have the ability to "learn" and alter their structure in much the same way that the neurons in our brain are altered with memory.[6]

Neural network architecture is structured in layers composed of interconnected nodes. Each node of the network performs a weighted sum of the input data that are subsequently passed to an activation function. Weights are dynamically optimized during the training phase. There are three different kinds of layers: (1) The input layer, which receives input data; (2) The output layer, which produces the results of data processing; and (3) The hidden layer(s), which extract the patterns within the data **(Fig. 2)**. The DL approach was developed to improve on the performance of a conventional ANN when using deep architectures. A deep ANN differs from the single hidden layer by having a large number of hidden layers, which characterize the depth of the network.[6] Among the different deep ANNs, convolutional neural networks (CNNs) have become popular in computer vision applications. In this class of deep ANNs, convolution operations are used to obtain feature maps in which the intensities of each pixel/voxel are calculated as the sum of each pixel/voxel of the original image and its neighbors, weighted by convolution matrices (also called kernels). Different kernels are applied for specific tasks, such as blurring, sharpening, or edge detection. CNNs are biologically

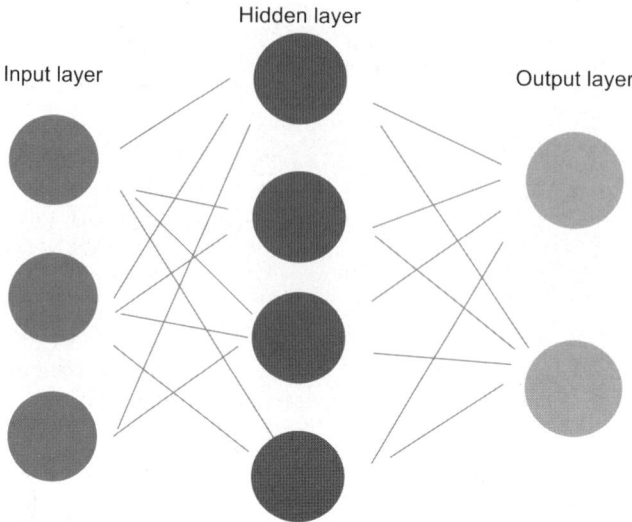

Fig. 2: Artificial neural networks with a single hidden layer.

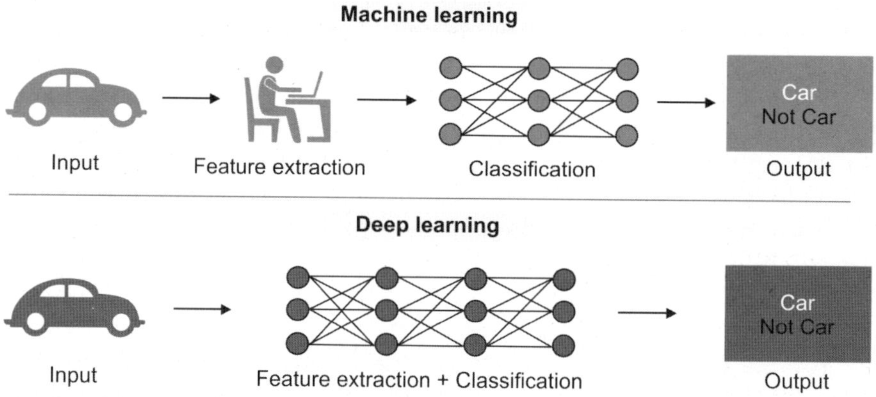

Fig. 3: Machine learning versus deep learning.

inspired networks mimicking the behavior of the brain cortex, which contains a complex structure of cells sensitive to small regions of the visual field. The architecture of deep CNNs allows for the composition of complex features (such as shapes) from simpler features (e.g., image intensities) to decode image raw data without the need to detect specific features **(Fig. 3)**. Hence, DL can both extract features and classify images without prior selection through a feature algorithm.

With increasing input of data from thousands of images of cars, DL is able to correctly recognize a car with increasing accuracy, while ML may hit a learning plateau much earlier. With the use of programmed algorithms, ML may take an early lead in performance but ultimately with an increasing amount of input data the performance of DL will far exceed that of ML **(Fig. 4)**.

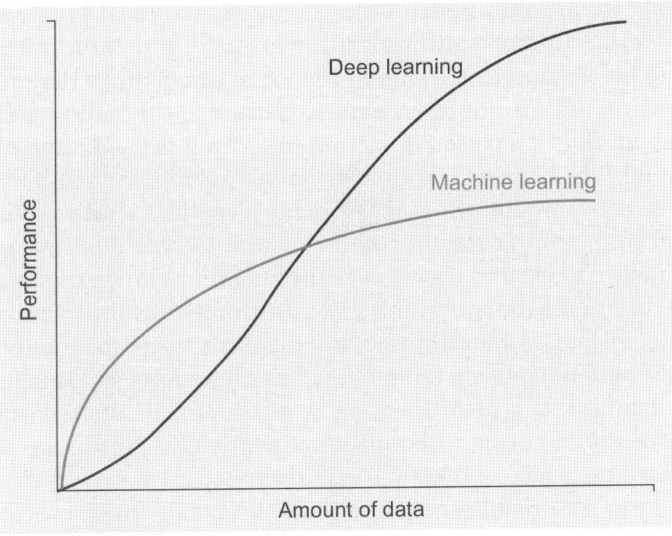

Fig. 4: Machine learning versus deep learning.

APPLICATION OF ARTIFICIAL INTELLIGENCE IN GASTROINTESTINAL RADIOLOGY

One of the first areas where DL is superior to ML is in the area of image recognition. Face recognition software has been the main driver. Images are by nature difficult to apply algorithms to as feature extraction requires difficult constructs. With DL, the convoluted neural nets "learn" by viewing hundreds of images and with each subsequent iteration the neural network, like human neurons, makes appropriate connections as it learns the features of say a car. Not dissimilar to a child who having been shown lots of images of "cars" would extract details of these images leading to image recognition when encountering similar, even cartoon images of cars.

Such technology would thus not unsurprisingly make its first forays into the medical arena in the area of medical imaging. Radiology trainees learn by viewing hundreds of images. Despite being taught a systematic way of reporting a chest X-ray or a CT scan, it is through viewing many images with an experienced radiologist that trainees gain the necessary experience. While a human may be able to view dozens of scans a day, a computer can view thousands.

The initial learning phase for AI may require an advanced computer or one of the supercomputers. These behemoths of the computer world can gobble up thousands of images and process them. But after the initial learning phase, the neural nets may be translated to a machine with far less processing power. In the case of AlphaZero, the chess DL program, the programmers used a supercomputer to run the self-play. Once its neural networks had been set, it needed no more than the equivalent of a laptop processor to play the game.

Today, there are hundreds of thousands of images of say liver lesions for the AI programmer to input and eventually one would expect the machine to be as good as a trained radiologist in making a diagnosis. One would imagine that AI posed an eminent threat to the radiologists' image interpretation skills. However, in its present form it is used as an aid rather than competition. AI may pick up a lesion in the lung or a mass in the liver and even give its probability of say this being a vascular lesion versus a mass lesion. But ultimately it requires a doctor to interpret the findings in the correct clinical context and thus inform the attending clinician as to the likely diagnosis and management plan.[7] AI's performance is thus similar to our natural intelligence; AI algorithms look at medical images to identify patterns after being trained using vast numbers of examinations and images. Those systems will be able to give information about the characteristics of abnormal findings, mostly in terms of conditional probabilities through Bayesian decision-making.[8]

So where can AI be of service to the GI physician? Experts emphasized AI's potential for improving the efficiency and productivity of radiologists, enabling them to deal with an increasing workload. By taking care of much of the drudgery and by automating routine tasks, AI may also free up radiologists to get more involved in direct patient care, working even more closely with clinicians. Many of AI most fervent supporters believe that taking on a higher profile role in the clinical care team will benefit patients and also ensure the survival of the specialty. The initial concern over the dire warnings, mainly by some AI luminaries outside of healthcare, that AI would soon replace radiologists has largely given way to excitement over the technology's promise for enhancing "radiology and augmenting radiologists," not displacing them.[9]

It is important to remember AI's potential not just for image analysis. DL algorithms are poised to benefit the entire imaging process, including speeding up scanning times, lowering radiation dose, and enabling optimized patient imaging protocols. Furthermore, AI may also uncover new imaging biomarkers that are too subtle for the human eye.

AI may also prescreen imaging studies to highlight urgent cases for radiologists to review and provide decision support to radiologists during the interpretation process. AI can also help to detect and characterize disease, such as improving lesion recognition, e.g., liver lesions as to the probability of them being benign, vascular, or malignant. Computers do not suffer fatigue or succumb to "search satisfaction" when detecting a lesion; the radiologist may become fatigued and fail to conduct a comprehensive survey of the images.

In many medical institutions, there is a cultural behavior of segregating specialties. The physician is the clinician who first interacts with the patient and orders the radiological examination while the radiologist remains cooped up in a dark room and may be reduced to merely being an image analyst. The clinical interpretation of the findings is left to the physicians. This is potentially dangerous for patients as nonradiologists may have a full understanding of the clinical situation but do not have the radiological knowledge. Where AI would have a direct and lasting role is to free the radiologist from the dark room and into the multidisciplinary arena where the clinical scenario could be jointly discussed with the relevant physicians. They would then genuinely be more involved in the clinical management of patients.

Where AI will excel in radiology is in its capacity to process vast numbers of radiological images. Like one giant brain, the more data available for it to process, the more accurate it becomes. This may lead to the possibility of the machine identifying lesions that the human eye cannot detect.[10] Radiology should move from a subjective perceptual skill to a more objective science. There will therefore be fewer missed lesions and reduction in attention to inter- and intrareader variability. Work to improve the repeatability and reproducibility of medical imaging over the past decades proves the need for reproducible radiological results.[11]

Finally, AI applications may enhance the development of technical protocols, improving image quality and decreasing radiation dose, decreasing MRI scanner time, and optimizing staffing and CT/MRI scanner utilization, thereby reducing costs. These applications will simplify and accelerate technicians' work, also resulting in an average higher technical quality of examinations.

In GI radiology, AI has the potential to replace many of the routine detection, characterization, and quantification tasks currently performed by radiologists as well as to accomplish the integration of data mining of its vast electronic medical records into the process.[12] This is highly valuable as the ability to characterize lesions, say in the liver, is often a besetting one. With its ability to mine data, radiomic features such as intensity, shape, texture, and wavelength can be extracted from medical images. The case in point is in the area of liver lesions. Here, computer-derived radiomics has borne fruit.[13,14]

Furthermore, ML can extend to follow-up images after chemotherapy of malignant lesions, eventually being able to discern the biological behavior of the cancer type and thus moving closer to the holy grail of "personalized" treatment of malignant diseases.[14] This would be of tremendous help to the GI oncologist as tumor response may be predicted based on improved characterization of the tumor lesion radiologically. Such an aspiration is realized in neuroradiology[15] and rapidly taken in by the GI radiological investigators.[16]

Focal Liver Lesion Detection

Deep learning algorithms combined with multiple imaging modalities have been widely used in the detection of focal liver lesions. Compared with visual assessment, this strategy may capture more detailed lesion features and make more accurate diagnosis. In an earlier study, Vivanti et al., by using DL models based on longitudinal liver CT studies, found that new liver tumors could be detected automatically with a true positive rate of 86%, while the standalone detection rate was only 72% and this method achieved a precision of 87% and an improvement of 39% over the traditional methods.[17] Currently, studies have reported improvement in detection accuracies using neural networks based on CT to detect liver tumors automatically. In the difficult task of predicting the primary source of a liver lesion, Ben-Cohen et al. developed a CNN model predicting the primary origin of liver metastases among four sites (melanoma, colorectal cancer, pancreatic cancer, and breast cancer) with CT images.[18] In this task of automatic multiclass categorization of liver metastatic lesions, the automated system was able to achieve a 56% accuracy for the primary sites. This is actually quite remarkable already, and as ML takes place with more data, these automated systems will eventually take away much of the guesswork in interpreting liver lesions.

Diffuse Liver Lesions

In transabdominal ultrasound for the diagnosis of fatty liver, AI programs have achieved accuracies of 100%.[19] In the area of liver cirrhosis diagnosis, accuracies of 97% were achieved with DL.[20] Further evaluation of positron emission tomography (PET) scans using neural networks has produced superior accuracies in detecting hepatic metastases.[21]

The way forward may be the use of multimodal imaging, integrating data, and using powerful Bayesian algorithms to aid diagnosis.

Is Artificial Intelligence a Threat to Radiologists?

There is an increasing awareness of the inevitability of technology to revolutionize many aspects of healthcare delivery. Many of the "backroom" engines of the modern health delivery system can be automated; however, at the "sharp end" are the clinician and the patient who will expect and require human-to-human interaction. Radiologists may reasonably feel some threat as they are often portrayed as sitting in dimly lit offices, viewing and reporting radiographic images. But that is to caricaturize the role of radiologists. They are highly trained doctors who understand clinical scenarios and are an integral, in fact vital, part of the diagnostic and therapeutic team that help construct a full picture of the patient's clinical condition and help formulate a management plan as part of a multidisciplinary team. Analyses of radiologists' workload suggest a surfeit of the more "routine" reporting of endless "normal" chest radiographs. AI will assist and enhance that role by reducing the drudgery of this and other aspects of reporting and reduce the number of errors that humans will make due to sheer fatigue.

The emergency departments of many hospitals are highly demanding environments. The modern hospital is a 24/7 establishment, but many hospitals do not have the staff numbers to run a comprehensive service.

However, anxious patients and relatives demand immediate answers. The reporting of "run-of-the-mill" radiology can be automated and relegated to the AI program. The computer never sleeps, and reports would be generated in minutes. Thus, the clinical radiological expertise can be diverted to the interventional side, specialist interpretation, and complex cases where their expertise may be better deployed.

ARTIFICIAL INTELLIGENCE IN GASTROINTESTINAL ENDOSCOPY

The other area where AI will have a significant impact in gastroenterology is in GI endoscopy.[22] Image capture technology can now allow endoscopists to focus on areas of interest and analyze prospective lesions. Lesion recognition is often difficult to a novice endoscopist and even experienced endoscopists may miss significant lesions.

Upper Gastrointestinal Endoscopy

In the area of upper GI, endoscopy, or esophagogastroduodenoscopy (EGD), Takiyama et al.[23] took 27,335 images from 1,750 patients as a training set for the recognition of anatomical locations of EGD images using neural nets and validated it with a set of 17,081 images from 435 patients and had accuracies of 99% in recognition of sites, thus proving how the technology works.

In the esophagus area, where AI has forays into endoscopy is in esophageal lesions, specifically Barrett's mucosa. van der Sommen et al.[24] used white light endoscopy to look at discrimination of early neoplastic lesions in Barrett's esophagus. They used retrospective 100 endoscopic images from 44 patients and demonstrated sensitivity of 83% and specificity of 83%. Such figures would improve with more image sets. In the diagnosis of esophageal cancer, Horie et al.[25] used a retrospective training set of 8,428 white-light images from 384 patients and validated against a set of 1,118 images from 97 patients and again with CNN demonstrated a sensitivity of 98% at detecting malignancy.

Studies in the stomach have concentrated on the diagnosis of gastric malignancy and refining it to look at estimation of invasion depth and detection of early cancers.[26-29] **Table 1** summarizes the current studies with new ones being produced in rapid succession. As the data sets increase, the accuracies in terms of sensitivity and specificity of computer-aided diagnosis will doubtless increase. Detection of early gastric cancers is particularly difficult. With the aid of CNN and magnifying endoscopy, a remarkable positive predictive value (PPV) of 98% could be achieved.[29]

It might be expected that in the area of capsule endoscopy, AI and CNN would be of greatest utility. The hours of video for every patient requires tedious viewing by the technician or have areas identified by rather primitive algorithms like presence of blood. However, the images from capsule endoscopy are of poor resolution and variable in quality as the capsule is

Table 1: Studies of artificial intelligence in the endoscopic detection of gastric cancer.

Reference	Year	Aim of study	Design of study	Number of subjects	Endoscopic modality	Outcomes
Kubota et al.[26]	2012	Diagnosis of depth of invasion in gastric cancer	Retrospective	902 images (10 times cross validation)	White-light endoscopy	Accuracy: 77.2%, 49.1%, 51.0%, and 55.3% for T1–4 staging, respectively
Hirasawa et al.[27]	2018	Detection of gastric cancers	Retrospective	Training set: 13,584 images, Test set: 2,296 images	White-light endoscopy, chromoendoscopy, NBI	Sensitivity: 92.2%, detection rate with a diameter of 6 mm or more: 98.6%
Zhu et al.[28]	2018	Diagnosis of depth of invasion in gastric cancer (mucosa/SM1/ deeper than SM1)	Retrospective	Training set: 790 images, Test set: 203 images	White-light endoscopy	Accuracy: 89.2%, AUROC: 0.94, sensitivity: 74.5%, specificity: 95.6%
Kanesaka et al.[29]	2018	Diagnosis of early gastric cancer using magnifying NBI images	Retrospective	Training set: 126 images, Test set: 81 images	Magnifying NBI	Accuracy: 96.3%, sensitivity: 96.7%, specificity: 95%, PPV: 98.3%

(AUROC: area under the receiver operating characteristic curve; NBI: narrow-band imaging; PPV: positive predictive value) driven by peristalsis. As a result, so far to date only very few studies have been performed. Leenhardt et al. developed a gastrointestinal telangiectasia detection model using segmentation images from capsule endoscopy. They used 600 control images and 600 typical telangiectasia images which were divided equally into training and test datasets.[30] Another looked at capsule endoscopy ability to identify coeliac mucosa.[31] As such, the usefulness of these two technologies is limited.

Lower Gastrointestinal Endoscopy

It is in the area of lower GI endoscopy that AI in endoscopy holds most promise of direct and imminent application in gastroenterology. One of the limitations of AI as especially DL is the need for vast quantities of data to improve accuracy. Polyps are a frequent finding at colonoscopy and detection of polyps is one of the major roles of diagnostic colonoscopy, especially when applied for screening for colorectal neoplasia. Hence, it is no surprise that a lot of recent attention has been directed in this area. There are two main aspects: (1) The detection of polyps from raw video images and (2) the characterization of polyps.

The first group of studies looked at the feasibility of AI in recognizing polyps. These use mainly white light endoscopy and show that it has a very good sensitivity and specificity. Depending on the training regimen, the results vary from 72 to 98% for sensitivity and 68 to 98% for specificity with the figures improving with higher numbers of training colonoscopies **(Table 2)**.[32-35]

Perhaps more useful is the use of AI to aid characterization of colonic polyps. Most colonoscopists use the Kudo pit pattern recognition which is complex, and the novice and many even very experienced colonoscopists get it wrong or require frequent comparisons with the pictures from atlases **(Figs. 5 and 6)**. The key is to differentiate between hyperplastic polyps that do not need excision and adenomas. Takemura et al. were among the first to use AI to aid pit pattern recognition.[36] More useful is to use the facilities of the modern colonoscope such as magnification and narrow-band imaging (NBI) to enhance and facilitate histological differentiation. This has been the breakthrough that could very soon revolutionize how we differentiate small polyps and aid the colonoscopist in making the important decision as to whether to excise the lesion or not. Here, studies have demonstrated the technology to be at least as good as expert operators. Kominami et al.[37] used a training set of 2,247 images from 1,262 colorectal lesions and a validation set of 118 colorectal lesions for the differentiation between hyperplastic and polyps and neoplastic ones. Using magnifying NBI images, they found an accuracy of 93.2%, sensitivity—93.0%, specificity—93.3%, with a PPV of 93% and an negative predictive value (NPV) of 93.3%. These are impressive results and with more numbers of images, the accuracy will only improve.

Table 2: Studies on artificial intelligence use in detecting colonic polyps.

Reference	Year	Aim of study	Design of study	Number of subjects	Endoscopic modality	Results
Fernandez-Esparrach et al.[32]	2016	Detection of colonic polyps	Retrospective	24 videos containing 31 polyps	White-light colonoscopy	Sensitivity: 70.4%, specificity: 72.4%
Misawa et al.[33]	2018	Detection of colonic polyps	Retrospective	546 short videos (training set: 105 polyp-positive videos and 306 polyp-negative videos, test set: 50 polyp-positive videos and 85 polyp-negative videos) from 73 full-length videos	White-light colonoscopy	Accuracy: 76.5%, sensitivity: 90.0%, specificity: 63.3%,
Urban et al.[34]	2018	Detection of colonic polyps	Retrospective	8,641 images with 20 colonoscopy videos	White-light colonoscopy with NBI	Accuracy: 96.4%, AUROC: 0.991
Wang et al.[35]	2018	Detection of colonic polyps	Retrospective	*Training set:* 5,545 images from 1,290 patients *Validation set A:* 27,113 images from 1,138 patients *Validation set B:* 612 images *Validation set C:* 138 video clips from 110 patients *Validation set D:* 54 video clips from 54 patients	White-light colonoscopy	*Dataset A:* AUROC—0.98 for at least one polyp detection, per-image sensitivity—94.4%, per-image specificity—95.2% *Dataset B:* Per-image sensitivity—88.2% *Dataset C:* Per-image sensitivity—91.6%, per-polyp sensitivity—100% *Dataset D:* Per-image specificity—95.4%

(AUROC: area under the receiver operating characteristic curve; NBI: narrow-band imaging)

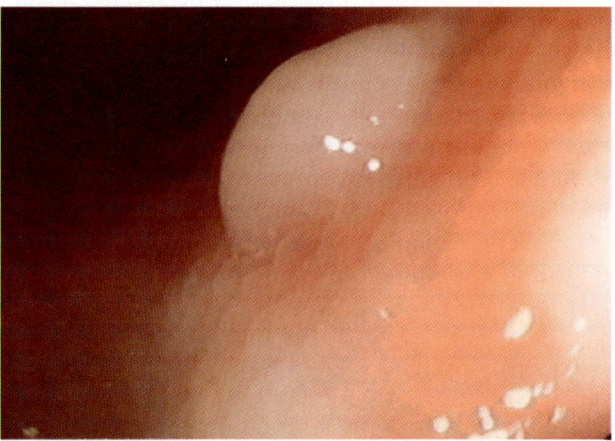

Fig. 5: Hyperplastic colonic polyp.

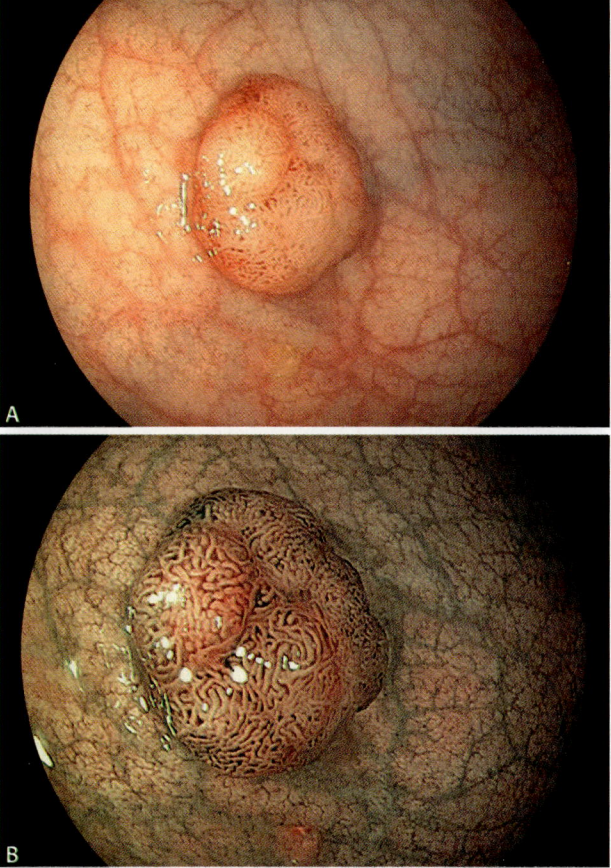

Figs. 6A and B: Colonic adenoma in (A) white light and (B) narrow-band imaging.

This technology is now available as a supplementary AI unit attached to the endoscopy stack and could well be incorporated into future endoscope systems. Further details will be discussed in Chapter 9.

Finally, AI in endoscopy will likely become a powerful audit tool of an endoscopist's performance and also thus soon could revolutionize endoscopic practice. Performance measures in colonoscopy such as cecal intubation rates and withdrawal times can be automated rather than just self-reporting. Adenoma detection rates can be validated by the machine. These developments would doubtless improve performance and could be used to revalidate the skills of the endoscopists.

KEY POINTS FOR CLINICAL PRACTICE

- AI is the use of computers to emulate human intelligence through algorithms, ML, and DL. Neural nets simulate the human neurons and convoluted networks are used in DL.
- Application of AI in image recognition is now widespread and application in radiology is increasing. In GI radiology, it is used in recognizing liver lesions.
- AI is increasingly used in GI endoscopy and in upper GI endoscopy in recognizing gastric malignancies.
- AI is perhaps most useful in recognition and characterization of colonic polyps.

REFERENCES

1. McCarthy J, Minsky ML, Rochester N, Shannon CE. A proposal for the Dartmouth summer research project on artificial intelligence, August 31, 1955. AI Mag. 2006;27:12-4.
2. Moore GE. Cramming more components onto integrated circuits. Electronics. 1965;114-7.
3. Goodman D, Keene R. Man versus machine: Kasparov versus deep blue. Cambridge, MA: H3 Inc; 1997.
4. Silver D, Hubert T, Schrittwieser J, Antonoglou I, Lai M, Guez A, et al. A general reinforcement learning algorithm that masters chess, shogi, and go through self-play. Science. 2018;362(6419):1140-4.
5. Samuel AL. Some studies in machine learning using the game of checkers. IBM J Res Dev. 1959;3:210-29.
6. LeCun Y, Bengio Y, Hinton G. Deep learning. Nature. 2015;521:436-4.
7. Pesapane F, Codari M, Sardanelli F. Artificial intelligence in medical imaging: Threat or opportunity? Radiologists again at the forefront of innovation in medicine. Eur Radiol Exp. 2018;2:35.
8. Litjens G, Kooi T, Bejnordi BE, Setio AAA, Ciompi F, Ghafoorian M, et al. A survey on deep learning in medical image analysis. Med Image Anal. 2017;42:60-88.
9. Chokshi FH, Flanders AE, Prevedello LM, Langlotz CP. Fostering a healthy AI ecosystem for radiology: conclusions of the 2018 RSNA summit on AI in radiology. Radiology: Artificial Intelligence. 2019;1(2).

10. Gillies RJ, Kinahan PE, Hricak H. Radiomics: Images are more than pictures, they are data. Radiology. 2016;278:563-77.
11. Sutton EJ, Huang EP, Drukker K, Burnside ES, Li H, Net JM, et al. Breast MRI radiomics: Comparison of computer- and human-extracted imaging phenotypes. Eur Radiol Exp. 2017;1:22.
12. Lakhani P, Prater AB, Hutson RK, Andriole KP, Dreyer KJ, Morey J, et al. Machine learning in radiology: Applications beyond image interpretation. J Am Coll Radiol. 2018;15:350-9.
13. Becker AS, Schneider MA, Wurnig MC, Wagner M, Clavien PA, Boss A. Radiomics of liver MRI predict metastases in mice. Eur Radiol Exp. 2018;2:11.
14. Aerts HJ, Velazquez ER, Leijenaar RT, Parmar C, Grossmann P, Carvalho S, et al. Decoding tumour phenotype by noninvasive imaging using a quantitative radiomics approach. Nat Commun. 2014;5:4006.
15. Peng SL, Chen CF, Liu HL, Lui CC, Huang YJ, Lee TH, et al. Analysis of parametric histogram from dynamic contrast-enhanced MRI: Application in evaluating brain tumor response to radiotherapy. NMR Biomed. 2013;26:443-50.
16. Zhou LQ, Wang JY, Yu SY, Wu GG, Wei Q, Deng YB, et al. Artificial intelligence in medical imaging of the liver. World J Gastroenterol. 2019;25(6):672-82.
17. Vivanti R, Szeskin A, Lev-Cohain N, Sosna J, Joskowicz L. Automatic detection of new tumors and tumor burden evaluation in longitudinal liver CT scan studies. Int J Comput Assist Radiol Surg. 2017;12(11):1945-57.
18. Ben-Cohen A, Klang E, Diamant I, Rozendorn N, Raskin SP, Konen E, et al. CT image-based decision support system for categorization of liver metastases into primary cancer sites: Initial results. Acad Radiol. 2017;24(12):1501-9.
19. Biswas M, Kuppili V, Edla DR, Suri HS, Saba L, Marinhoe RT, et al. Symtosis: A liver ultrasound tissue characterization and risk stratification in optimized deep learning paradigm. Comput Methods Programs Biomed. 2018;155:165-77.
20. Liu X, Song JL, Wang SH, Zhao JW, Chen YQ. Learning to diagnose cirrhosis with liver capsule guided ultrasound image classification. Sensors (Basel). 2017;17.
21. Preis O, Blake MA, Scott JA. Neural network evaluation of PET scans of the liver: A potentially useful adjunct in clinical interpretation. Radiology. 2011;258:714-21.
22. Yang YJ, Bang CS. Application of artificial intelligence in gastroenterology. World J Gastroenterol. 2019;25(14):1666-83.
23. Takiyama H, Ozawa T, Ishihara S, Fujishiro M, Shichijo S, Nomura S, et al. Automatic anatomical classification of esophagogastroduodenoscopy images using deep convolutional neural networks. Sci Rep. 2018;8:7497.
24. van der Sommen F, Zinger S, Curvers WL, Bisschops R, Pech O, Weusten BL, et al. Computer-aided detection of early neoplastic lesions in Barrett's esophagus. Endoscopy. 2016;48:617-24.
25. Horie Y, Yoshio T, Aoyama K, Yoshimizu S, Horiuchi Y, Ishiyama A, et al. Diagnostic outcomes of esophageal cancer by artificial intelligence using convolutional neural networks. Gastrointest Endosc. 2019;89:25-32.
26. Kubota K, Kuroda J, Yoshida M, Ohta K, Kitajima M. Medical image analysis: Computer-aided diagnosis of gastric cancer invasion on endoscopic images. Surg Endosc. 2012;26:1485-89.

27. Hirasawa T, Aoyama K, Tanimoto T, Ishihara S, Shichijo S, Ozawa T, et al. Application of artificial intelligence using a convolutional neural network for detecting gastric cancer in endoscopic images. Gastric Cancer. 2018;21:653-60.
28. Zhu Y, Wang QC, Xu MD, Zhang Z, Cheng J, Zhong YS, et al. Application of convolutional neural network in the diagnosis of the invasion depth of gastric cancer based on conventional endoscopy. Gastrointest Endosc. 2019;89:806-15.e1.
29. Kanesaka T, Lee TC, Uedo N, Lin KP, Chen HZ, Lee JY, et al. Computer-aided diagnosis for identifying and delineating early gastric cancers in magnifying narrow-band imaging. Gastrointest Endosc. 2018;87:1339-44.
30. Leenhardt R, Vasseur P, Li C, Saurin JC, Rahmi G, Cholet F, et al. A neural network algorithm for detection of GI angiectasia during small-bowel capsule endoscopy. Gastrointest Endosc. 2019;89:189-94.
31. Zhou T, Han G, Li BN, Lin Z, Ciaccio EJ, Green PH, et al. Quantitative analysis of patients with celiac disease by video capsule endoscopy: A deep learning method. Comput Biol Med. 2017;85:1-6.
32. Fernández-Esparrach G, Bernal J, López-Cerón M, Córdova H, Sánchez-Montes C, Rodríguez de Miguel C, et al. Exploring the clinical potential of an automatic colonic polyp detection method based on the creation of energy maps. Endoscopy. 2016;48:837-42.
33. Misawa M, Kudo SE, Mori Y, Cho T, Kataoka S, Yamauchi A, et al. Artificial intelligence-assisted polyp detection for colonoscopy: Initial experience. Gastroenterology. 2018;154:2027-9.e3.
34. Urban G, Tripathi P, Alkayali T, Mittal M, Jalali F, Karnes W, et al. Deep learning localizes and identifies polyps in real time with 96% accuracy in screening colonoscopy. Gastroenterology. 2018;155:1069-78.e8.
35. Wang H, Liang Z, Li LC, Han H, Song B, Pickhardt PJ, et al. An adaptive paradigm for computer-aided detection of colonic polyps. Phys Med Biol. 2015;60:7207-28.
36. Takemura Y, Yoshida S, Tanaka S, Onji K, Oka S, Tamaki T, et al. Quantitative analysis and development of a computer-aided system for identification of regular pit patterns of colorectal lesions. Gastrointest Endosc. 2010;72:1047-51.
37. Kominami Y, Yoshida S, Tanaka S, Sanomura Y, Hirakawa T, Raytchev B, et al. Computer-aided diagnosis of colorectal polyp histology by using a real-time image recognition system and narrow-band imaging magnifying colonoscopy. Gastrointest Endosc. 2016;83:643-9.

CHAPTER

9

Improving Polyp Detection at Colonoscopy

Sreedhari Thayalasekaran, Pradeep Bhandari

INTRODUCTION

Colorectal cancer remains a common cause of morbidity and mortality, with 525,048 deaths registered in England and Wales in 2016.[1] The majority of colorectal cancers are formed from the malignant transformation of adenomatous polyps via the adenoma-carcinoma sequence.[2,3]

Hyperplastic polyps are the other main type of colonic polyp but have a lower potential for malignant transformation. Sessile serrated polyps are a type of hyperplastic polyp that are usually located in the right side of the colon and can transform into malignancy via the alternative serrated pathway.[4] Approximately two-thirds of cancers arise from the left colon.[4] The majority (over 90%) of colorectal polyps are subcentimeter in size and have a low risk of advanced histology (villous/serrated/HGD or invasive component).[5] Colonoscopy and polypectomy are important therapeutic tools for the detection and prevention of colorectal carcinoma.[6]

The cecal intubation rate (CIR) is a key quality measure of colonoscopy.[7] An early nationwide audit in the UK published in 2004 showed a very low CIR of 77%, with CIR increasing to 92.3% in 2013, when the audit was repeated.[8,9] If the proximal colon is not reached during colonoscopic examination, there is an increased potential to miss right-sided neoplastic lesions. In a large observational study, the reported miss rates of right-sided colorectal cancer were 4%, with these patients undergoing a prior colonoscopy 6–36 months before their hospital admission.[10]

Despite colonoscopy remaining the gold standard investigation in the detection of colorectal adenoma, reported adenoma miss rates can be as high as 20%.[11] Therefore, in recent years, there has been considerable effort to improve quality of colonoscopy, resulting in the identification of key performance indicators and minimum targets in colonoscopy.[7] The ADR has been identified as a key performance indicator in colonoscopy.[7] The ADR is defined as the proportion of colonoscopies where at least one adenoma is detected. A large Polish study demonstrated that endoscopists with a minimum ADR of 20% had the lowest risk of interval colorectal cancer.[12] The current guidelines in the United Kingdom recommend endoscopists have a minimum 15% ADR, with 20% as an aspirational target.[7] Studies have shown that even a 1% increase in the ADR can result in a 3% reduction in the risk of interval colorectal cancer.[13] All these evidences highlight the importance of adenoma detection at colonoscopy.

In order to achieve a high ADR, endoscopists must possess a good withdrawal technique that involves careful inspection behind colonic folds and flexures, adequate cleansing of fecal residue, and luminal distension.[14] Furthermore, proximal colon polyps can often be very subtle and difficult to detect. A range of recent technological advances can help improve detection of colorectal polyps.

SIMPLE MEASURES

Good colonoscope handling is crucial in effective mucosal exposure. Simple techniques to increase polyp detection include the following:
- Adequate withdrawal time
- Dynamic position change on withdrawal
- Proximal colon retroflexion
- Use of Buscopan on withdrawal

Withdrawal Time

A benchmark paper confirmed that colonoscopists with a mean withdrawal time of 6 minutes or more had higher rates of adenoma detection (28.3% vs. 11.8%, $p < 0.001$).[15]

A recent study published from the BCSP cohort in the UK reported a statistically significant increase in the ADR when withdrawal times were >11 minutes [47.1% vs. 42.5%, when <7 minutes ($p < 0.001$)]. Regression analysis showed a minimal increase in ADR when withdrawal times were greater than 10 minutes. The authors proposed that the optimal withdrawal time is 10 minutes. If individuals are performing a meticulous colonic examination, it is likely that this correlates with longer withdrawal times. Current UK guidelines recommend minimum mean withdrawal time of 6 minutes (where polypectomy is not performed) and ideally 10 minutes.[7]

Dynamic Position Change on Withdrawal

Suggested position changes on withdrawal are as follows:
- Left lateral; cecum to hepatic flexure
- Supine; transverse colon
- Right lateral; splenic flexure and descending colon
- Left lateral; sigmoid colon and rectum.[16]

An early study on the benefits of position change during withdrawal showed that luminal distension improved on a nonvalidated scoring system.[17] The same group confirmed in a larger randomized controlled study that dynamic position change improved polyp and adenoma detection; 34% of patients where dynamic position change was performed had at least one adenoma detected compared to 23% examined in the left lateral position alone having at least 1 adenoma detected ($p = 0.01$).[16] One Canadian study found that prescribed dynamic position changes during colonoscope withdrawal did not affect ADR when the baseline ADR of endoscopists was above the recommended standard of 40%.[18] The largest multicenter study (1,072 patients) showed that dynamic position change compared to the left lateral position during colonoscope withdrawal increased the ADR from 33% to 42.4% ($p = 0.002$).[19]

Proximal Colon Retroflexion

Right-sided lesions are often flat, subtle, and easily missed. The technique of proximal colon retroflexion has shown to reduce the polyp miss rate. In a large (1,000 patient) observational cohort study, polyps in the right colon were removed on forward view. A repeat examination in retroflexion, once the cecum had been re-intubated occurred. The colonoscope was then withdrawn to the hepatic flexure, with polyps removed and sent separately for histological examination. In this study, retroflexion was successful in 94.4% of patients. A total of 634 polyps and 497 adenomas were identified in the proximal colon on forward view, with retroflexion identifying an additional 68 polyps and 54 adenomas.[20] The limitations of this study are that the examinations were performed by two operators in a single tertiary unit.[20] Cecal retroflexion with a standard colonoscope can be challenging and has the potential to cause significant discomfort and harm to patients, if performed by inexperienced endoscopists. The application of this technique by nonexperts is yet to be established. We believe that further evidence is required before this technique can be routinely recommended.

Buscopan

Buscopan is an anticholinergic drug that produces smooth muscle relaxation and decreases bowel spasm. It is used in colonoscopy to enhance mucosal visualization on withdrawal and increase the detection of adenoma. Caution should be used when considering Buscopan in patients who are already tachycardic or have pre-existing cardiac comorbidity, due to its anticholinergic effect which can precipitate tachycardia and hypotension. Monitoring of heart rates should be performed when administered during a procedure. Buscopan can infrequently trigger formerly undiagnosed asymptomatic acute closed-angle glaucoma. Advice should be given instructing patients to seek urgent medical attention if they develop painful red eye. Generally, Buscopan use is thought to be safe in open-angle glaucoma and also in closed-angle glaucoma who have had iridectomy.[21] A large observational study in the English Bowel Cancer Screening Programme found that the use of Buscopan increased adenoma detection by 30%.[22] However, statistically significant increases have not been confirmed in randomized controlled trials (RCTs).[23,24] A recent meta-analysis showed that Buscopan may provide a marginal improvement in the polyp and ADR, but due to heterogeneity in the data across the different studies, firm conclusion could not be drawn.[25] We recommend the use of low dose Buscopan in carefully selected patients to assist polyp detection on withdrawal.

WATER-ASSISTED COLONOSCOPY

Water-assisted colonoscopy is becoming increasingly popular and is broadly of two types:
1. *Water immersion* involves the infusion of water and air suction on intubation, without the removal of luminal contents.
2. *Water exchange* involves the insufflation of water and suction of air and dirty luminal contents in exchange for clean water.

Current evidence has shown that water exchange through improving bowel preparation improves the adenoma detection.[26-28] In one single center study on a screening population of 1,224 patients, randomization in a 1:1:1 method to water exchange, water immersion or air insufflation was performed. After cecal intubation was achieved, a different colonoscopist who was blinded to the intervention limb performed the withdrawal. Water exchange achieved a significantly higher ADR 49.3% versus 43.4% for water immersion and 40.4% for air insufflation, overall $p = 0.04$.[28] A recent meta-analysis of 17 RCTs, including 10,350 patients, showed that water exchange has a higher overall ADR, especially in the right colon, but prolongs insertion time by an additional 3-5 minutes.[27] Water exchange not only increases ADR, but also reduces patient discomfort, and is an option for experienced endoscopists.

COLONOSCOPY TECHNOLOGY

High-definition Colonoscopy

High-definition (HD) colonoscopy is the use of a HD monitor and colonoscope that produces more images per second with a higher resolution compared to standard definition (SD).[29] There has been a continuous improvement in the definition of white light endoscopy, with the initial video endoscopes consisting of approximately 50,000–100,000 pixels.[30] The current HD endoscopes contain up to 1.3 million pixels. In theory, HD colonoscopy should make the detection of subtle mucosal abnormalities, such as diminutive polyps, easier. Early studies comparing high-definition colonoscopy to SD did not report a significant increase in the ADRs.[31-33]

More recently, studies have shown a statistically significant increase in polyp and adenoma detection with HD compared to standard colonoscopy (SC).[34-36] The largest retrospective study of 2,430 patients showed a significantly higher ADR with high-definition white-light (HDWL) compared to SD (28.8% vs. 24.3%, $p = 0.012$). A meta-analysis has shown that HD colonoscopy produces a 2–4% gain in the ADR. This meta-analysis of five studies and 4,422 patients showed an incremental yield of 3.8% with a number needed to treat (NNT) of 26 for polyp detection and an incremental yield of 3.5% with an NNT of 28 for adenoma detection.[37] HD endoscopes are the current standard for most units in western countries.

Dye-based Chromoendoscopy

Chromoendoscopy is the application of dye to the gastrointestinal tract in a segmental fashion through the use of a spray catheter. Contrast agents are the nonabsorptive dyes that sit on the mucosa, highlighting raised areas and surface patterns.

Chromoendoscopy enhances the visualization of colonic mucosal patterns and can be used to increase the yield of colonoscopy for flat or depressed neoplasms. There has been a poor uptake of chromoendoscopy amongst Western endoscopists due to a combination of multiple factors—lack of training, increased procedural time, and equipment expense. Withdrawal times are unsurprisingly longer with the use of chromoendoscopy. Studies have shown an increase in adenoma detection with its use.[38,39] One two-center RCT of 1,008 patients found a significantly higher ADR with the use of chromoendoscopy (46.2%) compared to SC (36.3%), $p = 0.002$.[38] Studies have shown improved adenoma detection, with a more noticeable effect for diminutive adenomas in the proximal colon.[40,41] A systematic review concluded that chromoendoscopy was more likely to produce patients with at least one neoplastic lesion [OR 1.67 (CI 1.29–2.15)] and significantly more patients with three or more neoplastic lesions [OR 2.55 (CI 1.49–4.36)].[42] Dye-based chromoendoscopy is effective but is cumbersome and increasingly being replaced by virtual chromoendoscopy.

Virtual Chromoendoscopy

Endoscopy companies have developed their own virtual chromoendoscopy systems that provide the endoscopist with enhanced images through the switching on or off of a button on the endoscope. Virtual chromoendoscopy is an alternative to conventional chromoendoscopy and enhances the visualization of the mucosal surface and vasculature. The term "virtual chromoendoscopy" refers to narrow-band imaging (NBI) (Olympus, Tokyo, Japan), flexible spectral imaging color enhancement (FICE) (Fujinon, Saitama, Japan), i-scan (Pentax, Tokyo, Japan), and blue laser imaging (BLI) and linked color imaging (LCI) (Fujinon, Saitama, Japan). NBI, FICE, and i-scan are now widely available in clinical practice, but their use remains mostly in academic endoscopy units. Virtual chromoendoscopy has been shown to be beneficial in both lesion detection and lesion characterization. The advantage to virtual chromoendoscopy over traditional dye-spray chromoendoscopy is that it is less time-consuming and cumbersome, due to its push button approach.[43]

LCI has shown promising results in recent studies. Earlier studies of the other image enhancement technologies showed some benefit, but this has not been consistently shown in recent studies, particularly when used by endoscopists with high baseline ADRs.

Narrow-band Imaging

The majority of data on the use of virtual chromoendoscopy come from studies performed with the use of NBI. Most of the data has been done in expert settings, limiting conclusions that can be drawn in widespread practice. The principles of NBI depend on the principle of variable penetration of light. Red light penetrates deep into the submucosa but does not help with surface pattern. Blue and green light at a wavelength range of 415–540 nm do not penetrate deep but enhance mucosal vessel patterns. Blue light displays superficial capillary networks, while green light highlights subepithelial vessels. NBI uses a physical filter to block red light and to narrow the bandwidth of the blue and green light, resulting in a high-contrast image that improves visualization of surface patterns.[43] Initial studies showed greater polyp detection with the use of NBI compared to standard white light colonoscopy.[44,45] Subsequent studies, however, conflicted with these findings.[46,47] A Cochrane review of 11 RCTs and 3,673 patients in 2012 found no evidence to suggest that NBI was significantly better than SC at improving detection rates in average-risk populations.[48] A more recent meta-analysis of data from individual patients in 11 RCTs found that the ADR was higher with the use of NBI over white-light endoscopy (WLE), with the effect more noticeable when the bowel preparation was optimal.[49]

i-scan

i-scan (Pentax, Tokyo, Japan) is a digital contrast system that uses post-processing computer algorithms and a SD processor to regulate light reflected from the mucosa to enhance surface visualization. i-scan consists of three enhancement modalities: (1) Surface enhancement, (2) contrast enhancement, and (3) tone enhancement. Studies on the efficacy of i-scan compared to WLE have shown conflicting results. One RCT did not show a statistically significant difference in the ADR with i-scan compared to high-definition colonoscopy [31.9% (HDWL) vs. i-scan (36.5%), $p = 0.742$].[50] One large cohort study by Bowman et al. (1,936 patients) showed that polyps were detected more in the i-scan cohort, i.e., 56% compared to 47% in the control group ($p = 0.03$).[51] One RCT showed that HDWL + i-scan had a 25% greater adenoma detection than SC. This study was limited due to the i-scan limb being combined with HDWL, which could also potentially explain the greater ADR.[52] Further studies are needed to confirm beneficial effects of i-scan.

Flexible Spectral Imaging Color Enhancement and Blue Laser Imaging

Flexible spectral imaging color enhancement is the virtual chromoendoscopy system found on Fujifilm endoscopes. It is a post-processor technology that uses a charge coupled device to narrow the bandwidth of light and enhance mucosal visibility. FICE provides a selection of wavelengths for optimal views. Studies thus far have failed to demonstrate a noticeable benefit in the use of FICE with white light colonoscopy.[53] Two prospective, RCTs comparing FICE to WLE have not shown increased polyp or adenoma detection.[54-56] A recent meta-analysis showed no benefit to FICE over WLE.[57]

This technology has been superseded by BLI and LCI from Fujifilm. The newest image enhancement (Blue Light Imaging; Fujifilm) uses a 4-light emitting diode multi-light technology, which produces brighter images. BLI is the first technology to produce blue light in a narrow spectrum without the use of a filter. The most recent introduction to image-enhanced endoscopy has come from Fujinon and is called BLI. BLI is another form of image enhancement endoscopy that utilizes two lasers and a white light phosphor to enhance superficial blood vessels in the mucosa.[58] Contrary to NBI, there is the direct emission of blue light. In one small Japanese study, 182 patients were randomized to BLI or WLI. The study showed a significant improvement with the use of BLI over WLI with a polyp detection rate (PDR) of 59.8% versus 40%, respectively, $p = 0.008$. The ADR was also 46.2% versus 27.8%, respectively, with a p-value of 0.010.[58] In a large RCT from Japan, BLI was found to significantly increase the mean adenomas per patient (MAP); 1.27 compared to SC 1.01, $p = 0.008$, but not increase the ADR when compared to SC.[59] BLI is a relatively new technology and further studies are needed to make definitive conclusion.

Linked Color Imaging

Linked color imaging is a new virtual chromoendoscopy system, built into the Eluxeo 7000 Fujifilm series. LCI is designed to provide brighter images and improve subtle differences in red color, thereby providing clearer images of the vasculature and pit patterns.[60] In a recent multicenter RCT, a statistically significant improvement in the PDR was demonstrated for LCI over WL endoscopy, 91% versus 73% ($p < 0.0001$).[60] One recent Italian study showed that there was a statistically significant reduction in the miss rates of adenoma in the LCI limb compared to the WL endoscopy limb, 11.8% versus 30.6%, respectively ($p < 0.001$).[61] LCI and BLI are the newest image enhancement modalities, and therefore need further data to prove their superiority to the older modalities.

Device-assisted Colonoscopy

Two different technologies have been studied the most which are as follows:
1. Distal attachment devices (CAC/ECUFF/ERING)
2. Newer endoscopes designed to provide a wider field of view (G-EYE/FUSE and EWAVE).

Cap-assisted Colonoscopy

The transparent cap was the first distal attachment device to show promise in improving adenoma detection **(Fig. 1)**.[62] It was initially used as an adjunct to provide stabilization of the colonoscope when performing endoscopic mucosal resection.[63] Of all the distal attachment devices, the transparent cap has been around the longest, with the most research performed. It helps to improve mucosal visualization, by straightening the colonic haustra, keeping the colonic lumen open with minimal air insufflation.[64] The majority of cap-related studies have examined polyp, rather than adenoma detection. A large Dutch study where the baseline ADR of the endoscopists was >20% showed no statistically significant difference between cap-assisted colonoscopy (CAC) compared to SC, with an ADR 28% in SC versus 28% in CAC (RR 0.98; 95% CI 0.82–0.16).[65] A large RCT found that CAC improved PDR to 47% compared to standard colonoscopy 42.6% ($p = 0.03$). In a large RCT performed by experienced endoscopists with a baseline ADR of at least 20%, no beneficial effect with the use of a cap was reported; ADR 28% for both the CAC limb and SC limb.[65] A Cochrane systematic review concluded that CAC increased polyp detection compared to SC, but also reduced cecal intubation times.[66] A recent meta-analysis of 16 RCTs showed that CAC detected a marginal benefit over SC for polyp detection and shortened the cecal intubation time.[67] Proximal colon ADR has also been shown, in another meta-analysis, to be improved with the use of CAC.[68]

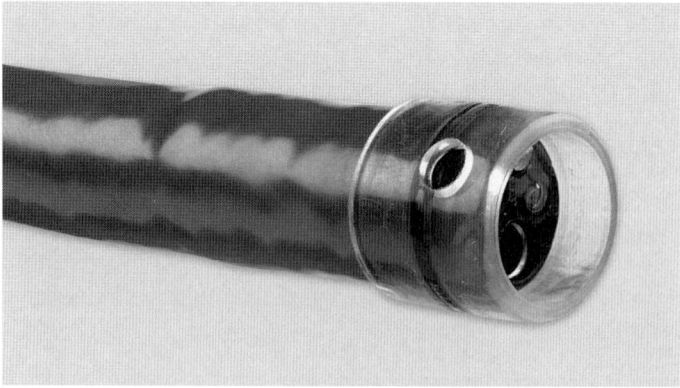

Fig. 1: Cap-assisted colonoscopy device.

EndoCuff

The EndoCuff (EC) (Arc medical, Leeds, United Kingdom) was originally designed to increase tip stability and improve access when performing therapeutic endoscopy but current evidence shows that it can increase the ADR **(Fig. 2)**.[69,70] The EC consists of soft side projections designed to remain flat on insertion and open on withdrawal, flattening out colonic folds, and preventing the accidental backward slipping of the colonoscope at colonic flexures. There have been two RCTs where the endoscopists had a high baseline ADR where no statistically significant benefit in ER colonoscopy compared to SC colonoscopy was shown. Both studies showed a reduction in withdrawal time in colonoscopy where polypectomy was not performed.[71,72] The shorter withdrawal time could be due to the EC providing good views and opening up folds and flexures, avoiding the need to do a double pass for complete examination.[71,72] The largest EC study to date by Ngu et al.[73] (1,772 patients) reported an increased ADR in the EC arm by 4.7% ($p = 0.02$) overall, with a significant increase in the BCSP cohort of 10.8% ($p \leq 0.001$).[73] This is in contrast to the studies by Bhattacharyya et al. and van Doorn et al.,[71,72] where no increase was seen in the screening population. A recent meta-analysis concluded that the use of the EC had the greatest improvement in ADR when used by endoscopists with low-to-moderate ADRs.[74]

EndoRings™

The EndoRings™ device is the newest distal attachment device, consisting of two layers of soft circular rings that evert mucosal folds on withdrawal, facilitating improved mucosal exposure **(Fig. 3)**. The EndoRings™ has a

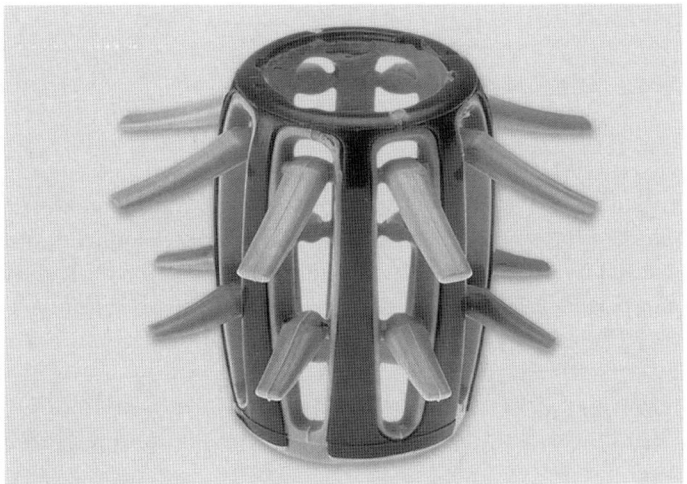

Fig. 2: EndoCuff.

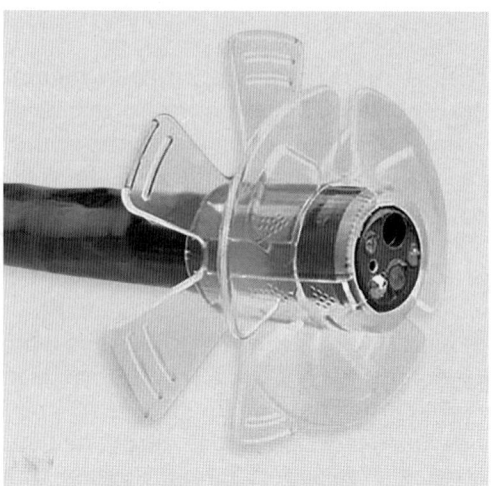

Fig. 3: EndoRings™ device.

larger, bulkier diameter than both the cap and the EC, so theoretically should flatten colonic folds. However, cecal intubation might be more challenging, with this design. In one large recent Italian study performed by experienced endoscopists in a fecal immunochemical test (FIT) positive population, no benefit with EndoRings™ colonoscopy compared to SC was shown.[75] One large study showed an increase in the mean number of adenomas per patient 1.46 (ER) versus 1.06 (SC) ($p = 0.025$), with a 9% removal rate of the device.[76] Another similar sized study showed a statistically significant increase in the mean number of polyps per patient 1.84 (SC) versus 2.25 (ER), $p = 0.004$, with a trend toward an increase in the mean number of adenomas per patient 1.22 (SC) versus 1.32 (ER), $p = 0.38$. A 27% removal rate for the device was found, with sigmoid diverticulosis as a common reason for removal.[77] Further studies are needed to clarify the role of ER colonoscopy.

Wide-angle Colonoscopy

Standard colonoscopes have a 140–170° field of view. The Extra-Wide-Angle View (EWAVE) colonoscope (Olympus Medical Systems) prototype was developed with one forward-viewing and two lateral backward-viewing lenses. A single image with a 235° field of view is obtained from both lenses simultaneously. In a pilot study on animal models, significantly more polyps were detected with EWAVE colonoscopy than standard colonoscopy (68% EWAVE vs. 51% SC, $p < 0.0001$).[78] In a recent international cohort study of 193 patients who underwent EWAVE colonoscopy, an ADR of 39.9% was demonstrated. This study was, however, terminated early owing to technical limitations with the EWAVE prototype and a new prototype is in development.[79]

G-EYE Colonoscopy

The G-EYE (Smart Medical Systems Ltd, Ra'anana, Israel) colonoscope contains a reusable balloon that is partly inflated on withdrawal once cecal intubation is achieved, enabling straightening of the colonic folds and centralizing the colonic lumen, with a reduction in bowel slippage. Initial studies showed an improvement in the ADR with the use of the G-EYE balloon.[80,81] A recent large multicenter international study that compared the G-EYE system to standard high-definition colonoscopy found a significantly higher yield in the ADR 48% (G-EYE) compared to SD (37.5%). There was also a greater detection of advanced flat and sessile serrated adenomas/polyps when compared with SC.[82]

Full-spectrum Endoscopy

The full-spectrum endoscopy (FUSE) system is a colonoscope that provides high definition, 330° field of view using three imagers and light-emitting diode groups found at the front and sides of the tip of the scope. Colon images are displayed on three, side-by-side, contiguous video monitors, thus providing the endoscopist with the 330° angle of view. After a pilot study in human subjects,[83] a randomized back-to-back study showed a significantly lower adenoma miss rate with FUSE (FUSE 7% vs. SC 41%, $p < 0.0001$).[84] A more recent study on a FIT positive population in 7 Italian centers randomised 658 subjects to either SC or FUSE; no statistically significant increase in the ADR was demonstrated with FUSE (43.6%) versus SC (45.5%) [OR 0.96, 95% CI 0.81–1.14]. The FUSE system is no longer available on the market, limiting conclusions on its current utility.

ARTIFICIAL INTELLIGENCE

The use of artificial intelligence (AI) in endoscopy has gained interest in lesion detection and diagnosis. In one large study involving 1,058 patients, Wang et al. randomized patients to undergo SC with or without the use of an automated polyp detection system that notifies via an alarm and visual notice when a polyp was detected.[85] Study found an increase in the detection of hyperplastic polyps 114 versus 52, $p < 0.001$. The study found that there was a statistically significant increase in the ADR (29.1% vs. 20.3%, $p < 0.001$) and mean number of adenomas per patient (0.53 vs. 0.31, $p < 0.001$). An increased number of diminutive polyps were found 185 versus 102, $p < 0.001$, without significant increase in larger adenomas 77 versus 58, $p = 0.075$.[85] Kominami et al.[86] evaluated the performance of a real-time image recognition system in making an in vivo diagnosis of colorectal polyps against a diagnosis made by NBI and correlated the results with the actual histological diagnosis. 118 colorectal lesions were evaluated; 93.0% sensitivity, 93.3% specificity, 93.0% positive predictive value (PPV), and 93.3% negative predictive value (NPV) was shown.[86] Two other studies to date have reported similar positive findings with the use of AI-based support systems, with both reporting a NPV of 90% for the diagnosis of diminutive adenomas.[87,88]

CONCLUSION

Chromoendoscopy, virtual and dye-based, newer endoscope designs, and distal attachment devices have shown mixed results with the majority of studies performed in tertiary centers, limiting conclusion that can be drawn on their routine clinical use. It is an exciting time in endoscopic innervation, especially with initial studies on the use of AI showing some promise. However, in the current economic climate, it is unlikely that such technology will be available for routine use by all practicing endoscopists in the near future. Improving withdrawal and mucosal exposure by focusing on simple measures such as minimum withdrawal time, use of Buscopan, and dynamic position change that can be achieved by every individual, should be the priority.

REFERENCES

1. Deaths. Deaths broken down by age, sex, area and cause of death. Office for National Statistics; 2016.
2. Hill MJ, Morson BC, Bussey HJ. Aetiology of adenoma—carcinoma sequence in large bowel. Lancet. 1978;1(8058):245-7.
3. Hill M. Etiology of the adenoma-carcinoma sequence. Major Probl Pathol. 1978;10:153-62.
4. Cunningham D, Atkin W, Lenz HJ, Lynch HT, Minsky B, Nordlinger B, et al. Colorectal cancer. Lancet. 2010;375(9719):1030-47.
5. Lieberman D, Moravec M, Holub J, Michaels L, Eisen G. Polyp size and advanced histology in patients undergoing colonoscopy screening: implications for CT colonography. Gastroenterology. 2008;135(4):1100-5.
6. Winawer SJ, Zauber AG, Ho MN, O'Brien MJ, Gottlieb LS, Sternberg SS, et al. Prevention of colorectal cancer by colonoscopic polypectomy. The National Polyp Study Workgroup. N Engl J Med. 1993;329(27):1977-81.
7. Rees CJ, Thomas Gibson S, Rutter MD, Baragwanath P, Pullan R, Feeney M, et al. UK key performance indicators and quality assurance standards for colonoscopy. Gut. 2016;65(12):1923-9.
8. Bowles CJ, Leicester R, Romaya C, Swarbrick E, Williams CB, Epstein O. A prospective study of colonoscopy practice in the UK today: are we adequately prepared for national colorectal cancer screening tomorrow? Gut. 2004;53(2):277-83.
9. Gavin DR, Valori RM, Anderson JT, Donnelly MT, Williams JG, Swarbrick ET. The national colonoscopy audit: a nationwide assessment of the quality and safety of colonoscopy in the UK. Gut. 2013;62(2):242-9.
10. Bressler B, Paszat LF, Vinden C, Li C, He J, Rabeneck L. Colonoscopic miss rates for right-sided colon cancer: a population-based analysis. Gastroenterology. 2004;127(2):452-6.
11. van Rijn JC, Reitsma JB, Stoker J, Bossuyt PM, van Deventer SJ, Dekker E, et al. Polyp miss rate determined by tandem colonoscopy: a systematic review. Am J Gastroenterol. 2006;101(2):343-50.

12. Kaminski MF, Regula J, Kraszewska E, Polkowski M, Wojciechowska U, Didkowska J, et al. Quality indicators for colonoscopy and the risk of interval cancer. N Engl J Med. 2010;362:1795-803.
13. Corley DA, Jensen CD, Marks AR, Zhao WK, Lee JK, Doubeni CA, et al. Adenoma detection rate and risk of colorectal cancer and death. N Engl J Med. 2014;370(14):1298-306.
14. Rex DK. Polyp detection at colonoscopy: Endoscopist and technical factors. Best Pract Res Clin Gastroenterol. 2017;31(4):425-33.
15. Barclay RL, Vicari JJ, Doughty AS, Johanson JF, Greenlaw RL. Colonoscopic withdrawal times and adenoma detection during screening colonoscopy. N Engl J Med. 2006;355(24):2533-41.
16. East JE, Bassett P, Arebi N, Thomas-Gibson S, Guenther T, Saunders BP. Dynamic patient position changes during colonoscope withdrawal increase adenoma detection: a randomized, crossover trial. Gastrointest Endosc. 2011;73(3):456-63.
17. East JE, Suzuki N, Arebi N, Bassett P, Saunders BP. Position changes improve visibility during colonoscope withdrawal: a randomized, blinded, crossover trial. Gastrointest Endosc. 2007;65(2):263-9.
18. Ou G, Kim E, Lakzadeh P, Tong J, Enns R, Ramji A, et al. A randomized controlled trial assessing the effect of prescribed patient position changes during colonoscope withdrawal on adenoma detection. Gastrointest Endosc. 2014;80(2):277-83.
19. Lee SW, Chang JH, Ji JS, Maeong IH, Cheung DY, Kim JS, et al. Effect of dynamic position changes on adenoma detection during colonoscope withdrawal: a randomized controlled multicenter trial. Am J Gastroenterol. 2016;111(1):63-9.
20. Hewett DG, Rex DK. Miss rate of right-sided colon examination during colonoscopy defined by retroflexion: an observational study. Gastrointest Endosc. 2011;74(2):246-52.
21. Lee T, Anderson J, Thomas-Gibson S, Rees C. Use of intravenous hyoscine butyl-bromide (Buscopan) during gastrointestinal endoscopy. Frontline Gastroenterol. 2018;9(3):183-4.
22. Lee TJ, Rees CJ, Blanks RG, Moss SM, Nickerson C, Wright KC, et al. Colonoscopic factors associated with adenoma detection in a national colorectal cancer screening program. Endoscopy. 2014;46(3):203-11.
23. Corte C, Dahlenburg L, Selby W, Griffin S, Byrne C, Chua T, et al. Hyoscine butylbromide administered at the cecum increases polyp detection: a randomized double-blind placebo-controlled trial. Endoscopy. 2012;44(10):917-22.
24. de Brouwer EJ, Arbouw ME, van der Zwet WC, van Herwaarden MA, Ledeboer M, Jansman FG, et al. Hyoscine N-butylbromide does not improve polyp detection during colonoscopy: a double-blind, randomized, placebo-controlled, clinical trial. Gastrointest Endosc. 2012;75(4):835-40.
25. Madhoun MF, Ali T, Tierney WM, Maple JT. Effect of hyoscine N-butylbromide on adenoma detection rate: meta-analysis of randomized clinical trials. Dig Endosc. 2015;27(3):354-60.
26. Cadoni S, Hassan C, Frazzoni L, Ishaq S, Leung FW. Impact of water exchange colonoscopy on endoscopy room efficiency: a systematic review and meta-analysis. Gastrointest Endosc. 2019;89(1):159-67.e13.
27. Fuccio L, Frazzoni L, Hassan C, La Marca M, Paci V, Smania V, et al. Water exchange colonoscopy increases adenoma detection rate: a systematic review with network meta-analysis of randomized controlled studies. Gastrointest Endosc. 2018;88(4):589-97.e11.

28. Cadoni S, Falt P, Rondonotti E, Radaelli F, Fojtik P, Gallittu P, et al. Water exchange for screening colonoscopy increases adenoma detection rate: a multicenter, double-blinded, randomized controlled trial. Endoscopy. 2017;49(5):456-67.
29. Ngu WS, Rees C. Can technology increase adenoma detection rate? Therap Adv Gastroenterol. 2018;11:1756283X17746311.
30. Sivak MV Jr, Fleischer DE. Colonoscopy with a Video Endoscope: preliminary experience. Gastrointest Endosc. 1984;30(1):1-5.
31. Pellise M, Fernandez-Esparrach G, Cardenas A, Sendino O, Ricart E, Vaquero E, et al. Impact of wide-angle, high-definition endoscopy in the diagnosis of colorectal neoplasia: a randomized controlled trial. Gastroenterology. 2008;135(4):1062-8.
32. Longcroft-Wheaton G, Brown J, Cowlishaw D, Higgins B, Bhandari P. High-definition vs. standard-definition colonoscopy in the characterization of small colonic polyps: results from a randomized trial. Endoscopy. 2012;44(10):905-10.
33. East JE, Stavrindis M, Thomas-Gibson S, Guenther T, Tekkis PP, Saunders BP. A comparative study of standard vs. high definition colonoscopy for adenoma and hyperplastic polyp detection with optimized withdrawal technique. Aliment Pharmacol Ther. 2008;28(6):768-76.
34. Jrebi NY, Hefty M, Jalouta T, Ogilvie J, Davis AT, Asgeirsson T, et al. High-definition colonoscopy increases adenoma detection rate. Surg Endosc. 2017;31(1):78-84.
35. Bond A, O'Toole P, Fisher G, Subramanian S, Haslam N, Probert C, et al. New-generation high-definition colonoscopes increase adenoma detection when screening a moderate-risk population for colorectal cancer. Clin Colorectal Cancer. 2017;16(1):44-50.
36. Buchner AM, Shahid MW, Heckman MG, McNeil RB, Cleveland P, Gill KR, et al. High-definition colonoscopy detects colorectal polyps at a higher rate than standard white-light colonoscopy. Clin Gastroenterol Hepatol. 2010;8(4):364-70.
37. Subramanian V, Mannath J, Hawkey CJ, Ragunath K. High-definition colonoscopy vs. standard video endoscopy for the detection of colonic polyps: a meta-analysis. Endoscopy. 2011;43(6):499-505.
38. Pohl J, Schneider A, Vogell H, Mayer G, Kaiser G, Ell C. Pancolonic chromoendoscopy with indigo carmine versus standard colonoscopy for detection of neoplastic lesions: a randomised two-centre trial. Gut. 2011;60(4):485-90.
39. Kahi CJ, Anderson JC, Waxman I, Kessler WR, Imperiale TF, Li X, et al. High-definition chromocolonoscopy vs. high-definition white light colonoscopy for average-risk colorectal cancer screening. Am J Gastroenterol. 2010;105(6):1301-7.
40. Brooker JC, Saunders BP, Shah SG, Thapar CJ, Thomas HJ, Atkin WS, et al. Total colonic dye-spray increases the detection of diminutive adenomas during routine colonoscopy: a randomized controlled trial. Gastrointest Endosc. 2002;56(3):333-8.
41. Lapalus MG, Helbert T, Napoleon B, Rey JF, Houcke P, Ponchon T, et al. Does chromoendoscopy with structure enhancement improve the colonoscopic adenoma detection rate? Endoscopy. 2006;38(5):444-8.
42. Brown SR, Baraza W. Chromoscopy versus conventional endoscopy for the detection of polyps in the colon and rectum. Cochrane Database Syst Rev. 2010;(10):CD006439.
43. Longcroft-Wheaton G, Bhandari P. A review of image-enhanced endoscopy in the evaluation of colonic polyps. Expert Rev Gastroenterol Hepatol. 2014;8:267-81.
44. Inoue T, Murano M, Murano N, Kuramoto T, Kawakami K, Abe Y, et al. Comparative study of conventional colonoscopy and pan-colonic narrow-band imaging system in the detection of neoplastic colonic polyps: a randomized, controlled trial. J Gastroenterol. 2008;43(1):45-50.

45. Rastogi A, Bansal A, Wani S, Callahan P, McGregor D, Cherian R, et al. Narrow-band imaging colonoscopy—a pilot feasibility study for the detection of polyps and correlation of surface patterns with polyp histologic diagnosis. Gastrointest Endosc. 2008;67(2):280-6.
46. Kaltenbach T, Friedland S, Soetikno R. A randomised tandem colonoscopy trial of narrow band imaging versus white light examination to compare neoplasia miss rates. Gut. 2008;57(10):1406-12.
47. Adler A, Pohl H, Papanikolaou IS, Abou-Rebyeh H, Schachschal G, Veltzke-Schlieker W, et al. A prospective randomised study on narrow-band imaging versus conventional colonoscopy for adenoma detection: does narrow-band imaging induce a learning effect? Gut. 2008;57(1):59-64.
48. Nagorni A, Bjelakovic G, Petrovic B. Narrow-band imaging versus conventional white light colonoscopy for the detection of colorectal polyps. Cochrane Database Syst Rev. 2012;(1):CD008361.
49. Atkinson NSS, Ket S, Bassett P, Aponte D, Aguiar S, Gupta N, et al. Narrow-band imaging for detection of neoplasia at colonoscopy: a meta-analysis of data from individual patients in randomized controlled trials. Gastroenterology. 2019;157(2):462-71.
50. Hong SN, Choe WH, Lee JH, Kim SI, Kim JH, Lee TY, et al. Prospective, randomized, back-to-back trial evaluating the usefulness of i-scan in screening colonoscopy. Gastrointest Endosc. 2012;75(5):1011-21.
51. Bowman EA, Pfau PR, Mitra A, Reichelderfer M, Gopal DV, Hall BS, et al. High-definition colonoscopy combined with i-scan imaging technology is superior in the detection of adenomas and advanced lesions compared to high definition colonoscopy alone. Diagn Ther Endosc. 2015;2015:167406.
52. Hoffman A, Sar F, Goetz M, Tresch A, Mudter J, Biesterfeld S, et al. High-definition colonoscopy combined with i-scan is superior in the detection of colorectal neoplasias compared with standard video colonoscopy: a prospective randomized controlled trial. Endoscopy. 2010;42(10):827-33.
53. Chung SJ, Kim D, Song JH, Park MJ, Kim YS, Kim JS, et al. Efficacy of computed virtual chromoendoscopy on colorectal cancer screening: a prospective, randomized, back-to-back trial of Fuji Intelligent Color Enhancement versus conventional colonoscopy to compare adenoma miss rates. Gastrointest Endosc. 2010;72(1):136-42.
54. Aminalai A, Rosch T, Aschenbeck J, Mayr M, Drossel R, Schröder A, et al. Live image processing does not increase adenoma detection rate during colonoscopy: a randomized comparison between FICE and conventional imaging (Berlin Colonoscopy Project 5, BECOP-5). Am J Gastroenterol. 2010;105(11):2383-8.
55. Pohl J, Lotterer E, Balzer C, Sackmann M, Schmidt K-D, Gossner L, et al. Computed virtual chromoendoscopy versus standard colonoscopy with targeted indigocarmine chromoscopy: a randomised multicentre trial. Gut. 2009;58(1):73-8.
56. Yoshida Y, Matsuda K, Sumiyama K, Kawahara Y, Yoshizawa K, Ishiguro H, et al. A randomized crossover open trial of the adenoma miss rate for narrow band imaging (NBI) versus flexible spectral imaging color enhancement (FICE). Int J Colorectal Dis. 2013;28(11):1511-6.
57. Omata F, Ohde S, Deshpande GA, Kobayashi D, Masuda K, Fukui T. Image-enhanced, chromo, and cap-assisted colonoscopy for improving adenoma/neoplasia detection rate: a systematic review and meta-analysis. Scand J Gastroenterol. 2014;49(2):222-37.

58. Ang TL, Li JW, Wong YJ, Tan YJ, Fock KM, Tan MTK, et al. A prospective randomized study of colonoscopy using blue laser imaging and white light imaging in detection and differentiation of colonic polyps. Endosc Int Open. 2019;7(10):E1207-13.

59. Ikematsu H, Sakamoto T, Togashi K, Yoshida N, Hisabe T, Kiriyama S, et al. Detectability of colorectal neoplastic lesions using a novel endoscopic system with blue laser imaging: a multicenter randomized controlled trial. Gastrointest Endosc. 2017;86(2):386-94.

60. Min M, Deng P, Zhang W, Sun X, Liu Y, Nong B. Comparison of linked color imaging and white-light colonoscopy for detection of colorectal polyps: a multicenter, randomized, crossover trial. Gastrointest Endosc. 2017;86(4):724-30.

61. Paggi S, Mogavero G, Amato A, Rondonotti E, Andrealli A, Imperiali G, et al. Linked color imaging reduces the miss rate of neoplastic lesions in the right colon: a randomized tandem colonoscopy study. Endoscopy. 2018;50(4):396-402.

62. Matsushita M, Hajiro K, Okazaki K, Takakuwa H, Tominaga M. Efficacy of total colonoscopy with a transparent cap in comparison with colonoscopy without the cap. Endoscopy. 1998;30(5):444-7.

63. Inoue H, Takeshita K, Hori H, Muraoka Y, Yoneshima H, Endo M. Endoscopic mucosal resection with a cap-fitted panendoscope for esophagus, stomach, and colon mucosal lesions. Gastrointest Endosc. 1993;39(1):58-62.

64. Sumiyama K, Rajan E. Endoscopic caps. Techniques in Gastrointestinal Endoscopy. 2006;8(1):28-32.

65. de Wijkerslooth TR, Stoop EM, Bossuyt PM, Mathus-Vliegen EMH, Dees J, Tytgat KMAJ, et al. Adenoma detection with cap-assisted colonoscopy versus regular colonoscopy: a randomised controlled trial. Gut. 2012;61(10):1426-34.

66. Morgan J, Thomas K, Lee-Robichaud H, Nelson RL, Braungart S. Transparent cap colonoscopy versus standard colonoscopy to improve caecal intubation. Cochrane Database Syst Rev. 2012;(12):CD008211.

67. Ng SC, Tsoi KK, Hirai HW, Lee YT, Wu JCY, Sung JSY, et al. The efficacy of cap-assisted colonoscopy in polyp detection and cecal intubation: a meta-analysis of randomized controlled trials. Am J Gastroenterol. 2012;107(8):1165-73.

68. Desai M, Sanchez-Yague A, Choudhary A, Pervez A, Gupta N, Vennalaganti P, et al. Impact of cap-assisted colonoscopy on detection of proximal colon adenomas: systematic review and meta-analysis. Gastrointest Endosc. 2017;86(2):274-1.

69. Lenze F, Beyna T, Lenz P, Heinzow HS, Hengst K, Ullerich H. Endocuff-assisted colonoscopy: a new accessory to improve adenoma detection rate? Technical aspects and first clinical experiences. Endoscopy. 2014;46(7):610-4.

70. Tsiamoulos ZP, Saunders BP. A new accessory, endoscopic cuff, improves colonoscopic access for complex polyp resection and scar assessment in the sigmoid colon (with video). Gastrointest Endosc. 2012;76(6):1242-5.

71. van Doorn SC, van der Vlugt M, Depla A, Wientjes CA, Mallant-Hent RC, Siersema PD, et al. Adenoma detection with Endocuff colonoscopy versus conventional colonoscopy: a multicentre randomised controlled trial. Gut. 2017;66(3):438-45.

72. Bhattacharyya R, Chedgy F, Kandiah K, Fogg C, Higgins B, Haysom-Newport B, et al. Endocuff-assisted vs. standard colonoscopy in the fecal occult blood test-based UK Bowel Cancer Screening Programme (E-cap study): a randomized trial. Endoscopy. 2017;49(11):1043-50.

73. Ngu WS, Bevan R, Tsiamoulos ZP, Bassett P, Hoare Z, Rutter MD, et al. Improved adenoma detection with Endocuff Vision: the ADENOMA randomised controlled trial. Gut. 2019;68(2):280-8.

74. Williet N, Tournier Q, Vernet C, Dumas O, Rinaldi L, Roblin X, et al. Effect of Endocuff-assisted colonoscopy on adenoma detection rate: meta-analysis of randomized controlled trials. Endoscopy. 2018;50(9):846-60.
75. Hassan C, Senore C, Manes G, Fuccio L, Iacopini F, Ricciardiello L, et al. Diagnostic yield and miss rate of EndoRings in an organized colorectal cancer screening program: the SMART (Study Methodology for ADR-Related Technology) trial. Gastrointest Endosc. 2019;89(3):583-90.
76. Rex DK, Kessler WR, Sagi SV, Rogers NA, Fischer M, Bohm ME, et al. Impact of a ring-fitted cap on insertion time and adenoma detection: a randomized controlled trial. Gastrointest Endosc. 2020;91(1):115-20.
77. Thayalasekaran SBR, Chedgy F, Bhandari P. EndoRings-assisted colonoscopy versus standard colonoscopy for polyp detection in symptomatic and asymptomatic patients: a randomized controlled trial. Gastrointest Endosc. 2019;89(6):AB88.
78. Uraoka T, Tanaka S, Matsumoto T, Matsuda T, Oka S, Moriyama T, et al. A novel extra-wide-angle view colonoscope: a simulated pilot study using anatomic colorectal models. Gastrointest Endosc. 2013;77(3):480-3.
79. Bronzwaer MES, Dekker E, Weingart V, Groth S, Pioche M, Rivory J, et al. Feasibility, safety, and diagnostic yield of the extra-wide-angle view (EWAVE) colonoscope for the detection of colorectal lesions. Endoscopy. 2018;50(1):63-8.
80. Gralnek IM, Suissa A, Domanov S. Safety and efficacy of a novel balloon colonoscope: a prospective cohort study. Endoscopy. 2014;46(10):883-7.
81. Halpern Z, Gross SA, Gralnek IM, Shpak B, Pochapin M, Hoffman A, et al. Comparison of adenoma detection and miss rates between a novel balloon colonoscope and standard colonoscopy: a randomized tandem study. Endoscopy. 2015;47(3):238-44.
82. Shirin H, Shpak B, Epshtein J, Karstensen JG, Hoffman A, de Ridder R, et al. G-EYE colonoscopy is superior to standard colonoscopy for increasing adenoma detection rate: an international randomized controlled trial (with videos). Gastrointest Endosc. 2019;89(3):545-53.
83. Gralnek IM, Segol O, Suissa A, Siersema PD, Carr-Locke DL, Halpern Z, et al. A prospective cohort study evaluating a novel colonoscopy platform featuring full-spectrum endoscopy. Endoscopy. 2013;45(9):697-702.
84. Gralnek IM, Siersema PD, Halpern Z, Segol O, Melhem A, Suissa A, et al. Standard forward-viewing colonoscopy versus full-spectrum endoscopy: an international, multicentre, randomised, tandem colonoscopy trial. Lancet Oncol. 2014;15(3):353-60.
85. Wang P, Berzin TM, Glissen Brown JR, Bharadwaj S, Becq A, Xiao X, et al. Real-time automatic detection system increases colonoscopic polyp and adenoma detection rates: a prospective randomised controlled study. Gut. 2019;68(10):1813-9.
86. Kominami Y, Yoshida S, Tanaka S, Sanomura Y, Hirakawa T, Raytchev B, et al. Computer-aided diagnosis of colorectal polyp histology by using a real-time image recognition system and narrow-band imaging magnifying colonoscopy. Gastrointest Endosc. 2016;83(3):643-9.
87. Byrne MF, Chapados N, Soudan F, Oertel X, Pérez ML, Kelly R, et al. Real-time differentiation of adenomatous and hyperplastic diminutive colorectal polyps during analysis of unaltered videos of standard colonoscopy using a deep learning model. Gut. 2019;68(1):94-100.
88. Chen PJ, Lin MC, Lai MJ, Lin JC, Horng-Shing LH, Tseng VS. Accurate classification of diminutive colorectal polyps using computer-aided analysis. Gastroenterology. 2018;154(3):568-75.

CHAPTER

10

Post-endoscopic Retrograde Cholangiopancreatography Pancreatitis

Arjun Sugumaran

INTRODUCTION

Since the first endoscopic pancreatogram in 1968 and description of biliary sphincterotomy for management of bile duct pathologies in 1974,[2] the procedure has evolved from a diagnostic endoscopic modality to mostly therapeutic intervention for hepatobiliary-pancreatic disorders. It is now a commonly performed endoscopic test even in small regional hospitals by trained endoscopists that may be gastroenterologists, surgeons, radiologists or nurse endoscopists as practicing in some large tertiary centers. The technique has undergone various adaptations and modifications over the years from experts to make it as safe a surgical treatment as possible and prevent major complications.

The indication for endoscopic retrograde cholangiopancreatography (ERCP) comprises commonly to treat the two major pathologies—bile duct stones (choledocholithiasis) and obstructing bile duct or pancreatic tumors. Other reasons for referral to ERCP can include postoperative bile leak, benign bile duct strictures, and suspected sphincter of Oddi dysfunction (SOD). With modern radiological modalities available widely, most of the cases will have ultrasound (US), computed tomography (CT) or magnetic resonance cholangiopancreatography (MRCP) scans suggesting an obstructed bile duct system along with the relevant blood test biomarkers especially jaundice, cholestatic liver function, abnormal coagulation or elevated tumor markers.

In many occasions, ERCPs are done as day case procedures unless patients are acutely unwell when they are performed on hospital inpatients. Patients are sometimes transferred to central or tertiary hospitals to have their scopes done depending on endoscopist or operation theater facility and availability. There are guidelines recommending timeframes for intervention based on how unwell patients are with their cholangitis or pancreatitis and also planned surgery for stone diseases.[3,4] Most centers observe patients for up to 4 hours post procedure to pick up any early complication and recommendation for nil by mouth or other treatment comes from the surgeon.

COMPLICATIONS FOLLOWING AN ERCP

Whilst obtaining consent from any patient undergoing ERCP, senior endoscopists ideally spend 10-15 minutes explaining the proceedings and risks involved in detail. Not uncommonly we find some patients decline the procedure after fully understanding ERCP risks and we have to offer alternate modalities that may include radiological interventions like percutaneous transhepatic cholangiography (PTC) or surgery where bile duct exploration and cholecystectomy can be carried out in selected patients. The complications can be mild, moderate or severe. Abdominal discomfort and nausea can be common post procedure but mostly settle after 2-3 hours. But the most often encountered and serious complication is post-ERCP pancreatitis (PEP). The other not uncommon procedure-related risks include failure to locate or cannulate the papilla needing repeat procedure or other interventions, bleeding post sphincterotomy, cholangitis, perforation, and adverse sedation effects in some patients. Some of these complications can be serious but we will cover only PEP in this chapter.

POST-ERCP PANCREATITIS

It is unfortunate to see any complication from a surgery but most ERCPists will agree it is always frustrating and not uncommon to see PEP develop on a patient despite the procedure performed flawlessly and all appropriate precautions undertaken. But every ERCPist should be aware of the common risk factors for PEP as it is the most common and potentially life-threatening complication following ERCP. There are American[5] and European guidelines[6,7] on prophylaxis to prevent PEP that are very helpful to avoid complications if incorporated in daily clinical practice.

Definition

The definition of pancreatitis has varied widely but the two most debated and discussed definitions in the concept of PEP were from Peter Cotton et al. and the 2012 revised Atlanta classification and definition. Cotton's consensus workshop group from 1991 definition[8] includes "clinical pancreatitis with amylase at least three times the upper limit of normal at more than 24 hours after the procedure, requiring hospital admission or a prolongation of planned admission". There has been lot of studies contradicting the statement based on the amount of amylase elevation, timing of the test, and the severity of diagnosis being based on primarily the duration of symptoms. Studies comparing serum lipase to amylase have demonstrated more positive yield with using lipase in early PEP.[9]

Atlanta 2012 definition of pancreatitis[10] warrants two of the following three criteria—symptoms of new epigastric pain radiating to back indicating pancreatitis, lipase or amylase blood levels more than three times normal following the procedure, and contrast CT findings confirming features of new pancreatic inflammation. Also the severity of the pancreatitis based on this paper is classified as mild, moderate, or severe. The mild form (interstitial edematous pancreatitis) has no organ failure, local or system complications, and usually resolves in the first week. If there is transient (<48 hours) organ failure, local complications or exacerbation of comorbid disease, it is classified as moderate. Patients with persistent (>48 hours) organ failure have the severe form of the disease.

Both these definitions were not primarily proposed for PEP and studies have not shown any good correlation with utilization of these definitions in course of disease or outcome of patients.[11]

The PANCREA (Pancreatitis Across Nations Clinical Research and Education Alliance) group has defined four grades of severity for pancreatitis based on presence or absence of complications, both local (necrosis of the pancreas and/or peripancreatic tissue) and systemic (cardiovascular, renal, or respiratory organ failure).[12]

These are definitions for guidance but we see lot of variation when symptoms are more severe with mild elevations in enzyme levels or very high enzymes or worrying CT features but with minimal symptoms. The primary aim will be to treat the patient and not scans or blood tests but the degrees of pancreatitis severity can guide targeted therapy.

Incidence

The incidence of PEP in retrospective and prospective studies has been reported anywhere between 1% and 15% in literature.[13,14] Most PEP patients (80–85%) will develop a mild disease course (self-limited, mortality <1–3%), but around 20% will have a moderate or severe episode of pancreatitis with mortality rate from 13% to 35%.[15] This can vary largely and in some terms based on patient factors, procedure factors, hospital and proceduralist expertise, and technique. We will discuss each in detail below.

Patient Risk Factors

Careful patient selection for ERCP should be the key factor in prevention of unnecessary complications. ERCP-related complications have proven to cost up annually to USD 150 million in the US and so there has been trend to concentrate more on therapeutic biliary intervention rather on diagnostic or pancreatic indications over the past decades.[16] There are many patient factors studied that may pose higher risk for post-procedure pancreatitis that every ERCPist should take into consideration.

Female sex is a risk factor for PEP for not properly understood reason. A study found longer cannulation time and alternate devices used in female but no significant correlation to PEP.[17] A meta-analysis found relative risk for female gender to be OR: 1.84, 95% CI: 1.25–2.70, $p = 0.002$.[18] But other studies have not found similar risk figures.

Age <60 years has been shown at increased risk and one study found <50 years of age to pose highest risk.[19] A meta-analysis evaluating five patient-related risk factors demonstrated a relative risk for PEP with suspected SOD of 4.09 (95% CI: 1.93–3.12, $p < 0.001$) and female gender of 2.23 (95% CI: 1.75–2.84; $p < 0.001$).[20]

Patients with suspected SOD are at highest risk for PEP.[21] This has been confirmed in many studies so whenever possible it will be good to adopt to alternative means or conservative management.

The EPISOD prospective study looked into the causes for the high incidence in this specific subset of patients and found that the sphincterotomy or the pancreatic ductal stenting did not affect the outcome so SOD on own as suspected diagnosis unfortunately presents a high risk.[22] When we do decide to perform the ERCP for patients with suspected SOD, we recommend procedure performed in the hands of an experienced endoscopist and all precautions still to be undertaken. Pancreatic ductal stenting should be achieved whenever possible and there is some evidence for reduction in PEP rates through injection of botulinum toxin into the residual pancreatic sphincter.[23]

Another high-risk group for PEP comprises patients who have history of recurrent acute pancreatitis and previous ERCP-induced pancreatitis.[14,18,20,24] Retrospective and prospective studies have confirmed higher rates of PEP in this subgroup so extreme vetting of patients and other protective measures should be exercised.

Normal bilirubin and normal caliber bile duct on cannulation in some studies have proven to increase risk of PEP but many of the patients with elective planned outpatient ERCP are not jaundiced and with cholestatic liver function. It would certainly prove to be difficult cannulation if there is normal caliber bile duct thereby increasing the PEP rates probably.

Proceduralist-related Risk Factors

In different hospitals, ERCPs are performed by gastroenterologists, surgeons or radiologists and in some tertiary centers, by advanced nurse endoscopists. It has been shown in some studies that risk of complications can be associated with lack of experience or suboptimal skill level of the proceduralist. But recent studies have found that proceduralist volume has not been statistically found to have direct association to PEP risk.[25] There have been lot of discussions about standard and validated accreditation policies to approve of endoscopists to perform ERCPs but there is no universal agreed minimum competency, quality requirement criteria to practice ERCPs independently in most countries.

Hospital ERCP volume has been thought to correlate to the rates of PEP and a large study showed more pancreatitis in centers performing <200 ERCP cases a year, though other studies have not confirmed similar figures.[26]

Having a trainee or fellow present in the endoscopy list has been revealed to increase risk of complications though again not confirmed in other studies.[24]

A good endoscopist carefully selects patients for ERCP and knows when to give up or refer to alternate means of management of the obstructed bile system. Many new therapeutic endoscopists are also skilled in endoscopic ultrasound (EUS) and many tertiary centers now have lower threshold to embark on EUS-guided bile duct intervention when a difficult papillary cannulation is anticipated or encountered. More data is emerging every day regarding good safety and effectiveness of EUS and avoiding ERCP-related PEP. A recent systemic review found PEP rates in patients with malignant biliary decompression achieved via ERCP versus EUS-guided techniques at 9.2% versus 0%, the difference being significant [risk ratio (RR) = 8.5; 95% CI: 1.03–69.91, $p = 0.05$].[27]

Procedure and Technique Factors

The less attempts at and shorter time taken for bile duct cannulation have been shown to help prevent PEP. The theory is to avoid much trauma to the papilla during cannulation that is the proposed cause for pancreatitis precipitated by chemical, hydrostatic, mechanical, enzymatic, and thermal factors.

Most centers throughout the world are now practicing the short-wire technique and though one study showed trend to shorter procedure time, fluoroscopy time, and time to cannulation[28] using short-wire compared to long-wire system, there have been no reports of different PEP rates between the two techniques.

Difficult bile duct cannulation is a well-recognized risk factor for PEP.[29] It has been quoted in studies as cannulation time involving more than 5–10 minutes and more than 6–15 attempts as "difficult"[30] and can be due to abnormal papillary, biliopancreatic duct or duodenal anatomy, position of papilla in duodenum, periampullary diverticulum, and operator skills.

Historically ERCP cannulas using contrast and guided through the duodenoscope were used to gain bile duct entry. But the method via sphincterotome with wire-guided technique and avoiding contrast-aided cannulation has proven to improve successful primary cannulation and decrease PEP. A large meta-analysis comprising 12 randomized controlled trials (RCTs) and 3,450 patients found significant reduction in rates of PEP [RR 0.51; 95% CI: 0.32–0.82) with greater primary cannulation success (RR 1.07; 95% CI: 1.00–1.15)[31] so in most practices, this technique has been adopted the first line approach.

In case of inadvertent pancreatic duct (PD) wire cannulation, normal practice is to retrieve the wire and aim at direction of bile duct but recurrent PD wire passes increase the chances of pancreatitis—more than five passes have been shown to increase this risk.[32]

With preferential PD access and inability to achieve bile duct entry, next steps are usually to trial different guidewires, perform precut biliary or small pancreatic sphincterotomy or trial double-wire technique.

There are angled and finer wires that have been used in this scenario and a large study on >700 patients showed no significant difference in rates of pancreatitis when used a 0.025-inch or 0.035-inch hydrophilic wire (7.8% vs. 9.3%, $p = 0.5$).[33]

Holding the wire in the PD and straightening the angle of the duct, biliary duct cannulation can sometimes be gained by introducing another guidewire through the scope and aiming higher using the PD wire as anchor. Successful bile duct access can be achieved using this technique [Double Guidewire Cannulation (DGC)] but there has been high rates of PEP reported using this method (18% vs. 4% without DGC, $p < 0.005$).[34]

At times of inadvertent PD wire cannulation, some endoscopists perform a small pancreatic sphincterotomy and then aim the sphincterotome higher into the opening to locate the bile duct entry for cannulation. This has been shown to affect PEP so ERCPists have to be aware to avoid large sphincterotomies involving the pancreatic duct.

Precut sphincterotomies are performed not uncommonly to aid bile duct access when there is difficult cannulation and mostly using a needle knife. Precuts ideally have to be done in expert hands as there is high chance for bleeding and previously thought to increase rates of PEP. But many recent studies and guidelines support early precut sphincterotomies as most of the PEP are presumed due to the multiple attempts of cannulation prior to the precut and the rates are especially lower in patients who have PD stents inserted following precut sphincterotomies.[35,36]

Sphincteroplasty or endoscopic bile duct balloon dilatation (EBDBD) performed to remove large biliary stones has been linked to PEP and there is conflicting evidence to support or refute this approach currently. The American and European guidelines differ in their recommendation.[5-7] Some evidence points to better outcomes when EBDBD follows a sphincterotomy or combined with pancreatic duct stenting.

Pancreatic duct stenting can prevent pancreatitis and studies support short and less caliber plastic stents—3, 4 or 5 Fr.[37] One of the strong recommendations from societies is to remove the stents in 2–3 weeks so a routine X-ray or endoscopy follow-up is advised.

There are also reports suggesting irritation from stents can lead to pancreatic ductal and parenchymal changes in more than 50% of patients. Chronic pancreatitis may develop as consequence of PD stenting.[38] In another study, acute pancreatitis occurred after prophylactic pancreatic stent (PPS) removal in 3% of cases, none of them severe.[39]

Medical Prophylaxis to Prevent PEP

Medications to prevent pancreatitis have gained lot of interest recently and there is increasing evidence that they help. These are drugs that decrease pancreatic inflammation, decrease sphincter of Oddi pressure, attenuate systemic inflammation, decrease pancreatic stimulation or interrupt the activity of proteases.[40]

Nonsteroidal anti-inflammatory drugs (NSAIDs) have been studied in concept of PEP prevention with very positive outcomes. The first randomized trial on 602 patients with high-risk for PEP received single dose of 100 mg rectal indomethacin or placebo immediately after ERCP. In this study, PD stenting was performed at the discretion of the endoscopist. PEP occurred in 9.2% of the indomethacin group versus 16.9% of the placebo group ($p < 0.01$). Furthermore, those receiving indomethacin were less likely to develop moderate-to-severe pancreatitis compared with those receiving placebo (4.4% vs. 8.8%; $p < 0.05$).[41] Diclofenac has also been shown in improvement of pancreatitis figures with number needing to treat patients ranging between 11 and 17. Rectal preparations before or after the procedure have been shown to be equally effective.[42] Initially suggested to consider rectal NSAIDs for high-risk patients, literature now supports administration of these agents to low-risk patients for PEP as well.[43]

Corticosteroids[44] and antibiotics[45] were trialed in peri-ERCP situations but did not correlate to improved PEP rates.

Somatostatin[46] and octreotide[47] are potential inhibitors of exocrine pancreatic secretion and evidence has been conflicting regarding their use in the setting of prevention of PEP. Andriulli et al. meta-analysis showed less postoperative hyperamylasemia but no prevention of PEP.

Sublingual and transdermal nitroglycerine were tried in view of their effect on reduction of pressure in the Sphincter of Oddi. Though initial studies showed some promise, recent data do not show statistical evidence for regular usage in ERCP.[48] More studies are needed.

Gabexate maleate has also been studied in ERCP.[46] It is a protease inhibitor and along with ulinastatin has been used previously for PEP prevention. But recent evidence not revealing any advantage in PEP prevention precludes routine usage.[49]

Interleukin 10 (IL-10) has been an interesting anti-inflammatory cytokine shown to decrease PEP in a single study but follow-up studies have not yielded such positive results.[50]

Intravenous Hydration

A pilot study of 62 patients that randomized patients to aggressive intravenous (IV) hydration with lactated Ringer's (LR) solution versus standard hydration demonstrated significant reduction in PEP (0% vs. 17%; $p < 0.05$). Patients in the aggressive hydration group received 3 mL/kg/h during the procedure, a 20 mL/kg bolus immediately after the procedure, and 3 mL/kg/h for 8 hours after the procedure.[51] This approach may certainly hold promise and further studies are needed to check on role of other electrolyte solutions or hydration status in perioperative patients.

Treatment

The discussion about treatment of PEP was not aim of this chapter. The management of PEP is same as therapy of any acute pancreatitis. The APACHE-II score has been validated and used extensively to assess patients with acute pancreatitis and recommends treatment targeted according to the severity.[52]

CONCLUSION

A popular survey published in the Frontline Gastroenterology in 2014 confirmed UK ERCPists not taking appropriate precautions. Less than 53% of practitioners use prophylactic pancreatic stenting or consider NSAIDs to protect against PEP.[53] Similar practice is noted in US as well with poor compliance with recommendation from societies to consider NSAIDs in perioperative period of ECP.[54]

Multiple risk factors have a synergistic effect and so increase risk of PEP further.[29] Endoscopists should use several approaches to mitigate the risk of PEP, including guidewire-assisted cannulation, pancreatic stent placement, and rectal NSAIDs use for high-risk patients. The exact role of aggressive hydration and combination therapies needs to be further investigated.[55] A table of evidence-based risk factors for PEP is summarized below. We hope that being aware of the common patient and technique risk factors and taking appropriate prevention or prophylaxis should help prevent some of the PEP thus avoiding morbidity and mortality.

Definitely contributes	Likely contributes	Can contributes
Suspected sphincter of Oddi dysfunction (SOD)	Pancreatic duct wire passage > once	Pancreatic sphincterotomy
Previous PEP	Minor papilla cannulation	Bile duct sphincteroplasty
Pancreatic duct dye injection	Female	Low annual ERCP hospital volume
Multiple cannulation attempts (>10 minutes)	<60 years of age	Trainee presence in endoscopy list
	Double guidewire cannulation	Less operator experience
	Normal bilirubin	
	Normal caliber bile duct	

REFERENCES

1. Thaker AM, Mosko JD, Berzin TM. Post-endoscopic retrograde cholangiopancreatography pancreatitis. Gastroenterol Rep (Oxf). 2015;3(1):32-40.
2. Peel AL, Hermon-Taylor J, Ritchie HD. Technique of transduodenal exploration of the common bile duct. Duodenoscopic appearances after biliary sphincterotomy. Ann R Coll Surg Engl. 1974;55(5):236-44.

3. Buxbaum JL, Fehmi A, Sultan S, Fishman DS, Qumseya BJ, Cortessis VK, et al. ASGE guideline on the role of endoscopy in the evaluation and management of choledocholithiasis. Gastrointest Endosc. 2019;89(6):1075-105.
4. Tenner S, Baillie J, DeWitt J, Vege SS; American College of Gastroenterology. American College of Gastroenterology Guideline: Management of acute pancreatitis. Am J Gastroenterol. 2013;108(9):1400-15.
5. ASGE Standards of Practice Committee, Chandrasekhara V, Khashab MA, Muthusamy VR, D Acosta R, Agrawal D, et al. Adverse events associated with ERCP. Gastrointest Endosc. 2017;85(1):32-47.
6. Dumonceau JM, Andriulli A, Deviere J, Mariani A, Rigaux J, Baron TH, et al. European Society of Gastrointestinal Endoscopy (ESGE) guideline: prophylaxis of post-ERCP pancreatitis. Endoscopy. 2010;42(6):503-15.
7. Dumonceau JM, Andriulli A, Elmunzer BJ, Mariani A, Meister T, Deviere J, et al. Prophylaxis of post-ERCP Pancreatitis: European Society of Gastrointestinal Endoscopy (ESGE) Guideline - Updated June 2014. Endoscopy. 2014;46(9):799-815.
8. Cotton PB, Lehman G, Vennes J, Geenen JE, Russell RC, Meyers WC, et al. Endoscopic sphincterotomy complications and their management: an attempt at consensus. Gastrointest Endosc. 1991;37(3):383-93.
9. Tadehara M, Okuwaki K, Imaizumi H, Kida M, Iwai T, Yamauchi H, et al. Usefulness of serum lipase for early diagnosis of post-endoscopic retrograde cholangiopancreatography pancreatitis. World J Gastrointest Endosc. 2019;11(9):477-90.
10. Banks PA, Bollen TL, Dervenis C, Gooszen HG, Johnson CD, Sarr MG, et al. Classification of acute pancreatitis—2012: revision of the Atlanta classification and definitions by international consensus. Gut. 2013;62(1):102-11.
11. Artifon EL, Chu A, Freeman M, Sakai P, Usmani A, Kumar A, et al. A comparison of the consensus and clinical definitions of pancreatitis with a proposal to redefine post-endoscopic retrograde cholangiopancreatography pancreatitis. Pancreas. 2010;39(4):530-5.
12. Dellinger EP, Forsmark CE, Layer P, Lévy P, Maraví-Poma E, Petrov MS, et al. Determinant-based classification of acute pancreatitis severity: an international multidisciplinary consultation. Ann Surg. 2012;256(6):875-80.
13. Gottlieb K, Sherman S. ERCP and biliary endoscopic sphincterotomy-induced pancreatitis. Gastrointest Endosc Clin N Am. 1998;8(1):87-114.
14. Andriulli A, Loperfido S, Napolitano G, Niro G, Valvano MR, Spirito F, et al. Incidence rates of post-ERCP complications: a systematic survey of prospective studies. Am J Gastroenterol. 2007;102(8):1781-8.
15. Banks PA, Freeman ML; Practice Parameters Committee of the American College of Gastroenterology. Practice guidelines in acute pancreatitis. Am J Gastroenterol. 2006;101(10):2379-400.
16. Mazen Jamal M, Yoon EJ, Saadi A, Y Sy T, Hashemzadeh M. Trends in the utilization of endoscopic retrograde cholangiopancreatography (ERCP) in the United States. Am J Gastroenterol. 2007;102(5):966-75.
17. Vihervaara H, Salminen P, Hurme S, Gullichsen R, Laine S, Grönroos JM, et al. Female gender and post-ERCP pancreatitis: is the association caused by difficult cannulation? Scand J Gastroenterol. 2011;46(12):1498-502.
18. Wang P, Li ZS, Liu F, Ren X, Lu N-H, Fan Z-N, et al. Risk factors for ERCP-related complications: a prospective multicenter study. Am J Gastroenterol. 2009;104(1):31-40.

19. Christoforidis E, Goulimaris I, Kanellos I, Tsalis k, Demetriades C, Betsis D, et al. Post-ERCP pancreatitis and hyperamylasemia: patient-related and operative risk factors. Endoscopy. 2002;34(4):286-92.
20. Masci E, Mariani A, Curioni S, Testoni PA. Risk factors for pancreatitis following endoscopic retrograde cholangiopancreatography: a meta-analysis. Endoscopy. 2003;35(10):830-4.
21. Cotton P, Garrow D, Gallagher J, Romagnuolo J. Risk factors for complications after ERCP: a multivariate analysis of 11,497 procedures over 12 years. Gastrointest Endosc. 2009;70(1):80-8.
22. Yaghoobi M, Pauls Q, Durkalski V, Romagnuolo J, Fogel EL, Tarnasky PR, et al. Incidence and predictors of post-ERCP pancreatitis in patients with suspected sphincter of Oddi dysfunction undergoing biliary or dual sphincterotomy: results from the EPISOD prospective multicenter randomized sham-controlled study. Endoscopy. 2015;47(10):884-90.
23. Gorelick A1, Barnett J, Chey W, Anderson M, Elta G. Botulinum toxin injection after biliary sphincterotomy. Endoscopy. 2004;36(2):170-3.
24. Cheng CL, Sherman S, Watkins JL, Barnett J, Freeman M, Geenen J, et al. Risk factors for post-ERCP pancreatitis: a prospective multicenter study. Am J Gastroenterol. 2006;101:139-47.
25. Testoni PA, Mariani A, Giussani A, Vailati C, Masci E, Macarri G, et al. Risk factors for post-ERCP pancreatitis in high- and low-volume centers and among expert and non-expert operators: a prospective multicenter study. Am J Gastroenterol. 2010;105(8):1753-61.
26. Loperfido S, Angelini G, Benedetti G, Chilovi F, Costan F, De Berardinis F, et al. Major early complications from diagnostic and therapeutic ERCP: a prospective multicenter study. Gastrointest Endosc. 1998;48(1):1-10.
27. Li DF, Zhou CH, Wang LS, Yao J, Zou DW. Is ERCP-BD or EUS-BD the preferred decompression modality for malignant distal biliary obstruction? A meta-analysis of randomized controlled trials. Rev Esp Enferm Dig. 2019;111(12):953-60.
28. Draganov P, Kowalzyk L, Fazel A, Moezardalan K, Pan JJ, Forsmark CE. Prospective randomized blinded comparison of a short wire ERCP system with traditional long wire devices. Dig Dis Sci. 2010;55(2):510-5.
29. Freeman ML, Guda NM. Prevention of post-ERCP pancreatitis: a comprehensive review. Gastrointest Endosc. 2004;59(7):845-64.
30. Halttunen J, Meisner S, Aabakken L, Arnelo U, Grönroos J, Hauge T, et al. Difficult cannulation as defined by a prospective study of the Scandinavian Association for Digestive Endoscopy (SADE) in 907 ERCPs. Scand J Gastroenterol. 2014;49(6):752-8.
31. Tse F, Yuan Y, Moayyedi P, Leontiadis GI. Guidewire-assisted cannulation of the common bile duct for the prevention of post-endoscopic retrograde cholangiopancreatography (ERCP) pancreatitis. Cochrane Database Syst Rev. 2012;12:CD009662.
32. Lee TH, Park do H, Park JY, Kim EO, Lee YS, Park JH, et al. Can wire-guided cannulation prevent post-ERCP pancreatitis? A prospective randomized trial. Gastrointest Endosc. 2009;69(3, pt 1):444-9.
33. Bassan MS, Sundaralingam P, Fanning SB, Lau J, Menon J, Ong E, et al. The impact of wire caliber on ERCP outcomes: a multicenter randomized controlled trial of 0.025-inch and 0.035-inch guidewires. Gastrointest Endosc. 2018;87(6):1454-60.

34. Krill JT, DaVee T, Edwards JS, Slaughter JC, Yachimski PS. Risk of postendoscopic retrograde cholangiopancreatography pancreatitis after double-guidewire biliary cannulation in an average-risk population. Pancreas. 2018;47(6):748-52.
35. Sundaralingam P, Masson P, Bourke MJ. Early precut sphincterotomy does not increase risk during endoscopic retrograde cholangiopancreatography in patients with difficult biliary access: a meta-analysis of randomized controlled trials. Clin Gastroenterol Hepatol. 2015;13(10)1722-9.
36. Bailey AA, Bourke MJ, Kaffes AJ, Byth K, Lee EY, Williams SJ. Needle-knife sphincterotomy: factors predicting its use and the relationship with post-ERCP pancreatitis (with video). Gastrointest Endosc. 2010;71(2):266-71.
37. Freeman ML. Pancreatic stents for prevention of postendoscopic retrograde cholangiopancreatography pancreatitis. Clin Gastroenterol Hepatol. 2007;5(11): 1354-65.
38. Sherman S, Hawes RH, Savides TJ, Gress FG, Ikenberry SO, Smith MT, et al. Stent-induced pancreatic ductal and parenchymal changes: correlation of endoscopic ultrasound with ERCP. Gastrointest Endosc. 1996;44(3):276-82.
39. Moffatt DC, Coté GA, Fogel EL, Watkins JL, McHenry L, Lehman GA, et al. Acute pancreatitis after removal of retained prophylactic pancreatic stents. Gastrointest Endosc. 2011;73(5):980-6.
40. Badalov N, Tenner S, Baillie J. The prevention, recognition and treatment of post-ERCP pancreatitis. JOP. 2009;10(2):88-97.
41. Elmunzer BJ, Scheiman JM, Lehman GA, Chak A, Mosler P, Higgins PDR, et al. A randomized trial of rectal indomethacin to prevent post-ERCP pancreatitis. N Engl J Med. 2012;366:1414-22.
42. Sethi S, Sethi N, Wadhwa V, Garud S, Brown A. A meta-analysis on the role of rectal diclofenac and indomethacin in the prevention of post-endoscopic retrograde cholangiopancreatography pancreatitis. Pancreas. 2014;43(2):190-7.
43. Thiruvengadam NR, Forde KA, Ma GK, Ahmad N, Chandrasekhara V, Ginsberg GG, et al. Rectal indomethacin reduces pancreatitis in high- and low-risk patients undergoing endoscopic retrograde cholangiopancreatography. Gastroenterology. 2016;151(2):288-97.
44. Wiener GR, Geenen JE, Hogan WJ, Catalano MF. Use of corticosteroids in the prevention of post-ERCP pancreatitis. Gastrointest Endosc. 1995;42(6):579-83.
45. Ishigaki T, Sasaki T, Serikawa M, Kobayashi K, Kamigaki M, Minami T, et al. Evaluation of antibiotic use to prevent post-ERCP pancreatitis and cholangitis. Hepatogastroenterology. 2015;62(138):417-24.
46. Andriulli A, Leandro G, Federici T, Ippolito A, Forlano R, Iacobellis A, et al. Prophylactic administration of somatostatin or gabexate does not prevent pancreatitis after ERCP: an updated meta-analysis. Gastrointest Endosc. 2007;65(4):624-32.
47. Andriulli A, Leandro G, Niro G, Mangia A, Festa V, Gambassi G, et al. Pharmacologic treatment can prevent pancreatic injury after ERCP: a meta-analysis. Gastrointest Endosc. 2000;51(1):1-7
48. Kaffes AJ, Bourke MJ, Ding S, Alrubaie A, Kwan V, Williams SJ. A prospective, randomized, placebo-controlled trial of transdermal glyceryl trinitrate in ERCP: effects on technical success and post-ERCP pancreatitis. Gastrointest Endosc. 2006;64(3):351-7.

49. Ueki T, Otani K, Kawamoto K, Shimizu A, Fujimura N, Sakaguchi S, et al. Comparison between ulinastatin and gabexate mesylate for the prevention of post-endoscopic retrograde cholangiopancreatography pancreatitis: a prospective, randomized trial. J Gastroenterol. 2007;42(2):161-7.
50. Devière J, Le Moine O, Van Laethem JL, Eisendrath P, Ghilain A, Severs N, et al. Interleukin 10 reduces the incidence of pancreatitis after therapeutic endoscopic retrograde cholangiopancreatography. Gastroenterology. 2001;120(2):498-505.
51. Buxbaum J, Yan A, Yeh K, Lane C, Nguyen N, Laine L. Aggressive hydration with lactated Ringer's solution reduces pancreatitis after endoscopic retrograde cholangiopancreatography. Clin Gastroenterol Hepatol. 2014;12:303-7.
52. Larvin M, McMahon MJ. APACHE-II score for assessment and monitoring of acute pancreatitis. Lancet. 1989;2(8656):201-5.
53. Hanna MS, Portal AJ, Dhanda AD, Przemioslo R, et al. UK wide survey on the prevention of post-ERCP pancreatitis. Frontline Gastroenterol. 2014;5(2):103-10.
54. Avila P, Holmes I, Kouanda A, Arain M, Dai SC, et al. Practice patterns of post-ERCP pancreatitis prophylaxis techniques in the United States: a survey of advanced endoscopists. Gastrointest Endosc. 2019.
55. Zhang H, Cho J, Buxbaum J. Update on the prevention of post-ERCP pancreatitis. Curr Treat Options Gastroenterol. 2018;16(4):428-40.

CHAPTER

11

Management of Nonalcoholic Fatty Liver Disease

Stephen Malnick, Ali Abdullah

INTRODUCTION

Nonalcoholic fatty liver disease (NAFLD) is the hepatic manifestation of the metabolic syndrome.[1] The metabolic syndrome is defined by the presence of three out of the following five criteria:[2]
1. Elevated waist circumference (population- and country-specific definitions)
2. Elevated serum triglycerides ≥ 150 mg/dL
3. Reduced high-density lipoprotein cholesterol (HDL-C) < 40 mg/dL in men and 50 mg/dL in women (or drug treatment for a reduced HDL)
4. Elevated blood pressure, systolic ≥ 130 and/or diastolic ≥ 85 mm Hg, or antihypertensive drug treatment in a patient with a history of hypertension
5. Elevated fasting serum glucose ≥ 100 mg/dL (or drug treatment of elevated glucose)

Concomitant with the epidemic of obesity, the prevalence of the metabolic syndrome is now >39% of adults in the United States.[3] More than 25% of adults worldwide have hepatic steatosis. Following effective measures for prevention of chronic hepatitis [hepatitis C virus (HCV)] and the development of direct-acting antivirals,[1] NAFLD has replaced HCV as the major problem for modern hepatology. NAFLD progresses from simple steatosis to steatohepatitis [nonalcoholic steatohepatitis (NASH)] and fibrosis. The consequences of NAFLD include progression to cirrhosis and its complications including liver failure and hepatocellular carcinoma.[1] The strongest predictor of mortality in prospective studies of NAFLD has been shown to be the stage of hepatic fibrosis.[4,5] Fibrosis can now be accurately assessed by noninvasive methods,[6] although liver biopsy is still the gold standard for diagnosing NASH and staging liver fibrosis.[7] There are some problems with the use of noninvasive score in those aged >65 years.[8]

Nonalcoholic fatty liver disease develops as a result of many factors including diet consisting of processed food and fructose, physical activity, genetic variation, adipokines, and body fat distribution.[9]

In this chapter, we will discuss the current state of treatment for NAFLD.

DIETARY CHANGES

The recommendations for the treatment of NASH include weight loss, limiting the consumption of fructose-enriched beverages, limiting the consumption of alcohol to less than one drink per day for women and two for men, and drinking more than two cups of coffee per day.[10] In addition, what kind of food or drink is consumed is important. Population studies such as the United States multiethnic cohort have found a connection between NAFLD and consumption of red meat, processed meat, poultry, and cholesterol.[11] In addition, ultraprocessed diets have been shown to cause excess caloric intake and weight gain.[12] Recently, it has been suggested by the NutriRECS (Nutritional Recommendations) consortium that adults can continue on their current consumption of meat, both processed and unprocessed.[13]

The importance of dietary treatment of disease was recognized early on. The Jewish Philosopher and physician Rambam (1138-1204) declared that "No disease that can be treated by diet should be treated with any other means."

Initially, the first trials examined the effect of very low-calorie diets which result in a large weight loss. There was no discussion, however, regarding the effect of the components of the diet, despite there being a decrease in steatosis. In patients with type 2 diabetes mellitus (DM), moderate weight reduction has been shown to improve hepatic insulin resistance and reverse hepatic steatosis. In addition, too rapid a weight loss has detrimental effects including hepatic inflammation and increased fibrosis.[14] It seems that a maximum weekly weight loss of 1.6 kg is necessary to avoid a histological deterioration.

The central component of diet as treatment of NAFLD is a fiber-rich diet that is low in complex carbohydrates and avoidance of fructose.[15] More recently, the Mediterranean diet has been suggested as treatment for both NAFLD and the metabolic syndrome.[16] The Mediterranean diet improves weight, waist circumference, hepatic fat accumulation, serum transaminases, lipid profile, and insulin resistance. The current recommendations for diet include reduction of body weight within 6 months of 5-7% in patients with NAFLD and of 7-10% in patients with NASH, rate of weight loss from 0.5-1 to >1.5 kg/week in severe obesity, and total calorie content of 1,200-1,500 kcal/day for women and 1,500-1,800 kcal/day for men.

Sacks et al.[17] assigned 811 overweight patients to four different diets with different amounts of energy derived from fat, protein, and carbohydrates. At 6 months, there was an average weight loss of 6 kg, but they began to regain weight after 12 months. The average weight loss among the 80% of participants who completed the trial was 4 kg, and there was an improvement in lipid-related risk factors and fasting insulin levels, regardless of which macronutrients were dominant.

The DASH (dietary approaches to stop hypertension) diet is a sodium-restricted diet rich in vegetables, fruits, whole grains, and low-fat dairy and low in saturated fats, cholesterol, refined grains, and sweets. A total of 60 NAFLD patients (diagnosed by elevated liver enzymes and steatosis on ultrasound) were treated for 8 weeks with either the DASH diet or the control diet and 350–7,000 kcal less than the calculated energy requirement. The patients in the DASH group had greater decreases in body mass index (BMI), insulin, alanine aminotransferase (ALT) levels, serum triglycerides, and total to HDL cholesterol ratio.[18] There was no assessment of fibrosis in this study.

There seems to be a protective effect of vitamins C and E on the development of NASH but no effect on fibrosis.[19]

In addition, rapid weight loss is usually not maintained in the long term—this is termed the yo-yo effect.[20] Thus, it is more beneficial to consider diet when combined with physical activity, which we will define as lifestyle changes.

LIFESTYLE CHANGES

The evidence for a beneficial effect of lifestyle changes on NAFLD has been summarized in a review from 2014.[21] Both aerobic and resistance training have been shown to reduce hepatic fat content.[22-24] A Cuban study of 293 patients with histologically proven NASH, who were in a 1-year program of lifestyle modification consisting of a low-fat hypocaloric diet that was 750 kcal/day less than their daily energy need and were encouraged to walk 200 min/week, showed a histological improvement on repeat liver biopsy. A total of 72 (25%) of the patients achieved resolution of steatohepatitis, 138 (47%) had a reduction in the NAFLD activity score (NAS), and 56 (19%) had fibrosis regression. Comparing those patients who lost >5% of their body weight to those who lost less found a larger number with NASH resolution and a 2-point reduction in NAS. For those patients who lost >10% of their body weight, 100% had reduction in the NAS, 90% had NASH resolution, and 45% had fibrosis regression.[22] Hallsworth et al. reported a small study of 19 sedentary adults with clinically defined NAFLD who were assigned to 8 weeks of resistance exercise (11 patients) and compared to 8 who continued on standard treatment. Resistance training was associated with a decrease in hepatic lipid as assessed by magnetic resonance spectroscopy. There was also an improvement in lipid oxidation, glucose control, and HOMA-IR (Homeostatic Model Assessment of Insulin Resistance). There was no effect on body weight, visceral adipose tissue, or body fat mass.[23]

The benefits of moderate to vigorous physical activity has been shown in a study of 169 obese middle-aged men in a 12-week program of weight reduction compared the effects of dietary restrictions and aerobic exercise. The exercise was divided into three groups: <150, 150–250, and >250 min/week. Those patients performing >250 min/week had lower levels of hepatic steatosis without detectable weight reduction. There was also a reduction in inflammation and oxidative stress levels and changes in fatty acid metabolism.[24]

Weight loss also improves the quality of life of patients with NAFLD regardless of biochemical improvement. For every 5-point decrease in the BMI, there is a 10% increase in the adjusted quality of life.[25] The patients without diabetes, active NASH, and advanced fibrosis were the most likely to improve, and this group is the majority of the NAFLD population.

Drinking coffee features as a core recommendation for the treatment of NAFLD.[10] Coffee consumption of more than four cups per day has been shown to be related to a decrease in progression of both cirrhotic and noncirrhotic NAFLD.[26] The data were derived from the United States multiethnic cohort including 2,786 cases of NAFLD. In addition, a study of >500,000 people from 10 European countries followed for a mean of 16.4 years found that consumption of more than four cups of coffee per day resulted in a highly significant decrease in mortality of 12% for men and 7% for women after adjusting for multiple variables.[27] A decrease in mortality in African Americans, Japanese Americans, Latinos, and Whites was also found in a study from the United States multiethnic cohort.[28] The recent consensus guidelines of the International Liver Transplantation Society emphasizes the central role of lifestyle changes.[29]

BARIATRIC SURGERY

Bariatric surgery has an established role in the management of severe obesity with >113,000 operations performed per year in the USA.[30] Bariatric surgery can reduce insulin resistance and even the resolution of type 2 DM.[31] The beneficial effects of bariatric surgery in NAFLD include an improvement of histological features of NAFLD such as steatosis and fibrosis.[32] In addition, gastric bypass surgery is associated with a long-term decrease in total mortality and mortality from diabetes, heart disease, and cancer.[33] The possibility of endoscopic procedures for weight loss has recently been shown by a study that showed endoscopic sleeve gastroplasty and low-intensity lifestyle change to be superior to high-intensity lifestyle change after 12 months of follow-up.[34]

MEDICAL THERAPY OF NONALCOHOLIC FATTY LIVER DISEASE

Since weight loss is an essential element of treating the metabolic syndrome and NAFLD, the pharmacological treatment of obesity may be of value for NAFLD. At present, there is little data published regarding weight loss medications for NAFLD.

Orlistat

Orlistat was approved by the Food and Drug Administration (FDA) in 1999 for treating long-term obesity. It is a reversible inhibitor of gastric and pancreatic lipases. It is an effective drug for weight loss with an average of 2–3 kg weight loss; it is associated with a high level of discontinuation due to its side effect profile of oily spotting, flatus with discharge, fecal urgency, and bloating. A study of 50 overweight (BMI ≥ 27 kg/m^2) subjects with NASH on biopsy, who were treated with a 1,400 kcal/day diet, 800 IU of vitamin E, and with or without orlistat 120 mg TID for 36 weeks and then rebiopsy, found that there was no enhancement of weight loss or improvement of liver enzymes, insulin resistance, or hepatic histopathology.[35] There was, however, improvement in insulin resistance and hepatic steatosis in those losing >5% of their body weight and an improvement in hepatic histopathology in those losing >9% of body weight.

Liraglutide

Liraglutide is a glucagon-like peptide-1 (GLP-1) analog and is FDA approved for the treatment of overweight and obese patients. Liraglutide stimulates gastrointestinal (GI) peptides which stimulate glucose-dependent insulin secretion and inhibit glucagon release and gastric emptying. A placebo-controlled phase II study of 26 patients with biopsy-proven NASH from four centers in the United Kingdom received 48 weeks of treatment of liraglutide 1.8 mg subcutaneous (SC) injection daily or placebo. Repeat liver biopsies were performed at 48 weeks. Only nine (23%) of the patients receiving liraglutide had resolution of the NASH versus two (9%) receiving placebo. In addition, only two (9%) of the patients receiving liraglutide had progression of the fibrosis compared to eight (36%) in the placebo group.[36]

Off-label Use of Approved Pharmacological Agents

One of the components of the metabolic syndrome is diabetes, and several antidiabetic medicines have been examined for possible benefit in NAFLD.

Metformin

Metformin is a first-line treatment of DM. It reduces hepatic gluconeogenesis and intestinal glucose absorption. In addition, it is linked to weight loss and decreases insulin resistance.[37] An open-label trial of 15 patients with histologically confirmed NAFLD received 20 mg/kg of metformin daily for a year. Although in the first 3 months of treatment there was a decrease in ALT and aspartate aminotransferase (AST) levels, this was not sustained at 1 year. Only 10 of the 15 patients had a repeat liver biopsy at 1 year, two (20%) had an improvement in the inflammation score, and one (10%) in the fibrosis score. Similar results were found in a placebo-controlled study of 48 patients for 6 months.[38] Another study from Turkey with 36 patients did not detect a histological improvement after 6 months of treatment with metformin.[39] A study of 19 patients randomized to lifestyle changes and metformin compared to lifestyle changes alone showed similar histology in both groups.[40] There may be a beneficial effect on all-cause mortality in diabetic patients with cirrhosis who continued metformin therapy.[41] In this study of 250 patients with diabetes and end-stage liver disease, the median survival of those continuing metformin therapy as compared to those who discontinued therapy was 11.8 years versus 5.6 years.

A recent report of the combination of N-acetylcysteine with or without ursodeoxycholic acid with metformin in an open-label study of 53 patients with biopsy-proven NASH showed no improvement in fibrosis but a decrease in the NAS score in the group receiving N-acetylcysteine and metformin.[42]

Thiazolidinediones

Thiazolidinediones activate peroxisome proliferator-activated receptor γ (PPAR-γ) in liver, muscle, and adipose tissues and increase insulin sensitivity mainly by stimulating adipocyte differentiation.[43] The resulting increase in adiponectin secretion and a decrease in free fatty acid (FFA) secretion from adipocytes are thought to be the mechanism for a beneficial effect in NAFLD. The improvement on insulin-mediated suppression of FFA precedes decrease in liver fat content.[44] The FLIRT (Fatty Liver Improvement with Rosiglitazone Therapy) trial included 63 patients with biopsy-proven NASH who were treated with either placebo or rosiglitazone 8 mg/day for 1 year. The patients receiving rosiglitazone had a four times higher rate of ALT normalization and improvement in insulin sensitivity as compared to the placebo group. These changes, however, resolved 4 months after stopping the treatment. There was no improvement in hepatic fibrosis. There was no additional benefit upon extending the study by 2 years in the FLIRT 2 trial.[45]

The PIVENS (Pioglitazone vs. Vitamin E vs. Placebo for the Treatment of Non-Diabetic Patients with Nonalcoholic Steatohepatitis) trial examined the effect of treatment with pioglitazone and vitamin E in biopsy-proven NASH patients without type 2 DM.[46] A total of 247 patients were divided into three groups—pioglitazone 30 mg/day, vitamin E 800 IU/day, or placebo for a total of 96 weeks. Both the pioglitazone and the vitamin E groups achieved a decrease in hepatic steatosis and lobular inflammation. A larger percentage of the pioglitazone patients had NASH resolution (47% vs. 21% in the placebo group, $p < 0.001$). There was, however, no significant improvement in fibrosis. A meta-analysis of eight RCTs (five with pioglitazone and three with rosiglitazone) including a total of 516 patients with biopsy-proven NASH followed-up from 6 to 24 months did find an improvement in fibrosis of any stage and also advanced fibrosis.[47] All these effects were due to pioglitazone use and were present even in patients without diabetes. There was no evidence on clinical outcomes, however.

The adverse effects of TZDs include fluid retention, weight gain, bone fractures, and an increase in cardiovascular events. Thus, it remains to be seen if these agents will be of long-term clinical benefit.

Glucagon-like Peptide-1 Receptor Agonists

These medications have been discussed above as agents for weight loss. The recent guidance statement of the AASLD (American Association for the Study of Liver Diseases) states, "it is premature to consider GLP1 agonists to specifically treat liver disease in patients with NAFLD or NASH."[7]

Dipeptidyl Peptidase-4 Inhibitors

These inhibitors block the dipeptidyl peptidase-4 (DPP4) enzyme which itself inactivates incretins including GLP1 and glucose-dependent insulinotropic polypeptide (GIP). This results in an increase in insulin secretion, lowers hepatic glucose output, and suppresses glucagon release.[48] The hepatic expression of DPP4 is higher in NAFLD patients compared to healthy controls, and DPP4 inhibitors have been investigated as treatment for NAFLD.[49] Sitagliptin is one of the earliest available DPP4 inhibitors. A single arm study of 12 patients with type 2 DM and NASH receiving 100 mg of sitagliptin versus placebo was carried out for 1 year. There were paired liver biopsies. There was a significant decrease in ballooning and NASH scores, BMI, and AST and ALT levels. There was no effect on reducing fibrosis.[50]

A 24-week, randomized placebo-controlled study of 50 patients with NAFLD as assessed by hepatic steatosis on magnetic resonance imaging (MRI)-proton density fat fraction was conducted. In addition, fibrosis was assessed by MR elastography and FIBROSpect II. There was no statistically significant improvement histologically in this study.[51] Another 24-week study of 12 patients with biopsy-proven NASH found no advantage to sitagliptin (100 mg) for either fibrosis or NAS.[52]

A 12-month, nonrandomized multicenter single-arm study of NAFLD patients identified by ultrasound with type 2 DM showed that alogliptin reduced NAFLD progression as assessed by the NAFIC score (a composite of NASH, ferritin, insulin, and type IV collagen 7S).[53] A 6-month randomized placebo-controlled double-blind trial of vildagliptin 50 mg BID in well-controlled [mean hemoglobin A1c (HbA1c) of 6.4 ± 0.1%] found a reduction of 27% in ultrasound-assessed liver triglyceride content and improvement in ALT levels.[54]

In summary, there is at present insufficient evidence to make firm recommendations for treating NAFLD with DPP4 inhibitors.

Sodium-glucose Cotransporter-2 Inhibitors

These medications inhibit glucose reabsorption in the kidney by blocking the sodium-glucose cotransporter (SGLT) channels in the proximal convoluted tubules. This results in glucosuria. Since their mechanism of action is independent of insulin, they are of value in patients with a limited pancreatic β-cell reserve. The increasingly important role of SGLT2 inhibitors in NAFLD treatment has recently been reviewed.[55]

The resulting glycosuria results in an energy loss, a suppression of insulin release, and an increase in pancreatic glucagon secretion. In addition, there appears to be a direct neurogenic effect that enhances hepatic gluconeogenesis lipolysis.

There are several SGLT2 inhibitors for patients with type 2 DM. *Canagliflozin* is the most commonly prescribed. An initial retrospective study from Japan of 24 patients with biopsy-proven NAFLD with type 2 DM compared treatment for 24 weeks of canagliflozin 100 mg/day or ipragliflozin 50 mg/day to sitagliptin 100 mg/day. There were similar reductions in serum transaminases, but the BMI and fasting plasma glucose decreased in the group receiving SGLT2 inhibitors.[56] A small, nonrandomized, open-label study of only five patients with biopsy-proven NAFLD who had type 2 DM from Japan examined the effect of canagliflozin 100 mg/day for 24 weeks. Along with a decrease in serum fasting glucose, gamma-glutamyl transferase (GGT), ferritin, and type IV collagen 7S, there was a decrease in waist circumference. In addition, there was a decrease in the NAS score in all the patients, two of whom had a decrease in fibrosis.[57]

A recent study of nine patients with type 2 DM receiving canagliflozin 100 mg OD for 24 weeks and assessed by comparing baseline liver biopsies to biopsies performed after 24 weeks of treatment found a histological improvement. Specifically, there was a decrease in the scores of steatosis by 78%, lobular inflammation by 33%, and ballooning by 22%. There was also a decrease in the fibrosis stage by 33%.[58] Another prospective open-label pilot study of 35 NAFLD patients treated with canagliflozin 100 mg OD for 6 months found significant reductions in AST, ALT, GGT, triglycerides HBA1c, and body weight. In addition, there was a significant decrease in the Fibrosis-4 (FIB-4) index.[59]

Ipragliflozin (50 mg OD) was examined in 21 Japanese patients with type 2 DM. After 16 weeks of treatment, there was a significant decrease in the fatty liver index (FLI) from 70.1 to 60.3 as well as a decrease in body weight, visceral adipose tissue, subcutaneous adipose tissue, and fat mass.[60] It appears that ipragliflozin may be superior to pioglitazone for treating NAFLD. An open-label RCT of 66 patients with type 2 DM and NAFLD received either ipragliflozin 50 mg OD or pioglitazone 15–30 mg OD for 24 weeks. The primary outcome was a change from baseline in the liver-to-spleen attenuation ratio (L/S ratio) assessed at 24 weeks. The L/S ratio was increased similarly in both groups, and the ALT, AST, HBA1c, and fasting glucose levels were similarly reduced. There was, however, significant reduction in body weight and visceral fat only in the ipragliflozin group.[61]

A comparison of ipragliflozin administered to 11 Japanese NAFLD patients with abnormal ALT levels who were already treated with GLP1 analogs or compared to 13 already treated with DPP4 inhibitors for 320 days and compared to 13 patients improved glycemic control and a reduction in body weight, normalization of ALT levels, and a reduction in the FIB-4 index.[62] A multicenter prospectively enrolled trial of 43 patients with type 2 DM and NAFLD (12 with biopsy-proven NASH and 31 diagnosed by ultrasound) showed significant decreases in AST, ALT, HBA1c, body weight, and steatosis.[63]

Dapagliflozin is a highly selective competitive inhibitor of SGLT2. In a randomized controlled open-label study of 57 patients with type 2 DM and NAFLD (diagnosed by ultrasound), the patients were treated with dapagliflozin 5 mg OD (33 patients) or standard treatment (24 patients) for 24 weeks. Hepatic steatosis and fibrosis were measured via transient elastography to determine controlled attenuation parameter (CAP) and liver stiffness, respectively. There was a significant decrease in CAP in the dapagliflozin group versus none in the control group receiving standard therapy. Liver stiffness measurements had a trend to decrease in the dapagliflozin group, and in 14 patients with more advanced fibrosis (≥8.0 kPa), there was a significant decrease in liver stiffness.[64]

In addition, there is a suggestion from experiments on mice that SGLT2 inhibitors may reduce the development of hepatocellular carcinoma.[55,65] In humans, there is evidence for a beneficial effect on cardiovascular morbidity and mortality.[66] Recently, there has been a report of a reduced risk of worsening heart failure or cardiovascular mortality in a phase III multicenter, placebo-controlled trial of 4,744 type 2 diabetics with an ejection fraction <40%.[67] There seems to be some association with euglycemic diabetic ketoacidosis with this class of agents,[68] and thus caution is necessary before recommending widespread use, especially in nondiabetic patients.

Statins

Statins are used extensively for both primary and secondary treatment of cardiovascular diseases. Data from more than 11,000 patients on clinical follow-up after completion of trials have found a beneficial effect for atorvastatin improve both hepatic histology and cardiovascular events in NAFLD and NASH patients and rosuvastatin in NASH patients.[69] It seems that these medications are as safe in NAFLD patients as in the general population. Recently, a protective effect of statins on the development of hepatocellular carcinoma in NAFLD patients has been reported.[70]

Emerging Therapies for Nonalcoholic Fatty Liver Disease

There is a massive investment of resources in trying to develop pharmacological therapies for NAFLD.

Obeticholic acid, elafibranor, selonsertib, and cenicriviroc are now in phase III trials.

Obeticholic Acid

Lipophilic bile acids have been shown to bind to the farnesoid X nuclear receptor, decreasing hepatic gluconeogenesis and increasing insulin sensitivity.[71] In a multicenter, double-blind placebo-controlled trial of patients with biopsy-proven noncirrhotic NASH, the patients were treated with obeticholic acid 25 mg OD for 72 weeks. The end-point was a decrease in NAS of at least 2 points without a worsening of fibrosis. About 45% of the 110 patients receiving obeticholic acid had an improvement in hepatic histology after 72 weeks of treatment compared to 21% of 109 patients in the control group. There was, however, a high incidence of pruritus related to treatment (23% in those receiving obeticholic acid vs. 6% in the control group). In addition, there was an increase in total serum cholesterol and low-density lipoprotein (LDL) cholesterol, together with a decrease in HDL-C.[72] There were three cases of serious cardiovascular events in the obeticholic acid group compared to the placebo group, but this did not reach statistical significance.

Elafibranor

Elafibranor is a PPARα/δ dual agonist. PPARα lessens steatosis and inflammation, and PPARδ can lessen hepatic fibrosis.[73] A study of 93 patients with noncirrhotic NASH treated with elafibranor 80 mg OD compared to 91 patients with elafibranor 120 mg OD and 92 patients with placebo for 52 weeks in a multicenter randomized double placebo-controlled trial found that those receiving 120 mg/day had NASH resolution with no fibrosis worsening. Those patients with NASH resolution had reduced liver fibrosis stages.[74] There is currently an ongoing phase III trial that is examining the effect of 120 mg of elafibranor on NASH patients with NAS ≥ 4 and stage 2/3 fibrosis (RESOLVE-IT study, NTC 02704403).

Selonsertib

Selonsertib is an apoptosis signal-regulating kinase 1 (ASK1) inhibitor. ASK1 is activated by hyperglycemia, among other agents, to induce apoptosis and fibrosis via P38 and JNK (c-Jun N-terminal kinases). An upregulation of ASK1 JNK-1 increases insulin resistance, steatosis, and inflammation.[75] In a phase II trial, selonsertib was shown to improve NASH activity and fibrosis.[75] There are ongoing phase III trials for stage 3 fibrotics (STELLAR 3) and cirrhotic (STELLAR 4) NASH patients.

Cenicriviroc

Cenicriviroc is a C-C motif chemokine receptor (CCR) 2/5 antagonist. A phase IIb randomized controlled multicenter of patients with a NAS > 4 and liver fibrosis stages 1–3 has been reported. 289 patients were in the study and received either cenicriviroc 150 mg OD or placebo for 1 year. There was no improvement in the NAS, and resolution of steatohepatitis was similar in both groups (16% cenicriviroc vs. 19% placebo). There was no worsening of fibrosis in 20% of the cenicriviroc versus 10% in the control group ($p = 0.02$). In some of the patients there was an improvement in the fibrosis stage, which the authors state as being "paradigm-shifting" in that fibrosis can be improved without improving the metabolic abnormality.[76]

The treatments available for NAFLD are summarized in **Table 1**.

There are many investigational agents and they are summarized in **Table 2**. In a search on the *clinicaltrials.gov* site of the National Institutes of Health (NIH) database of clinical trials for NAFLD, there are a total of 111 completed interventional studies in phase 2, 3, or 4 on patients aged 18 years and over. In addition, there are 66 studies that are active and recruiting or not yet recruiting.

Microbiome Manipulation

The central role of the intestinal microbiome in the pathogenesis of NAFLD is slowly becoming apparent.[77] There has been an attempt to transplant feces from lean donors to overweight patients. A report of nine male patients receiving donor stool via a duodenal tube found an improvement in insulin sensitivity and an increase in butyrate-producing intestinal microbiota.[78] In order to preserve this effect in mice, repeated donor transfusions were performed. The availability of fecal capsules that are easily swallowed enables repeat stool transplants in human studies to be performed more easily. In an unpublished study of stool transplantation from lean donors to 10 obese patients undergoing screening colonoscopy, there was found a slower increase in weight loss after 1 year, but the study was limited by a large number of patients who dropped out of the trial (Malnick, Abdullah, Melzer, unpublished observations).

WHERE DO WE GO FROM HERE?

Nonalcoholic fatty liver disease is a huge public health issue. There needs to be a major investment in prevention by emphasizing the need for lifestyle

Table 1: Treatments available for NAFLD.

Treatment	Advantages	Disadvantages
Lifestyle changes—energy restriction, body weight reduction, physical activity, change in diet composition	Cheap, universally available, effective for prevention, fibrosis regression, endorsed by professional guidelines	High relapse rate
Coffee	Cheap, available, decreases overall mortality in both genders and multiple ethnic groups, endorsed by some authorities	
Aspirin	Daily use decreases rate of fibrosis progression over 10 years, cheap, available, many patients already receiving for comorbidities	Uncertain use in primary prevention, GI bleeding
Metformin	Consider use in nondiabetic NASH on biopsy	Not beneficial, not recommended by most professional organizations
Vitamin E	Consider use in nondiabetic	Not beneficial, not recommended by most professional organizations Increased risk of prostate cancer after 3 years
PPARγ agonists	Resolution of NASH	Did not improve fibrosis, weight gain is a side effect
Elafibranor (PPARα/δ agonist)	Resolution of fibrosis in patients with NASH	Not endorsed
Obeticholic acid	Improvement in fibrosis (EASL Meeting 2019)	Increase in cholesterol, pruritus, not endorsed by professional bodies
Liraglutide (GLP-1 receptor agonists)	Decreased progression, fibrosis and improvement of NASH, weight loss	Premature to recommend High rate of GI side effects
Selonsertib	Improves NASH and fibrosis	Ongoing phase III Not endorsed
Cenicriviroc	Improvement in fibrosis	Phase IIb study reported
Statins	Improve liver histology Decrease cardiovascular events	Not endorsed

(EASL: European Association for the Study of the Liver; GI: gastrointestinal; GLP-1: glucagon-like peptide-1; NAFLD: nonalcoholic fatty liver disease; NASH: nonalcoholic steatohepatitis; PPAR: peroxisome proliferator-activated receptor)

Table 2: Phase 2, 3 and 4 trials of pharmacological treatment of NAFLD.

Title	Medication	Primary endpoint	Enroll-ment	Period of study	Dates	Phase	Status
The Effect of NS-0200 versus Placebo on Hepatic Fat Content in Patients with Nonalcoholic Fatty Liver Disease (NAFLD)	Leu-Met-Sil 0.5 Leu-Met-Sil 1.0 Placebo	Change in hepatic fat and laboratory tests	91	112 days	09.2015–05.2018	Phase 2	Completed
Study to Assess the Efficacy, Safety and Tolerability of LCQ908 in NAFLD Patients	Placebo Pradigastat (LCQ908) 5 mg/10mg Pradigastat (LCQ908) 10 mg/20mg	Change in percentage of fat in the liver	52	24 weeks	03.2013–02.2016	Phase 2	Completed
A Study of IDN-6556 in Subjects with NAFLD and Raised Transaminases	IDN-6556 Placebo	Change in laboratory tests	38	28 days	03.2014–03.2015	Phase 2	Completed
6-week Safety and PD Study in Adults with NAFLD	Placebo PF-06835919 low dose 75 mg PF-06835919 high dose 300 mg	Percent change in whole liver fat	53	6 weeks	27.9.2017–27.4.2018	Phase 2	Completed
Sitagliptin versus Placebo in the Treatment of Non alcoholic Fatty Liver Disease	Placebo Sitagliptin 100 mg	Percentage change in liver fat	50	24 weeks	01.2014–01.2016	Phase 2	Completed
Adding Exenatide to Insulin Therapy for Patients with Type 2 Diabetes and Non Alcoholic Fatty Liver Disease	Exenatide	Hepatic steatosis	24	6 months	01.2008–12.2009	Phase 4	Completed

Contd...

Title	Medication	Primary endpoint	Enroll-ment	Period of study	Dates	Phase	Status
Prevalence of Non alcoholic Fatty Liver Disease (NAFLD) in Hispanics with Type 2 Diabetes Mellitus (T2DM) and Role of Treatment (VA NASH)	Pioglitazone-placebo Pioglitazone Dietary supplement: Vitamin E Vitamin E-placebo	Liver histology	105	18 months	06.2010–12.2016	Phase 4	Completed
Study to Investigate the Effects of Different Doses of S-adenosyl-L-methionine (SAMe) in Subjects with Nonalcoholic Fatty Liver Disease and Non-treated Matched Healthy Volunteers as Control Group (EXPO)	SAMe 1000 mg, 1,500 mg, 2,000 mg	Methionine elimination half-life measured in blood	108	7 weeks	12.2012–09.2014	Phase 3	Completed
Farnesoid X Receptor (FXR) Ligand Obeticholic Acid in NASH Treatment (FLINT) Trial	Obeticholic acid Placebo	Hepatic histological improvement in nonalcoholic fatty liver disease (NAFLD) Activity Score (NAS)	283	72 week	03.2011–09.2014	Phase 2	Completed
University of Texas H.S.C. San Antonio Pioglitazone in Nonalcoholic Steatohepatitis Trial (UTHSCSA NASH Trial)	Pioglitazone study drug Placebo Pioglitazone Open Label	Liver histology	176	18 months	12.2008–12.2014	Phase 4	Completed

Contd...

Title	Medication	Primary endpoint	Enroll-ment	Period of study	Dates	Phase	Status
A Double-blind Randomized Placebo-controlled Study Comparing Epanova and Fenofibrate on Liver Fat in Overweight Subjects	Placebo Omega-3 carboxylic acid Fenofibrate 200 mg	Geometric mean ratio of % liver fat as assessed by MRI	78	12 weeks	09.2015–05.2016	Phase 2	Completed
Role of Exenatide in NASH-a Pilot Study (NAFLD)	Exenatide	Liver histology	8	28 weeks	08.2006–08.2010	Phase 2-3	Completed
Clinical Protocol to Investigate the Efficacy of Recombinant Human Leptin (Metreleptin) in Nonalcoholic Steatohepatitis (NASH) or Nonalcoholic Fatty Liver Disease (NAFLD) Associated with Lipodystrophy	Metreleptin	Liver histopathology	23	1 year	10.2012–07.2016	Phase 2	Completed
Evaluating the Safety, Tolerability, and Efficacy of GS-9674 in Participants with Nonalcoholic Steatohepatitis	GS-9674 Placebo to match GS-9674	Percentage of participants experiencing treatment-emergent adverse events	140	24 weeks	10.2016–01.2018	Phase 2	Completed
Pentoxifylline in Patients with Nonalcoholic Steatohepatitis	Pentoxifylline Placebo	Histological improvement	55	1 year	12.2006–12.2010	Phase 2	Completed
Double-Blind, Placebo-controlled Study of Two Doses of EPA-E in Patients with Nonalcoholic Steatohepatitis (NASH)	Placebo capsule EPA-E 300 mg capsule	Histological response	243	1 year	01.2010–10.2012	Phase 2	Completed

Contd...

Contd...

Title	Medication	Primary endpoint	Enrollment	Period of study	Dates	Phase	Status
Pentoxifylline/Nonalcoholic Steatohepatitis (NASH) Study: The Effect of Pentoxifylline on NASH	Pentoxifylline Placebo	Change in laboratory tests	26	12 months	05.2005–09.2009	Phase 2 Phase 3	Completed
JKB-121 for the Treatment of Nonalcoholic Steatohepatitis	JKB-121: 5 mg twice daily JKB-121: 10 mg twice daily Placebo	Analysis of MRI-PDFF change	65	24 weeks	08.2015–09.2017	Phase 2	Completed
Safety, Tolerability, and Efficacy of GS-4997 Alone or in Combination with Simtuzumab (SIM) in Adults with Nonalcoholic Steatohepatitis and Fibrosis Stages F2–F3	SEL SIM - Simtuzumab	Experienced treatment-emergent adverse events	72	28 weeks	01.2015–10.2016	Phase 2	Completed
Ezetimibe versus Placebo in the Treatment of Nonalcoholic Steatohepatitis	Ezetimibe	Change in liver fat as measured by MRI-PDFF	50	24 weeks	01.2013–09.2014	Phase 2	Completed
Phase II Trial of Silymarin for Non-Cirrhotic Patients with Nonalcoholic Steatohepatitis (SyNCH)	Placebo Silymarin 700 mg Silymarin 420 mg	Efficacy - improvement by at least 2 points in histology (NAS)	78	50 weeks	04.2008–11.2012	Phase 2	Completed
Recombinant Leptin Therapy for Treatment of Nonalcoholic Steatohepatitis	Metreleptin	Nonalcoholic steatohepatitis score as determined by liver histopathology	9	1 year	02.2006–03.2009	Phase 2	Completed

Contd...

Title	Medication	Primary endpoint	Enroll-ment	Period of study	Dates	Phase	Status
Efficacy and Safety Study of Cenicriviroc for the Treatment of Nonalcoholic Steatohepatitis in Adult Participants with Liver Fibrosis (CENTAUR)	Cenicriviroc Placebo	Histological improvement	289	1 year	09.2014–01.2017	Phase 2	Completed
Pioglitazone vs Vitamin E vs Placebo for Treatment of Non-diabetic Patients with Nonalcoholic Steatohepatitis (PIVENS)	Pioglitazone Dietary Supplement: Vitamin E Matching placebo	Number of participants with improvement in non-alcoholic fatty liver disease (NAFLD) activity	247	96 weeks	01.2005–06.2009	Phase 3	Completed
Treating Nonalcoholic Steatohepatitis with Metformin	Metformin	Change in the histological NASH Activity Index and laboratory tests	28	48 weeks	06.2003–03.2008	Phase 2	Completed
Treating Nonalcoholic Steatohepatitis With Pioglitazone	Actos (Pioglitazone)	Number of patients with improvement in liver histology	18	3 years	06.2003–02.2009	Phase 2	Completed
A Preliminary Study to Evaluate Cysteamine Therapy in Human Subjects With Nonalcoholic Steatohepatitis	Cysteamine	Normalization or >50% of serum ALT levels	13	6 months	10.2008–01.2010	Phase 1 Phase 2	Completed
Polyunsaturated Fatty Acids (PUFA) in Diabetic Fatty Liver	Polyunsaturated fatty acid (Opti- EPA) Placebo	Number of participants with improvement of ≥2 points in NAFLD Activity Score (NAS)	37	48 weeks	04.2006–12.2011	Phase 2	Completed

Contd...

Title	Medication	Primary endpoint	Enrollment	Period of study	Dates	Phase	Status
Ezetimibe-Ursodiol Combination Therapy on Biomarkers of Liver Function and Sterol Balance in Subjects with NAFLD	EZ-Urso combination therapy	Reduction in serum alanine transaminase (ALT), increase in plasma lathosterol, and reduction in hepatic fat fraction	2(12)	6 months	09.2014 to Failure to recruit	Phase 2	Terminated
Metformin for the Treatment of Nonalcoholic Fatty Liver Disease	Glucophage (Metformin) Placebo	Measurements of insulin sensitivity, hepatic insulin clearance, and altered parameters of lipid metabolism, changes in the histological features that define NAFLD, and quantitative measurements of visceral and peripheral fat increase in plasma lathosterol	11(66)	24 months	04.2009	Phase 4	Terminated
Fatty Liver Study in Patients With Type II Diabetes Mellitus	DPP4 inhibitor Pioglitazone Lantus insulin	Change in hepatic lipid content	5 (75)	6 months	02.2015	Phase 4	Terminated
Effects of Exenatide on Liver Biochemistry, Liver Histology and Lipid Metabolism in Patients with Fatty Liver Disease	Exenatide	Reduction in serum ALT from baseline and changes in components of liver histology	1 (20)	24 weeks	10.2007	Phase 2	Terminated

Contd...

Contd...

Title	Medication	Primary endpoint	Enrollment	Period of study	Dates	Phase	Status
Safety and Efficacy of Roflumilast and Pioglitazone in Treating Adults With Nonalcoholic Steatohepatitis	Roflumilast Pioglitazone Placebo	Percent change in serum ALT, serum AST and change in liver fat content	20 (75)	4 months	06.2013	Phase 2	Terminated
Fish Oil and Diet for the Treatment of Nonalcoholic Steatohepatitis (NASH)	Omega-3-acid ethyl esters (Lovaza) Placebo	Omega-3 fatty acid supplementation and its effect on hepatic steatosis and other factors associated with the development of nonalcoholic steatohepatitis	12 (24)	24 weeks	3.2006	Phase 2	Terminated
Safety and Efficacy of Simtuzumab (SIM, GS-6624) in Adults With Advanced Liver Fibrosis but not Cirrhosis Secondary to Nonalcoholic Steatohepatitis	Placebo Biological: SIM	Change from baseline in morphometric quantitative collagen (MQC) on liver biopsy	222 (225)	96 weeks	12.2012–12.2016	Phase 2	Terminated
Simtuzumab (SIM, GS-6624) in the Treatment of Cirrhosis due to NASH	Placebo Biological: SIM	Change from baseline in hepatic venous pressure gradient (HVPG)	259 (225)	96 weeks	10.2012–01.2017	Phase 2	Terminated

changes including dietary change and exercise at an early age. At present, there is an epidemic of both pediatric obesity and NAFLD. As physicians, we need to remind ourselves that the aim of medical treatment is to increase both the quality and the quantity of the patient's life. In most of the studies reported above, cardiovascular mortality is the major cause of death of the NAFLD patients. It has been suggested that histological endpoints are the best predictors of clinical outcome.[79] Most of the chronic liver disease patients die from complications of cirrhosis. The situation is not so clear regarding NAFLD. In the study by Ekstedt et al.,[4] there was no data available regarding the metabolic syndrome, smoking, and medications. One-third of the patients in Sweden are overweight, and thus it is likely that many patients in the control group had NAFLD. Furthermore, the risk for overall mortality was not observed when diabetic patients were excluded. The study by Angulo et al.[5] found advanced fibrosis to be the only histologic feature associated with the end-point of death and liver-related complications. Again, the majority of the end-points were from cardiovascular complications (38.3%). Furthermore, as distinct from cirrhosis, stage 1, 2, or 3 fibrosis does not cause a patient's death. The patient will not realize a major benefit to treatment of disease if there is a major cardiovascular event while enjoying the benefit of a decrease in the stage of fibrosis **(Fig. 1)**.

It also needs to be emphasized that the majority of patients diagnosed with NAFLD do not have advanced fibrosis. A multicenter study from Europe of more than 136,000 NAFLD patients found only 4.7% with advanced FIB-4 scores.[80] It is therefore likely that pharmacological therapy will not be appropriate for the vast majority of patients with the disease.

The most impressive medication in reducing the progression of fibrosis has recently been published. A prospective cohort study of 361 adults with biopsy-proven NAFLD were followed up every 3–12 months from 2006 to 2015, and advanced fibrosis was checked for by either the FIB-4 score, the

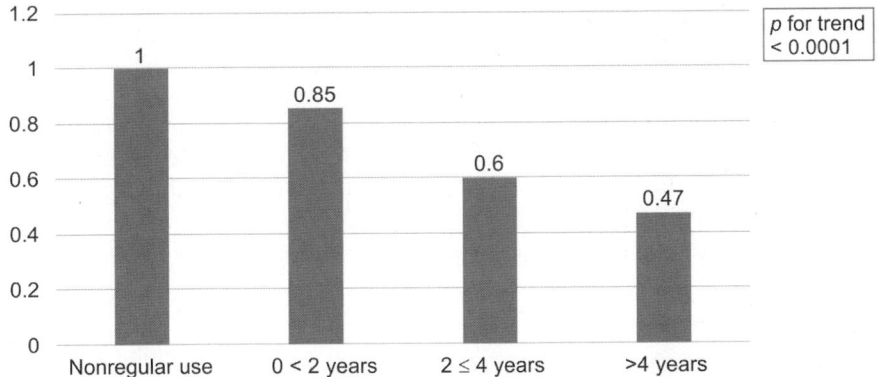

Fig. 1: Hazard ratio for risk of developing advanced fibrosis among patients with nonalcoholic fatty liver disease (NAFLD) fibrosis stage 0–2 at enrollment stratified by duration of daily aspirin use.[81]

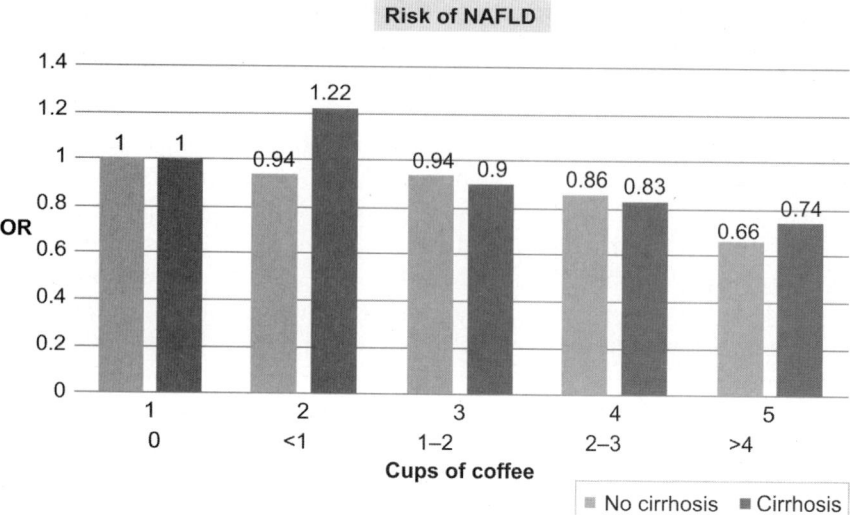

Fig. 2: Effect of coffee consumption on risk of developing NAFLD.[26] (NAFLD: nonalcoholic fatty liver disease; OR: odds ratio)

NAFLD fibrosis score, or the APRI (AST to Platelet Ratio Index) ratio.[81] Daily aspirin use resulted in a 37% reduction in the risk for developing advanced fibrosis. This finding may impact the recently revised guidelines regarding the nonrecommendation of aspirin for primary prevention of cardiovascular disease.[82]

In addition to aspirin, coffee consumption has been shown to decrease the progression of fibrosis.[26] Furthermore, coffee consumption has been linked to an overall decrease in mortality,[27,28] and consumption of soft drink consumption has been linked with an increase in mortality **(Fig. 2)**.[83]

The evaluation of the effect of medication is complicated by the finding of a placebo effect of pharmacotherapy in NAFLD trials with significant histological, radiological, and biochemical responses.[84]

In our opinion, there is a need for a robust comparison of the placebo arm in trials of pharmacological agents for treatment of NAFLD. This will need to include lifestyle changes with supervised diet, physical activity, consumption of four cups of coffee per day, avoidance of soft drinks, and consumption of aspirin daily. The effect of trials of pharmacotherapy needs to be compared to the best available alternative. Furthermore, the major issue facing hepatology today is how to avoid the development of NAFLD and the other complications of obesity and for this lifestyle changes are the only viable option.

REFERENCES

1. Sanyal AJ. Past, present and future perspectives in nonalcoholic fatty liver disease. Nature Rev Gastroenterol Hepatol. 2019;16(6):377-86.
2. Alberti KG, Eckel RH, Grundy SM, Zimmet PZ, Cleeman JI, Donato KA, et al. Harmonizing the metabolic syndrome: a joint interim statement of the international

diabetes federation task force on epidemiology and prevention; National heart, lung, and blood institute; American heart association; World heart federation; International. Circulation. 2009;120:1640-5.

3. Ford ES. Prevalence of the metabolic syndrome defined by the International Diabetes Federation among adults in the U.S. Diabetes Care. 2005;28:2745-9.

4. Ekstedt M, Hagström H, Nasr P, Fredrikson M, Stål P, Kechagias S, et al. Fibrosis stage is the strongest predictor for disease-specific mortality in NAFLD after up to 33 years of follow-up. Hepatology. 2015;61:1547-54.

5. Angulo P, Kleiner DE, Dam-Larsen S, Adams LA, Bjornsson ES, Charatcharoenwitthaya P, et al. Liver fibrosis, but no other histologic features, is associated with long-term outcomes of patients with nonalcoholic fatty liver disease. Gastroenterology. 2015;149:389-97.

6. Leoni S, Tovoli F, Napoli L, Serio I, Ferri S, Bolondi L, et al. Current guidelines for the management of non-alcoholic fatty liver disease: a systematic review with comparative analysis. World J Gastroenterol. 2018;24:3361-73.

7. Chalasani N, Younossi Z, Lavine JE, Charlton M, Cusi K, Rinella M, et al. The diagnosis and management of nonalcoholic fatty liver disease: practice guidance from the American Association for the Study of Liver Diseases. Hepatology. 2018;67:328-57.

8. McPherson S, Hardy T, Dufour JF, Petta S, Romero-Gomez M, Allison M, et al. Age as a confounding factor for the accurate non-invasive diagnosis of advanced NAFLD fibrosis. Am J Gastroenterol. 2017;112:740-51.

9. De Nooijer A, Vreugdenhil A, Karnebeek K, van Hasselt PM, Fuchs SA. A narrative review of factors associated with the development and progression if non-alcoholic fatty liver disease. Gastro Hep. 2019;1(4)180-91.

10. Diehl AM. Cause pathogenesis and treatment of nonalcoholic steatohepatitis. N Engl J Med. 2017;337:2063-72.

11. Noureddin M, Zelber-Sagi S, Wilkens LR, et al. Diet associations with nonalcoholic fatty liver disease in an ethnically diverse population: the multiethnic cohort. Hepatology. 2020;71(6):1940-52. doi: 10.1002/hep.30967.

12. Hall KD, Ayuketah A, Brychta R, Cai H, Cassimatis T, Chen KY, et al. Ultra-processed diets cause excess calorie intake and weight gain: an inpatient randomized controlled trial of Ad libitum food intake. Cell Metab. 2019; 30(1):67-77.e3.

13. Johnston BC, Zeraatkar D, Han MA, Vernooij RWM, Valli C, El Dib R, et al. Unprocessed red meat and processed meat consumption: dietary guideline recommendations From the NutriRECS Consortium; 2019. doi:10.7326/M19-1621.

14. Andersen T, Gluud C, Franzmann MB, Christoffersen P. Hepatic effects of dietary weight toss in morbidly obese subjects. J Hepatol. 1991;12:224-9.

15. Asrih M, Jornayvaz FR. Diets and nonalcoholic fatty liver disease: the good and the bad. Clin Nutr. 2014;33:186-90.

16. Abenavoli L, Boccuto L, Federico A, Dallio M, Loguercio C, Di Renzo L, et al. Diet and non-alcoholic fatty liver disease: the Mediterranean way. Int J Environ Res Public Health. 2019;16:3011.

17. Sacks FM, Bray GA, Carey VJ, Smith SR, Ryan DH, Anton SD, et al. Comparison of weight-loss diets with different compositions of fat, protein, and carbohydrates. N Engl J Med. 2009;360:859-73.

18. Razavi ZM, Telkabadi MH, Bahmani F, Salehi B, Farshbaf S, Asemi Z, et al. The effects of DASH diet on weight loss and metabolic status in adults with non-alcoholic fatty liver disease: A randomized clinical trial. Liver Int. 2026;36:563-71.
19. Ivancovsky-Wajcman D, Fliss-Isakov N, Salomone F, Webb M, Shibolet O, Kariv R, et al. Dietary vitamin E and C intake is inversely associated with the severity of nonalcoholic fatty liver disease. Dig Liver Dis. 2019;51(12):1698-705.
20. Force NT. Weight cycling definitions. JAMA. 1994;272:1196-202.
21. Nseir W, Hellou E, Assy N. Role of diet and lifestyle changes in nonalcoholic fatty liver disease. World J Gastroenterol. 2014;20:9338-44.
22. Vilar-Gomez E, Martinez-Perez Y, Calzadilla-Bertot L, Torres-Gonzalez A, Gra-Oramas B, Gonzalez-Fabian L, et al. Weight loss through lifestyle modification significantly reduces features of nonalcoholic steatohepatitis. Gastroenterology. 2015;149: 367-78.e5.
23. Hallsworth K, Fattakhova G, Hollingsworth KG, Thoma C, Moore S, Taylor R, et al. Resistance exercise reduces liver fat and its mediators in non-alcoholic fatty liver disease independent of weight loss. Gut. 2011;60:1278-83.
24. Oh S, Shida T, Yamagishi K, Tanaka K, So R, Tsujimoto T, et al. Moderate to vigorous physical activity volume is an important factor for managing nonalcoholic fatty liver disease: a retrospective study. Hepatology. 2015;61:1205-15.
25. Tapper EB, Lai M. Weight loss results in significant improvements in quality of life for patients with nonalcoholic fatty liver disease: a prospective cohort study. Hepatology. 2016;63:1184-9.
26. Setiawan VW, Porcel J, Wei P, Stram DO, Noureddin N, Lu SC, et al. Coffee drinking and alcoholic and nonalcoholic fatty liver diseases and viral hepatitis in the multiethnic cohort. Clin Gastroenterol Hepatol. 2017;15:1305-7.
27. Gunter MJ, Murphy N, Cross AJ, Dossus L, Dartois L, Fagherazzi G, et al. Coffee drinking and mortality in 10 European countries: a multinational cohort study. Ann Intern Med. 2017;167:236-47.
28. Park SY, Freedman ND, Haiman CA, Le Marchand L, Wilkens LR, Setiawan VW, et al. Association of coffee consumption with total and cause-specific mortality among nonwhite populations. Ann Intern Med. 2017;167:228-35.
29. Ratziu V, Ghabril M, Romero-Gomez M, Svegliati-Baroni G. Recommendations for management and treatment of nonalcoholic steatohepatitis. Transplantation. 2019;103:28-38.
30. Livingston EH. The incidence of bariatric surgery has plateaued in the U.S. Am J Surg. 2010;200:378-85.
31. Buchwald H, Avidor Y, Braunwald E, Jensen MD, Pories W, Fahrbach K. Bariatric surgery. A systematic review and meta-analysis. JAMA. 2004;292:1724-37.
32. Bower G, Toma T, Harling L, Jiao LR, Efthimiou E, Darzi A, et al. Bariatric surgery and non-alcoholic fatty liver disease: a systematic review of liver biochemistry and histology. Obes Surg. 2015;25:2280-9.
33. 32. Adams TD, Gress RE, Smith SC, Halverson C, Simper SC, Rosamond WD, et al. Long-term mortality after gastric bypass surgery. N Engl J Med. 2007;357:753-61.
34. Fayad L, Adam A, Schweitzer M, Cheskin LJ, Ajayi T, Dunlap M, et al. Endoscopic sleeve gastroplasty versus laparoscopic sleeve gastrectomy: a case-matched study. Gastrointest Endosc. 2019;89:782-8.

35. Harrison SA, Fecht W, Brunt EM, Neuschwander-Tetri BA. Orlistat for overweight subjects with nonalcoholic steatohepatitis: a randomized, prospective trial. Hepatology. 2009;49:80-6.
36. Armstrong MJ, Gaunt P, Aithal GP, Barton D, Hull D, Parker R, et al. Liraglutide safety and efficacy in patients with non-alcoholic steatohepatitis (LEAN): a multicentre, double-blind, randomised, placebo-controlled phase 2 study. Lancet. 2016;387: 679-90.
37. An H, He L. Current understanding of metformin effect on the control of hyperglycemia in diabetes. J Endocrinol. 2016;228:R97-R106.
38. Haukeland JW, Konopski Z, Eggesbø HB, von Volkmann HL, Raschpichler G, Bjøro K, et al. Metformin in patients with non-alcoholic fatty liver disease: a randomized, controlled trial. Scand J Gastroenterol. 2009;44:853-60.
39. Uygun A, Kadayifci A, Isik AT, Ozgurtas T, Deveci S, Tuzun A, et al. Metformin in the treatment of patients with non-alcoholic steatohepatitis. Aliment Pharmacol Ther. 2004;19:537-44.
40. Shields WW, Thompson KE, Harrison SA, Coyle WJ. The effect of metformin and standard therapy versus standard therapy alone in nondiabetic patients with insulin resistance and nonalcoholic steatohepatitis (NASH): a pilot trial. Therap Adv Gastroenterol. 2009;2:157-63.
41. Zhang X, Harmsen WS, Mettler TA, Kim WR, Roberts RO, Therneau TM, et al. Continuation of metformin use after a diagnosis of cirrhosis significantly improves survival of patients with diabetes. Hepatology. 2014;60:2008-16.
42. Oliveira CP, Cotrim HP, Stefano JT, Siqueira AC, Salgado AL, Parise ER, et al. ORIGINAL N-acetylcysteine and/or ursodeoxycholic acid associated with metformin in non-alcoholic steatohepatitis: An open-label multicenter randomized controlled trial. Arq Gastroenterol. 2019;56(2):184-90.
43. Phielix E, Szendroedi J, Roden M. The role of metformin and thiazolidinediones in the regulation of hepatic glucose metabolism and its clinical impact. Trends Pharmacol Sci. 2011;32:607-16.
44. Phielix E, Brehm A, Bernroider E, Krssak M, Anderwald CH, Krebs M, et al. Effects of pioglitazone versus glimepiride exposure on hepatocellular fat content in type 2 diabetes. Diabetes Obes Metab. 2013;15:915-22.
45. Ratziu V, Charlotte F, Bernhardt C, Giral P, Halbron M, Lenaour G, et al. Long-term efficacy of rosiglitazone in nonalcoholic steatohepatitis: Results of the fatty liver improvement by rosiglitazone therapy (FLIRT 2) extension trial. Hepatology. 2010;51: 445-53.
46. Sanyal AJ, Chalasani N, Kowdley KV, McCullough A, Diehl AM, Bass NM, et al. Pioglitazone, vitamin E, or placebo for nonalcoholic steatohepatitis. N Engl J Med. 2010;362:1675-85.
47. Musso G, Cassader M, Paschetta E, Gambino R. Thiazolidinediones and advanced liver fibrosis in nonalcoholic steatohepatitis: a meta-analysis. JAMA Intern Med. 2017;177:633-40.
48. Nauck M. Incretin therapies: Highlighting common features and differences in the modes of action of glucagon-like peptide-1 receptor agonists and dipeptidyl peptidase-4 inhibitors. Diabetes Obes Metab. 2016;18:203-16.

49. Miyazaki M, Kato M, Tanaka K, Tanaka M, Kohjima M, Nakamura K, et al. Increased hepatic expression of dipeptidyl peptidase-4 in non-alcoholic fatty liver disease and its association with insulin resistance and glucose metabolism. Mol Med Rep. 2012;5:729-33.
50. Yilmaz Y, Yonal O, Deyneli O, Celikel CA, Kalayci C, Duman DG. Effects of sitagliptin in diabetic patients with nonalcoholic steatohepatitis. Acta Gastroenterol Belg. 2012;75:240-4.
51. Cui J, Philo L, Nguyen P, Hofflich H, Hernandez C, Bettencourt R, et al. Sitagliptin vs. placebo for non-alcoholic fatty liver disease: a randomized controlled trial. J Hepatol. 2016;65:369-76.
52. Joy TR, McKenzie CA, Tirona RG, Summers K, Seney S, Chakrabarti S, et al. Sitagliptin in patients with non-alcoholic steatohepatitis: a randomized, placebo-controlled trial. World J Gastroenterol. 2017;23:141-50.
53. Mashitani T, Noguchi R, Okura Y, Namisaki T, Mitoro A, Ishii H, et al. Efficacy of alogliptin in preventing non-alcoholic fatty liver disease progression in patients with type 2 diabetes. Biomed Reports. 2016;4:183-7.
54. Macauley M, Hollingsworth KG, Smith FE, Thelwall PE, Al-Mrabeh A, Schweizer A, et al. Effect of vildagliptin on hepatic steatosis. J Clin Endocrinol Metab. 2015;100:1578-85.
55. Dokmak A, Almeqdadi M, Trivedi H, Krishnan S. Rise of sodium-glucose cotransporter 2 inhibitors in the management of nonalcoholic fatty liver disease. World J Hepatol. 2019;11:562-73.
56. Seko Y, Sumida Y, Tanaka S, Mori K, Taketani H, Ishiba H, et al. Effect of sodium glucose cotransporter 2 inhibitor on liver function tests in Japanese patients with non-alcoholic fatty liver disease and type 2 diabetes mellitus. Hepatol Res. 2017;47:1072-8.
57. Akuta N, Kawamura Y, Watanabe C, Nishimura A, Okubo M, Mori Y, et al. Effects of a sodium-glucose cotransporter 2 inhibitor in nonalcoholic fatty liver disease complicated by diabetes mellitus: Preliminary prospective study based on serial liver biopsies. Hepatol Commun. 2017;1:46-52.
58. Akuta N, Kawamura Y, Watanabe C, Nishimura A, Okubo M, Mori Y, et al. Impact of sodium glucose cotransporter 2 inhibitor on histological features and glucose metabolism of non-alcoholic fatty liver disease complicated by diabetes mellitus. Hepatol Res. 2019;49:531-9.
59. Itani T, Ishihara T. Efficacy of canagliflozin against nonalcoholic fatty liver disease: a prospective cohort study. Obes Sci Pract. 2018;4:477-82.
60. Takase T, Nakamura A, Miyoshi H, Yamamoto C, Atsumi T. Amelioration of fatty liver index in patients with type 2 diabetes on ipragliflozin: an association with glucose-lowering effects. Endocr J. 2017;64:363-7.
61. Ito D, Shimizu S, Inoue K, Saito D, Yanagisawa M, Inukai K, et al. Comparison of ipragliflozin and pioglitazone effects on nonalcoholic fatty liver disease in patients with type 2 diabetes: a randomized, 24-week, open-label, active-controlled trial. Diabetes Care. 2017;40:1364-72.
62. Ohki T, Isogawa A, Toda N, Tagawa K. Effectiveness of ipragliflozin, a sodium-glucose co-transporter 2 inhibitor, as a second-line treatment for non-alcoholic fatty liver

disease patients with type 2 diabetes mellitus who do not respond to incretin-based therapies including glucagon-like pep. Clin Drug Investig. 2016;36:313-9.
63. Miyake T, Yoshida S, Furukawa S, Sakai T, Tada F, Sneba H, et al. Ipragliflozin ameliorates liver damage in non-alcoholic fatty liver disease. Open Med. 2018;13:402-9.
64. Shimizu M, Suzuki K, Kato K, Jojima T, Iijima T, Murohisa T, et al. Evaluation of the effects of dapagliflozin, a sodium-glucose co-transporter-2 inhibitor, on hepatic steatosis and fibrosis using transient elastography in patients with type 2 diabetes and non-alcoholic fatty liver disease. Diabetes Obes Metab. 2019;21:285-92.
65. Shiba K, Tsuchiya K, Komiya C, Miyachi Y, Mori K, Shimazu N, et al. Canagliflozin, an SGLT2 inhibitor, attenuates the development of hepatocellular carcinoma in a mouse model of human NASH. Sci Rep. 2018;8:1-12.
66. Skelley JW, Carter BS, Roberts MZ. Clinical potential of canagliflozin in cardiovascular risk reduction in patients with type 2 diabetes. Vasc Health Risk Manag. 2018;14: 419-28.
67. McMurray, Solomon SD, Inzucchi SE, Køber L, Kosiborod MN, Martinez FA, et al. Dapagliflozin in patients with heart failure and reduced ejection fraction. N Engl J Med. 2019;381(21):1995-2008.
68. Jhaveri U, Vardesh D. Sodium-glucose cotransporter-2 inhibitors and euglycaemic diabetic ketoacidosis in the perioperative period: case report. Cureus. 2019;11:8-12.
69. Doumas M, Imprialos K, Dimakopoulou A, Stavropoulos K, Binas A, Athyros VG. The role of statins in the management of nonalcoholic fatty liver disease. Curr Pharm Des. 2018;24:4587-92.
70. German MN, Lutz MK, Pickhardt PJ, Bruce RJ, Said A. Statin use is protective against hepatocellular carcinoma in patients with nonalcoholic fatty liver disease: a case-control study. J Clin Gastroenterol. 2019;00:1-8.
71. Porez G, Prawitt J, Gross B, Staels B. Bile acid receptors as targets for the treatment of dyslipidemia and cardiovascular disease. J Lipid Res. 2012;53:1723-37.
72. Neuschwander-Tetri, Loomba R, Sanyal AJ, Lavine JE, Van Natta ML, Abdelmalek MF, et al. Farnesoid X nuclear receptor ligand obeticholic acid for non-cirrhotic, non-alcoholic steatohepatitis (FLINT): a multicentre, randomised, placebo-controlled trial. Lancet. 2015;385(9972):956-65.
73. Tanaka N, Aoyama T, Kimura S, Gonzalez FJ. Targeting nuclear receptors for the treatment of fatty liver disease. Pharmacol Ther. 2017;179:142-57.
74. Ratziu V, Harrison SA, Francque S, Bedossa P, Lehert P, Serfaty L, et al. Elafibranor, an agonist of the peroxisome proliferator-activated receptor-α and -δ, induces resolution of nonalcoholic steatohepatitis without fibrosis worsening. Gastroenterology. 2016;150:1147-59.e5.
75. Schuster S, Feldstein AE. NASH: Novel therapeutic strategies targeting ASK1 in NASH. Nat Rev Gastroenterol Hepatol. 2017;14:329-30.
76. Friedman SL, Ratziu V, Harrison SA, Abdelmalek MF, Aithal GP, Caballeria J, et al. A randomized, placebo-controlled trial of cenicriviroc for treatment of nonalcoholic steatohepatitis with fibrosis. Hepatology. 2018;67:1754-67.
77. Abdul-Hai A, Abdallah A, Malnick SD. Influence of gut bacteria on development and progression of non-alcoholic fatty liver disease. World J Hepatol. 2015;7(12) 1679-84.

78. Vrieze A, Van Nood E, Holleman F, Salojärvi J, Kootte RS, Bartelsman JF, et al. Transfer of intestinal microbiota from lean donors increases insulin sensitivity in individuals with metabolic syndrome. Gastroenterology. 2012;143:913-6.e7.
79. Ratziu V. A critical review of endpoints for non-cirrhotic NASH therapeutic trials. J Hepatol. 2018;68:353-61.
80. Alexander M, Loomis AK, Fairburn-Beech J, van der Lei J, Duarte-Sallès T, Prieto-Alhambra D, et al. Real-world data reveal a diagnostic gap in non-alcoholic fatty liver disease. BMC Med. 2018;16:1-11.
81. Simon TG, Henson J, Osganian S, Masia R, Chan AT, Chung RT, et al. Daily aspirin use associated with reduced risk for fibrosis progression in patients with nonalcoholic fatty liver disease. Clin Gastroenterol Hepatol. 2019;17(13):2776-84.e4.
82. Wenger NK. Female-friendly focus: 2019 ACC/AHA Guideline on the Primary Prevention of Cardiovascular Disease. Clin Cardiol. 2019;42(8):706-9.
83. Mullee A, Romaguera D, Pearson-Stuttard J, Viallon V, Stepien M, Freisling H, et al. Association between soft drink consumption and mortality in 10 European countries. JAMA Intern Med. 2019;1-12. doi:10.1001/jamainternmed.2019.2478
84. Han MA, Altayar O, Hamdeh S, Takyar V, Rotman Y, Etzion O, et al. Rates of and factors associated with placebo response in trials of pharmacotherapies for nonalcoholic steatohepatitis: systematic review and meta-analysis. Clin Gastroenterol Hepatol. 2019;17:616-29.e26.

CHAPTER

12

Management of Hepatitis C

Soe Thiha Maung, Aung Hlaing Bwa, Si Thu Sein Win, Khin Maung Win

INTRODUCTION

Hepatitis C virus (HCV) was first characterized by Choo et al.[1] and Kuo et al.[2] in 1989. It was soon identified as the main causative agent of the disease previously known as post-transfusion non-A, non-B hepatitis virus infection. HCV is a major cause of liver disease worldwide and a potential cause of substantial morbidity and mortality in the future. The complexity and uncertainty related to the geographic distribution of HCV infection and chronic hepatitis C, determination of its associated risk factors, and evaluation of cofactors that accelerate its progression underscore the difficulties in global prevention and control of HCV.[3]

Globally, HCV has infected an estimated 130 million people, most of who are chronically infected. HCV-infected people serve as a reservoir for transmission to others and are at risk for developing chronic liver disease, cirrhosis, and primary hepatocellular carcinoma (HCC). It has been estimated that HCV accounts for 27% of cirrhosis and 25% of HCC worldwide.[4] The World Health Organization (WHO) estimated that in 2016, approximately 399,000 people died from hepatitis C, mostly from cirrhosis and HCC (primary liver cancer).[5] Progression to chronic disease occurs in the majority of HCV-infected persons, and infection with the virus has become the main indication for liver transplantation.[6]

EPIDEMIOLOGY

The total global prevalence of anti-HCV antibody (anti-HCV Ab) was estimated to be 1.6% (1.3–2.1%), corresponding to 115 (92–149) million past viremic infections. The majority of these infections, 104 (87–124) million, were among adults (defined as those older than 15 years) with an anti-HCV infection rate of 2.0% (1.7–2.3%). The viremic [ribonucleic acid (RNA) positive] prevalence was forecasted to be 1.1% (0.9–1.4%), corresponding to 80 (64–103) million viremic infections. Again, most of these viremic infections were among adults who accounted for 75 (62–89) million viremic infections or a viremic prevalence of 1.4% (1.2–1.7%).[7]

Genotype Distribution of Hepatitis C Virus Infection

Globally, genotype 1 was most common, accounting for 46% of all infections, followed by genotypes 3 (22%) and genotypes 2 and 4 (13% each). Subtype 1b accounted for 22% of all infections at the global level. There were significant variations across regions with genotype 1 dominating in Australasia, Europe, Latin America, and North America (53–71% of all cases) and G3 accounting for 40% of all infections in Asia. Genotype 4 was most common (71%) in North Africa and the Middle East, but when Egypt was excluded, it accounted for 34% while genotype 1 accounted for 46% of infections across the same region.[7] Genotype 6 is only prevalent in South-East Asia regions, especially Myanmar and Vietnam. Knowledge of the genotype is important because it has a predictive value in terms of the response to antiviral therapy—with better responses associated with genotypes 2 and 3 than with genotype 1 **(Fig. 1)**.[8]

PATHOGENESIS

Hepatitis C is caused by an RNA virus which belongs to the family of flaviviruses. The natural targets of HCV are hepatocytes and, possibly, B lymphocytes.[9] HCV encodes a single polyprotein of 3,011 amino acids, which is then processed into 10 mature structural and regulatory proteins

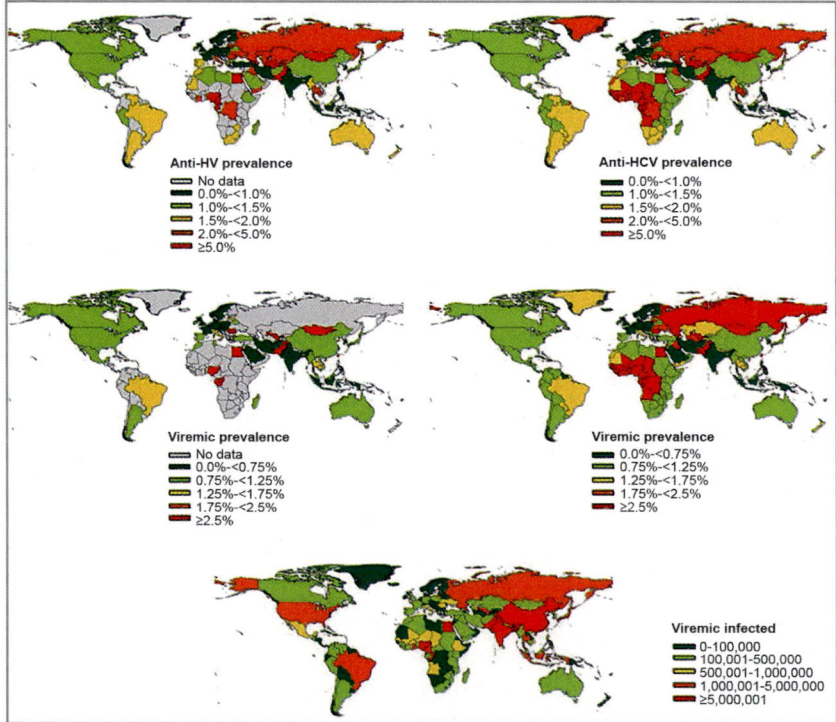

Fig. 1: Epidemiological distribution of hepatitis C virus (HCV) infection.
Source: Gower E, Estes C, Blach S, Razavi-Shearer K, Razavi H. Global epidemiology and genotype distribution of the hepatitis C virus infection. J Hepatol. 2014;61(1):S45-S57.

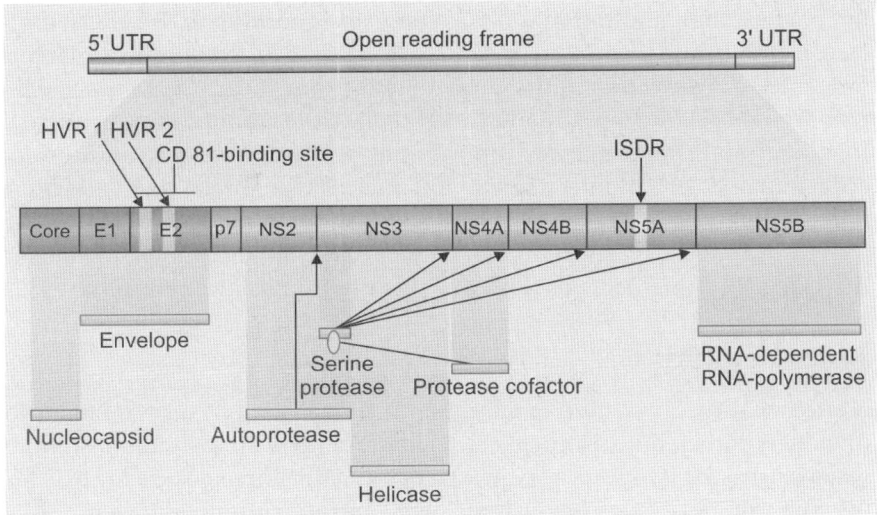

Fig. 2: Structure of HCV virus.
(CD81: cluster of differentiation 81; HCV: hepatitis C virus; HVR: hypervariable region; ISDR: interferon sensitivity determining region; NS2: nonstructural protein 2; NS4A: nonstructural protein 4A; NS4B: nonstructural protein 4B; NS5A: nonstructural protein 5A; UTR: untranslated region)
Source: Lauer G, Walker B. Hepatitis C virus infection. New Eng J Med. 2001;345(1):41-52.

(Fig. 2). Structural components include the core and two envelope proteins. Two regions of the envelope E2 protein, designated hypervariable regions 1 and 2, have an extremely high rate of mutation, believed to be the result of selective pressure by virus-specific antibodies. E2 also contains the binding site for CD81, a tetraspanin expressed on hepatocytes and B lymphocytes that is thought to function as a cellular receptor or co-receptor for the virus.[10]

Hepatitis C virus also encodes a virus-specific helicase, protease, and polymerase, and because of the critical function of these proteins in the viral life cycle, they represent attractive targets for antiviral therapy. Similarly, the untranslated regions at both ends of the viral RNA may show promise as therapeutic targets, since they are highly conserved and involved in critical stages of viral replication.[10] Therefore, every effort is being made to understand the pathogenesis of HCV infection to create a therapeutic model for an effective treatment against HCV.

CLINICAL PRESENTATIONS AND NATURAL HISTORY OF DISEASES

Transmission of Hepatitis C Virus Infection

The transmission of HCV is primarily through exposure to infected blood. Risks for transmission include blood transfusion before 1992, intravenous drug use, high-risk sexual activity, solid organ transplantation from an infected donor, occupational exposure, hemodialysis, household exposure, birth to an infected mother, and intranasal cocaine use. According to the US Centers for Disease Control and Prevention (CDC), the most common risk factors for acute HCV infection in the United States from 1991 to 1995 were high-risk drug (60%) and sexual behaviors (20%). Other modes of transmission (occupational, hemodialysis, household, and perinatal) accounted for approximately 10% of infections. A potential risk factor can be identified in approximately 90% of persons with HCV infection. In the remaining 10%, no recognized source of infection can be identified, although most persons in this category are associated with a low socioeconomic level **(Flowchart 1)**.[11]

Acute Hepatitis C

Acute hepatitis C infection is infrequently diagnosed because the majority of acutely infected individuals are asymptomatic. Clinical manifestations can occur, usually within 7–8 weeks (range, 2–26) after exposure to HCV, but the majority of persons have either no symptoms or only mild symptoms. Fulminant hepatitis has been described during this period, though it is very rare. In the transfusion setting, where acute onset of HCV infection has been best documented, 70–80% of cases were asymptomatic. The antibody to HCV, as detected by enzyme immunoassay (EIA), becomes positive near the onset of symptoms, approximately 1–3 months after exposure. Up to 30% of patients will test negative for anti-HCV at the onset of their symptoms, making anti-HCV testing unreliable in diagnosis of acute infection.[12]

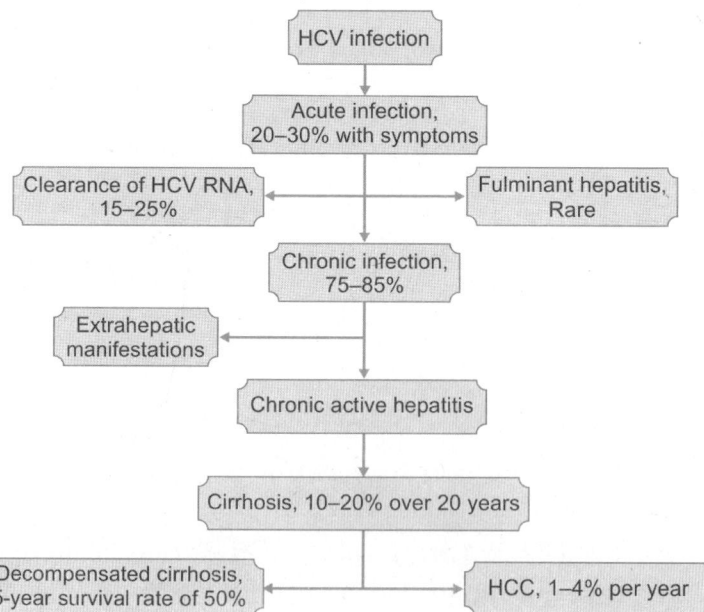

Flowchart 1: Natural history of hepatitis C virus (HCV) infection.

(HCC: hepatocellular carcinoma; RNA: ribonucleic acid)

Chronic Hepatitis C

Chronic hepatitis C is marked by the persistence of HCV RNA in the blood for at least 6 months after the onset of acute infection. HCV is self-limiting in only 15–25% of patients in whom HCV RNA in the serum becomes undetectable and alanine transaminase (ALT) levels return to normal. Approximately 75–85% of infected patients do not clear the virus by 6 months, and chronic hepatitis develops. In the setting of persistent hepatitis C viremia, the rate of progression of liver fibrosis varies widely. There have been extensive studies focusing on the natural course of disease progression from chronic hepatitis C to cirrhosis, HCC, and death. Cirrhosis develops in approximately 10–15% of individuals with chronic HCV infection.[12] The progression to cirrhosis is often clinically silent, and some patients are not known to have hepatitis C until they present with the complications of end-stage liver disease or HCC. The features of decompensated cirrhosis include the development of ascites, upper gastrointestinal bleeding secondary to varices or portal hypertensive gastropathy, hepatorenal syndrome, and hepatic encephalopathy. In the United States, deaths associated with chronic HCV are more likely to be caused from decompensated cirrhosis rather than HCC.[13]

DIAGNOSIS

Diagnostic tests for HCV infection are divided into:
- Serologic assays for antibodies
- Molecular tests for viral particles

Screening assays based on antibody detection have markedly reduced the risk of transfusion-related infection, and once persons seroconvert they usually remain positive for HCV antibodies.

Acute HCV infection is typically mild. It is often not diagnosed, and the infection may be recognized only when it becomes chronic.[14] The diagnostic procedures for HCV infection used in laboratories are based on the detection of anti-HCV Abs against recombinant HCV proteins using EIA and chemiluminescence immunoassay. In the setting of HCV infection diagnosis in clinical laboratories, only one ELISA (enzyme-linked immunosorbent assay) is necessary for the detection of anti-HCV Abs.[15]

Applications of molecular tests for detecting, quantifying, and characterization of the infecting virus became very important in the management of HCV infection.

Hepatitis C virus infection is diagnosed in two steps:
1. Testing for anti-HCV Abs with a serological test identifies people who have been infected with the virus.
2. If the test is positive for anti-HCV Abs, a nucleic acid test for HCV RNA is needed to confirm chronic infection because about 30% of people infected with HCV spontaneously clear the infection by a strong immune response without the need for treatment. Although no longer infected, they will still test positive for anti-HCV Abs.

Viral genotyping helps in predicting the outcome of therapy and also influences the choice of the therapeutic regimen. Different methods are available for the genotyping of HCV, most of which are based on amplification with the polymerase chain reaction (PCR) assay. Knowledge of the distribution of HCV genotypes has important clinical implications since the efficacy of current and new therapies differs by genotype. Until pan-genotypic therapies reach the market, sustained virologic response (SVR), duration of treatment, and cost of treatment will be impacted by the genotype distribution. To date, there are no published studies assessing HCV genotype at the global level; however, it is understood that there are notable geographical differences.[16]

No standardized tests for resistance of HCV to approved drugs are available as purchasable kits. Resistance testing mostly relies on in-house techniques based on population sequencing (Sanger sequencing) or deep sequencing. In addition, highly efficacious treatments are now available for patients with detectable pre-existing resistance-associated substitutions (RASs) at baseline. Thus, systematic testing for HCV resistance prior to treatment in direct-acting antivirals (DAA) drug-naïve individuals is not recommended.[7]

After a person has been diagnosed with chronic HCV infection, he/she should have an assessment of the degree of liver damage (fibrosis and cirrhosis). This can be done by liver biopsy or through a variety of noninvasive tests.

Histologic evaluation of a liver-biopsy specimen remains the gold standard for determining the activity of HCV-related liver disease, and histologic staging remains the only reliable predictor of prognosis and the likelihood of disease progression. A biopsy may also help to rule out other concurrent causes of liver disease. Therefore, biopsy is generally recommended for the initial assessment of persons with chronic HCV infection. However, a liver biopsy is not considered mandatory before the initiation of treatment, and some recommend a biopsy, only if treatment does not result in sustained remission.[17]

In chronic hepatitis C, noninvasive methods should be used instead of liver biopsy to assess liver disease severity prior to therapy. Liver stiffness measurement can be used to assess liver fibrosis and the presence of portal hypertension in patients with chronic hepatitis C. Both liver stiffness measurement and biomarkers perform well in the identification of cirrhosis or no fibrosis, but they perform less well in resolving intermediate degrees of fibrosis.

In low- and middle-income countries, as well as in settings where treatment expands outside of specialty clinics, aspartate aminotransferase to platelet ratio index (APRI) and fibrosis-4 (FIB4) are generally available, simple, and cheap, and the information they provide is reliable. Patients with cirrhosis must be identified, as their treatment regimen must be adjusted and post-treatment surveillance for HCC is mandatory. Post-treatment surveillance for HCC must also be performed in patients with advanced fibrosis (METAVIR score F3).[18]

TREATMENT

The goal of therapy is to cure HCV infection in order to:
- Prevent the complications of HCV-related liver and extrahepatic diseases, including hepatic necroinflammation, fibrosis, cirrhosis, decompensation of cirrhosis, HCC, severe extrahepatic manifestations, and death
- Improve quality of life and remove stigma
- Prevent onward transmission of HCV

The endpoint of therapy is an SVR, defined by undetectable HCV RNA in serum or plasma 12 weeks (SVR12) or 24 weeks (SVR24) after the end of therapy, as assessed by a sensitive molecular method with a lower limit of detection ≤15 IU/mL. Both SVR12 and SVR24 have been accepted as endpoints of therapy by regulators in Europe and the United States, given that their concordance is >99%.[19]

Undetectable HCV core antigen 12 weeks after the end of therapy may be used as an alternative to post-treatment HCV RNA testing to define the SVR12 in patients with detectable core antigen before treatment.[20]

Treatment for Acute Hepatitis C

Patients with acute hepatitis C are often asymptomatic or have nonspecific symptoms (e.g., fatigue, anorexia, mild or moderate abdominal pain, low-grade fever, nausea, and/or vomiting) that are frequently not recognized as being associated with acute HCV infection. A small proportion (<25%) of patients with acute HCV develop jaundice. Patients diagnosed with acute HCV should initially be monitored with hepatic panels [ALT, aspartate aminotransferase (AST), bilirubin, and international normalized ratio (INR) in the setting of an increasing bilirubin level] at 2- to 4-week intervals.[21]

Hepatitis C virus infection spontaneously clears in 20-50% of patients. In at least two-thirds of patients who spontaneous clear acute HCV infection, this occurs within 6 months of the estimated time of infection (median, 16.5 weeks). Only 11% of those who remain viremic at 6 months will spontaneously clear the infection at a later time. Thus, detectable HCV RNA at 6 months after the time of infection will identify most persons who need antiviral therapy.[22]

Data regarding the efficacy of the treatment of acute HCV infection are very limited, since the infection is seldom diagnosed during the acute phase. Given the high rate of progression to chronic infection and the relatively limited efficacy of therapy for chronic infection, the treatment of acute infection has been advocated.

In the interferon (IFN) era, the efficacy of acute HCV infection treatment (particularly for genotype 1), including abbreviated regimens, was superior to the treatment of chronic infection. There are emerging data on the treatment of acute HCV infection with shortened courses of all-oral, DAA regimens both in HCV monoinfection and in human immunodeficiency virus/HCV (HIV/HCV) coinfection. But as yet, there are insufficient data to support a particular regimen or treatment duration. Until more definitive data are available, monitoring for spontaneous clearance for a minimum of 6 months before initiating treatment is recommended. When the decision is made to initiate antiviral therapy after 6 months, treatment as described for chronic hepatitis C is recommended.[23]

Treatment for Chronic Hepatitis C

In principle, all patients with chronic HCV infection are candidates for antiviral therapy. All treatment-naïve and -experienced patients with HCV infection, who are willing to be treated and who have no contraindications for treatment, should be treated.[24] Treatment must be considered without delay in patients with significant fibrosis (METAVIR score F2 or F3) or cirrhosis (METAVIR score F4), including decompensated cirrhosis.[25] Patients with decompensated cirrhosis and an indication for liver transplantation with a MELD (model for end-stage liver disease) score ≥ 18–20 will benefit from transplantation first and antiviral treatment after transplantation, because the probability of significant improvement in liver function and delisting is low. However, patients with a MELD score ≥18–20 with a waiting time before transplantation expected to be >6 months can be treated for their HCV infection. Treatment is generally not recommended in patients with limited life expectancy because of non–liver-related comorbidities.[26]

The introduction of DAA agents will markedly change treatment options for individuals who have a chronic HCV infection **(Flowchart 2)**.

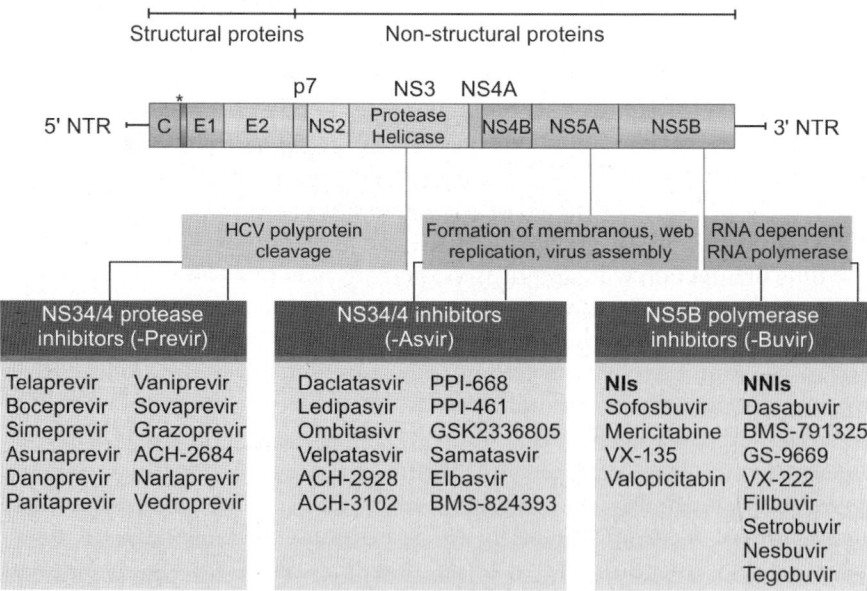

Flowchart 2: Different classes of direct-acting antivirals (DAAs).

(HCV: hepatitis C virus; NI: nucleoside/nucleotide inhibitor; NNI: non-nucleoside inhibitor; NS: nonstructural protein; NTR: nontranslated region; PPI: proton-pump inhibitor)
Source: Hofmann WP, Zeuzem S. A new standard of care for the treatment of chronic HCV infection. Nature Reviews Gastroenterology and Hepatology. 2011:8;257-64.

Several IFN-free combination trials were done with different DAAs that target multiple viral sites: NS3/4a protease inhibitors, NS5B polymerase inhibitors (NI and NNI), and NS5A inhibitors. There have been major advancements in the last several years with large numbers of trials with various DAAs showing increased SVR rates, favorable tolerability, and shortened treatment duration with all oral regimens. HCV drug development is shorter than, e.g., HIV drug development because of short treatment duration; the option of open-label studies without the need of a control arm and also the primary end point for efficacy is SVR12 (12 weeks' post-treatment follow-up).[27]

The recent advances in hepatitis C therapeutics have brought combinations of DAA medications that offer IFN-free, well-tolerated regimens with SVR rates >90% in clinical trials for many patient groups. The successes have prompted discussions regarding cure for all patients.[20]

In order for HCV to be eradicated, rates of SVR need to be higher than those of new HCV infections. Since 2011, the standard of care for chronic HCV infection has shifted from pegylated interferon (PEG-IFN)-based treatment to DAA-based therapy. In Asia, while PEG-IFN–based treatment is expensive and requires more intense follow-up of patients, it has resulted in SVR rates of approximately 70% for genotype 1, approximately 80–90% for genotype 2/3, and 80% for genotype 6–8. The introduction of pan-genotypic DAAs has led to significant increases in the tolerability and efficacy of chronic HCV treatment (>90% SVR rates for all genotypes).[28,29]

As such, the remaining challenges are identification of cases, education on transmission modes and prevention, and minimizing pretherapy assessment and on-treatment monitoring to be able to facilitate a broader implementation of an elimination strategy. Decreasing the cost of DAA-based therapy, especially in resource-constrained regions such as Myanmar, can increase rates of treatment and thus lead to lower transmission of infection rates. An example of the correlation between making DAAs more accessible and decreasing the new infection rate was seen in 2015 when the Netherlands introduced unrestricted access to DAAs for all newly infected HCV patients.[29]

While DAA-based HCV treatment is expensive in the Western world, several highly effective and safe pan-genotypic generic drugs have become available in resource-constrained areas, including Myanmar; bioequivalent data are only available for sofosbuvir (SOF).[30]

As HCV genotypes and treatment outcomes vary significantly based on the region, it is essential to study treatment strategies in context. This experience of pan-genotypic generic DAA SOF/VEL (SOF/velpatasvir) with or without ribavirin (RBV) reveals excellent rates of SVR (SVR 98.6%; $n = 354/359$) for HCV-infected patients in Myanmar, regardless of the genotype.[31]

The approval of Mavyret dual-combination therapy marks another milestone in the treatment of HCV infections. There had been a major effort to develop an all-oral combination therapy with activity against all genotypes. With the approval of Mavyret, this goal has been met. The newer generation inhibitors and various combinations provide treatment options for patients and improve SVR rates across all genotypes. For many cases, Mavyret has decreased the standard of care from 24 to 8 weeks. More importantly, treatment options for patients with compensated liver disease are now available. Given the excellent pan-genotypic response and safety profile in patients, Mavyret was approved for the treatment of genotypes 1–6 in patients without cirrhosis or with compensated cirrhosis. In patients with noncirrhotic chronic HCV who were treatment-naïve or had previously been treated with PEG-IFN or RBV, the SVR rate was 83–100% across all genotypes.[32] In treatment-naïve patients with compensated liver disease, about 99% of patients achieved SVR with a 12-week course. Mavyret was approved as an 8-week course for treatment-naïve patients without cirrhosis, shortening the previous standard of care by an additional 4 weeks.[33]

Thus, both components of Mavyret have good resistance profiles against wild-type genotypes and single-mutant variants of HCV. What needs to be considered is the emergence of double, triple or other multimutant variants that may have high levels of resistance to one or both components of this combination? Such multimutant variants potentially pose a threat to the longevity and success of HCV treatment.

Moving forward, it is important to minimize the number of steps it takes to diagnose HCV and implement treatment. A significant barrier to this goal is the lack of availability of rapid point-of-care HCV RNA testing. Without this technology, it can take multiple visits from the initial screening to implementation of HCV therapy.[34]

Treatment of Hepatitis C during Pregnancy

Pregnancy itself does not appear to negatively affect chronic HCV infection. In general, serum ALT levels decrease during the first and third trimesters of pregnancy and increase after delivery. HCV RNA levels rise during the first and third trimesters, reaching a peak during the third trimester, and decrease postpartum. These effects are likely due to the immunosuppressive effects of pregnancy. HCV-infected pregnant women have a higher incidence of intrahepatic cholestasis of pregnancy (ICP) [pooled odds ratio (OR) 20.40 {95% confidence interval (CI), 9.39–44.33, I2–55%}] based on a meta-analysis of three studies when compared to noninfected pregnant women. ICP is associated with an increased rate of adverse maternal and fetal outcomes; all patients with this syndrome should be immediately referred to a high-risk obstetrical specialist for monitoring and treatment.[35]

Although some studies show an increased risk of adverse perinatal outcomes (e.g., preterm delivery, low-birth weight infants, and congenital anomalies) with maternal HCV infection, these risks are confounded by comorbid conditions, such as substance use. However, pregnant women with cirrhosis are at increased risk for poor maternal outcomes (i.e., pre-eclampsia, cesarean section, hemorrhagic complication, and death) and neonatal outcomes (i.e., preterm delivery, low birth weight, and neonatal death).[36]

Women with cirrhosis should be counseled about these increased risks and care should be coordinated with specialists in maternal–fetal medicine. Hepatitis C mother-to-child transmission (MTCT) occurs at an overall rate of 5–15% with the number that progress to chronic infection being 3–5%. No specific risk factor predicts transmission and no specific intervention (e.g., antiviral, mode of delivery, or others) has been demonstrated to reduce transmission. Given the potential associated risk of MTCT, it is advisable to avoid invasive procedures (e.g., fetal scalp monitors and forceps delivery).[37]

It has been estimated that up to 29,000 HCV-infected women gave birth each year from 2011 to 2014. With the current increases in HCV among young adults including women of childbearing age, there is now a discussion about universal screening of pregnant women. To enhance mothers' health and address public health concerns, universal testing of pregnant women for the current HCV infection is recommended.[35]

Women of reproductive age with HCV should be counseled about the benefit of antiviral treatment prior to pregnancy to improve the health of the mother and eliminate the low risk of MTCT. The safety of DAAs in pregnancy is unknown, and there are no data on the effect of DAAs on male or female fertility. However, RBV is contraindicated in pregnancy due to its known teratogenicity. In addition, the risk for teratogenicity persists for up to 6 months after RBV cessation and applies to women-taking RBV and female partners of men-taking RBV. Women who become pregnant while on DAA therapy (with or without RBV) should discuss the risks versus benefits of continuing treatment with their physicians.[38]

Treatment of Hepatitis C in Children

Although the prevalence of chronic HCV is lower in children than adults, an estimated 5 million children worldwide have active HCV infection. Data from the National Health and Nutrition Examination Survey (NHANES) collected between 2003 and 2010 indicates that 0.2% of 6–11-year-olds (31,000 children) and 0.4% of 12–19-year-olds (101,000 adolescents) in the US are chronically infected with HCV.[39]

As birth to an HCV-infected mother is a known risk for infection, such offspring should be evaluated and tested for HCV. The rate of MTCT of HCV infection is approximately 5%, although rates are higher among women with inadequately controlled HIV coinfection, and women with higher HCV-RNA levels, or viral loads (>6 log IU/mL).[40]

In children, liver disease due to chronic HCV infection generally progresses slowly, and cirrhosis and liver cancer are infrequently encountered. Although elevated serum aminotransferase levels are often noted, HCV-infected children younger than 3 years of age virtually never have advanced liver disease.

If DAA regimens are available for a child's age groups, treatment is recommended for all HCV-infected children older than 3 years as they will benefit from antiviral therapy, independent of disease severity.[38]

Treatment of Hepatitis C in Patients with Chronic Kidney Disease

Chronic hepatitis C is independently associated with the development of chronic kidney disease (CKD). A meta-analysis published in 2015 demonstrated that chronic HCV infection was associated with a 51% increase in the risk of proteinuria and a 43% increase in the incidence of CKD. There is also a higher risk of progression to end-stage renal disease (ESRD) in persons with chronic HCV infection and CKD, and an increased risk of all-cause mortality in persons on dialysis.[41]

The C-SURFER (Hepatitis C: Study to Understand Renal Failure's Effect on Responses) trial evaluated the safety and efficacy of 12 weeks of the daily fixed-dose combination of elbasvir (50 mg)/grazoprevir (100 mg) versus placebo among genotype 1-infected patients with CKD stage 4 or 5 [estimated glomerular filtration rate (eGFR) < 30 mL/min]. The initial study randomized eligible patients to immediate or deferred treatment with elbasvir/grazoprevir. The delayed treatment arm initially received placebo and was later treated with elbasvir/grazoprevir. Notably, both elbasvir and grazoprevir are primarily hepatically metabolized and undergo minimal renal elimination. Based on these data, daily fixed-dose elbasvir/grazoprevir is recommended for the treatment of genotype 1 infection in patients with severely compromised renal function. Treatment with elbasvir/grazoprevir in persons with CKD has been shown to be cost effective in the United States.[42]

The EXPEDITION-4 trial evaluated the safety and efficacy of 12 weeks of the pan-genotypic NS3/NS4A protease inhibitor glecaprevir and the pan-genotypic NS5A inhibitor pibrentasvir for genotype 1, 2, 3, 4, 5, or 6 infection. The EXPEDITION-4 trial supports the efficacy and safety of glecaprevir/pibrentasvir in patients with CKD and ESRD. The recommended duration of therapy is the same as for patients without CKD.[43]

Treatment of Hepatitis C in Patients with HIV/HCV Coinfection

The HIV/HCV-coinfected patients suffer from more liver-related morbidity and mortality, nonhepatic organ dysfunction, and overall mortality than HCV-monoinfected patients.[44] Even in the potent HIV antiretroviral therapy era, HIV infection remains independently associated with advanced liver fibrosis and cirrhosis in patients with HIV/HCV coinfection.[45]

As such, treatment of HCV in HIV-infected patients should be a priority for providers, payers, and patients. However, if HCV treatment is delayed for any reason, liver disease progression should be monitored at routine intervals as recommended. With the availability of HCV DAAs, efficacy and adverse event rates among those with HIV/HCV coinfection are similar to those observed with HCV-monoinfection and many prior barriers have diminished. However, treatment of HIV/HCV-coinfected patients requires continued awareness and attention to the complex drug–drug interactions that can occur between DAAs and antiretroviral medications.[46]

The HIV/HCV coinfected patients should be treated and retreated the same as patients without HIV infection, after recognizing and managing interactions with antiretroviral medications. Daily daclatasvir plus SOF (400 mg) with or without RBV is the recommended regimen when antiretroviral regimen changes cannot be made to accommodate alternative HCV DAAs. Ledipasvir/SOF for 8 weeks is not recommended, regardless of the baseline HCV RNA level.[38]

REFERENCES

1. Choo QL, Kuo G, Weiner AJ, Overby LR, Bradley DW, Houghton M. Isolation of a cDNA clone derived from a blood-borne non-A, non-B viral hepatitis genome. J Hepatol. 2002;36(5):582-5.
2. Kuo G, Choo Q, Alter H, Gitnick GL, Redeker AG, Purcell RH, et al. An assay for circulating antibodies to a major etiologic virus of human non-A, non-B hepatitis. Science. 1989;244(4902):362-4.
3. Shepard C, Finelli L, Alter M. Global epidemiology of hepatitis C virus infection. Lancet Infect Dis. 2005;5(9):558-67.
4. Alter M. Epidemiology of hepatitis C virus infection. World J Gastroenterol. 2007;13(17):24-36.
5. World Health Organization. (2019) Key facts of hepatitis C. [online] Available from www.who.int › Newsroom › Fact sheets › Detail. [Last accessed January, 2020].
6. Lauer G, Walker B. Hepatitis C virus infection. New Eng J Med. 2001;345(1):41-52.
7. Gower E, Estes C, Blach S, Razavi-Shearer K, Razavi H. Global epidemiology and genotype distribution of the hepatitis C virus infection. J Hepatol. 2014;61(1):S45-S57.
8. Poynard T, Marcellin P, Lee SS, Niederau C, Minuk GS, Ideo G, et al. Randomised trial of interferon alpha2b plus ribavirin for 48 weeks or for 24 weeks versus interferon alpha2b plus placebo for 48 weeks for treatment of chronic infection with hepatitis C virus. Lancet. 1998;352:1426-32.
9. Okuda M, Hino K, Korenaga M, Yamaguchi Y, Katoh Y, Okita K. Differences in hypervariable region 1 quasispecies of hepatitis C virus in human serum, peripheral blood mononuclear cells and liver. Hepatology. 1999;29:217-22.
10. Kolykhalov AA, Mihalik K, Feinstone SM, Rice CM. Hepatitis C virus-encoded enzymatic activities and conserved RNA elements in the 3′ non-translated region are essential for virus replication in vivo. J Virol. 2000;74:2046-51.
11. Alter M. The epidemiology of acute and chronic hepatitis C. Clin Liver Dis. 1997;1(3):559-68.
12. McCaughan GW, McGuinness PH, Bishop GA, Painter DM, Lien AS, Tulloch R, et al. Clinical assessment and incidence of hepatitis C RNA in 50 consecutive RIBA-positive volunteer blood donors. Med J Aust. 1992;157(4):231-3.
13. National Institutes of Health Consensus Development Conference Statement: Management of hepatitis C: 2002-June 10-12, 2002. Hepatology. 2002;36(5B):s3-s20.
14. Fattovich G, Giustina G, Degos F, Tremolada F, Diodati G, Almasio P, et al. Morbidity and mortality in compensated cirrhosis type C: A retrospective follow-up study of 384 patients. Gastroenterology. 1997;112(2):463-72.

15. Moestrup T, Hansson B, Widell A, Nordenfelt E, Hagerstrand I. Long-term follow-up of chronic hepatitis B virus infection in intravenous drug abusers and homosexual men. BMJ. 1986;292(6524):854-7.
16. Pawlotsky J, Lonjon I, Hezode C, Raynard B, Darthuy F, Remire J, et al. What strategy should be used for diagnosis of hepatitis C virus infection in clinical laboratories? Hepatology. 1998;27(6):1700-2.
17. Pawlotsky J. Hepatitis C virus resistance to direct-acting antiviral drugs in interferon-free regimens. Gastroenterology. 2016;151(1):70-86.
18. Yano M. The long-term pathological evolution of chronic hepatitis C. Hepatology. 1996;23(6):1334-40.
19. EASL-ALEH Clinical Practice Guidelines: Non-invasive tests for evaluation of liver disease severity and prognosis. J Hepatol. 2015;63(1):237-64.
20. Martinot-Peignoux M, Stern C, Maylin S, Ripault MP, Boyer N, Leclere L, et al. Twelve weeks post-treatment follow-up is as relevant as 24 weeks to determine the sustained virologic response in patients with hepatitis C virus receiving pegylated interferon and ribavirin. Hepatology. 2009;51(4):1122-6.
21. Aghemo A, Degasperi E, De Nicola S, Bono P, Orlandi A, D'Ambrosio R, et al. Quantification of core antigen monitors efficacy of direct-acting antiviral agents in patients with chronic hepatitis C virus infection. Clin Gastroenterol Hepatol. 2016;14(9):1331-6.
22. Blackard J, Shata M, Shire N, Sherman K. Acute hepatitis C virus infection: a chronic problem. Hepatology. 2007;47(1):321-31.
23. Grebely J, Page K, Sacks-Davis R, van der Loeff MS, Rice TM, Bruneau J, et al. The effects of female sex, viral genotype, and IL28 Bgenotype on spontaneous clearance of acute hepatitis C virus infection. Hepatology. 2013;59(1):109-20.
24. Ghany M, Strader D, Thomas D, Seeff L. Diagnosis, management, and treatment of hepatitis C: An update. Hepatology. 2008;49(4):1335-74.
25. National Institutes of Health Consensus Development Conference Panel Statement: Management of hepatitis C. Hepatology. 1997;26(S3):2S-10S.
26. Charlton M, Everson G, Flamm S, Kumar P, Landis C, Brown RS Jr, et al. Ledipasvir and sofosbuvir plus ribavirin for treatment of HCV infection in patients with advanced liver disease. Gastroenterology. 2015;149(3):649-59.
27. Pascasio J, Vinaixa C, Ferrer M, Colmenero J, Rubin A, Castells L, et al. Clinical outcomes of patients undergoing antiviral therapy while awaiting liver transplantation. J Hepatol. 2017;67(6):1168-76.
28. Muir A, Naggie S. Hepatitis C virus treatment: Is it possible to cure all hepatitis C virus patients? Clin Gastroenterol Hepatol. 2015;13(12):2166-72.
29. Lok A, Chung R, Vargas H, Kim A, Naggie S, Powderly W. Benefits of direct-acting antivirals for hepatitis C. Ann Intern Med. 2017;167(11):812.
30. McQueen K. The burden of surgical conditions and access to surgical care in low- and middle-income countries. Bull World Health Organ. 2008;86(8):646-7.
31. Bwa A, Nangia G, Win S, Maung ST, Han KA, Htar SS, et al. Strategy and efficacy of generic and pan-genotypic sofosbuvir/velpatasvir in chronic hepatitis C virus: a Myanmar experience. J Clin Exp Hepatol. 2019;9(3):283-93.
32. Kwo P, Poordad F, Asatryan A, Wang S, Wyles DL, Hassanein T, et al. Glecaprevir and pibrentasvir yield high response rates in patients with HCV genotype 1–6 without cirrhosis. J Hepatol. 2017;67(2):263-71.

33. Forns X, Lee SS, Valdes J, Lens S, Ghalib R, Aguilar H, et al. Glecaprevir plus pibrentasvir for chronic hepatitis C virus genotype 1, 2, 4, 5, or 6 infection in adults with compensated cirrhosis (EXPEDITION-1): a single-arm, open-label, multicentre phase 3 trial. Lancet Infect Dis. 2017;17:1062-8.
34. Viganò M, Andreoni M, Perno C, Craxì A, Aghemo A, Alberti A, et al. Real life experiences in HCV management in 2018. Expert Rev Anti Infect Ther. 2019;17(2): 117-28.
35. Watts T, Stockman L, Martin J, Guilfoyle S, Vergeront J. Increased risk for mother-to-infant transmission of hepatitis C virus among Medicaid recipients—Wisconsin, 2011–2015. MMWR Morb Mortal Wkly Rep. 2017;66(42):1136-9.
36. Puljic A, Salati J, Doss A, Caughey A. Outcomes of pregnancies complicated by liver cirrhosis, portal hypertension, or esophageal varices. J Matern Fetal Neonatal Med. 2015;29(3):506-9.
37. Jhaveri R, Hashem M, El-Kamary S, Saleh DA, Sharaf SA, El-Mougy F, et al. Hepatitis C virus (HCV) vertical transmission in 12-month-old infants born to HCV-infected women and assessment of maternal risk factors. Open Forum Infect Dis. 2015;2(2):ofv089.
38. Chung R, Ghany M, Kim A, Marks KM, Naggie S, Vargas HE, et al. Hepatitis C Guidance 2018 Update: AASLD-IDSA Recommendations for testing, managing, and treating hepatitis C virus infection. Clin Infect Dis. 2018;67(10):1477-92.
39. Denniston MM, Jiles RB, Drobeniuc J, Klevens RM, Ward JW, McQuillan GM, et al. Chronic hepatitis C virus infection in the United States, National Health and Nutrition Examination Survey 2003 to 2010. Ann Intern Med. 2014;160(5):293-300.
40. Delotte J, Barjoan E, Berrébi A, Laffont C, Benos P, Pradier C, et al. Obstetric management does not influence vertical transmission of HCV infection: results of the ALHICE group study. J Matern Fetal Neonatal Med. 2014;27(7):664-70.
41. Rogal SS, Yan P, Rimland D, Lo Re V 3rd, Al-Rowais H, Fried L, et al. ERCHIVES (Electronically Retrieved Cohort of HCV Infected Veterans) Study Group. Incidence and progression of chronic kidney disease after hepatitis C seroconversion: results from ERCHIVES. Dig Dis Sci. 2016;61(3):930-6.
42. Elbasha E, Greaves W, Roth D, Nwankwo C. Cost-effectiveness of elbasvir/grazoprevir use in treatment-naive and treatment-experienced patients with hepatitis C virus genotype 1 infection and chronic kidney disease in the United States. J Viral Hepat. 2017;24(4):268-79.
43. Gane E, Lawitz E, Pugatch D, Papatheodoridis G, Bräu N, Brown A, et al. Glecaprevir and pibrentasvir in patients with HCV and severe renal impairment. N Engl J Med. 2017;377(15):1448-55.
44. Lo Re V, Kallan MJ, Tate JP, Localio AR, Lim JK, Goetz MB, et al. Hepatic decompensation in antiretroviral-treated patients co-infected with HIV and hepatitis C virus compared with hepatitis C virus-monoinfected patients: a cohort study. Ann Intern Med. 2014;160(6):369-79.
45. Fierer DS, Dieterich D, Fiel MI, Branch AD, Marks KM, Fusco DN, et al. Rapid progression to decompensated cirrhosis, liver transplant, and death in HIV-infected men after primary hepatitis C virus infection. Clin Infect Dis. 2013;56(7):1038-43.
46. Bhattacharya D, Belperio PS, Shahoumian TA, Loomis TP, Goetz MB, Mole LA, et al. Effectiveness of all-oral antiviral regimens in 996 human immunodeficiency virus/hepatitis C virus genotype 1-coinfected patients treated in routine practice. Clin Infect Dis. 2017;64(12):1711-20.

CHAPTER

13

Neurological Complications in Liver Diseases

J Zizzo, Z Rahaman, AR Jayakumar

INTRODUCTION

The liver is the largest glandular organ in the human body, comprising roughly 2-5% of body weight, and it plays a significant role in metabolic and immunological homeostasis. The liver is responsible for a spectrum of over 500 functions including energy production, detoxification, coagulation, storage, and hormonal balance. A healthy liver even possesses the ability to regenerate when damaged.[1]

Liver disease begins with the gradual onset of inflammation, resulting in tenderness and enlargement of the organ. Patients do not regularly notice any symptoms at this stage, in which successful treatment offers positive outlooks for most. Left untreated, the inflamed liver will then begin to scar, a process known as fibrosis, leaving scar tissue in place of healthy hepatic tissue. Scar tissue cannot carry out the normal functions of the liver, causing decreased blood flow and regulation. The next stage of liver disease, cirrhosis, typically requires an interval of 15-20 years to progress. Cirrhosis includes hard scar tissue replacing the soft tissue, eventually leading to liver failure and multiple potential complications including liver cancer and cognitive dysfunction due to insufficient toxin resistance.[2]

End-stage liver disease includes patients who have medically untreatable pathologies without imperative liver transplantation. Complications at this stage may include hepatic encephalopathy (HE), neoplasms, hepatitis, multiorgan failure (MOF), gastrointestinal (GI) bleeding, etc. An emerging paradigm is one in which neurological complications constitute a major issue in liver diseases based on clinical and experimental evidence. Neurological complications in liver disease, such as HE, represent an irreversible impairment of neuropsychiatric function.[3]

However, it is unclear whether all forms of liver disease have neurological complications since some liver disorders do not manifest neurological deficits [e.g., nonalcoholic fatty liver disease (NAFLD), congestive hepatopathy].[4] A neurological condition associated with a liver disease may be a complication of the disease or may be induced by factors that contribute to the liver disease itself (e.g., alcohol) or it may have no relation to the presence of the liver disease altogether (e.g., MOF). This chapter, therefore, summarizes the nature of various liver diseases and their involvement in neurological complications **(Table 1)**. This chapter also explores the possible direct link between hepatic ailments to neurological complications and more recent perspectives into why these correlations do not coincide with certain liver diseases.

HEPATIC ENCEPHALOPATHY

Hepatic encephalopathy is the neurological complication associated with mild-moderate or severe liver disease that occurs in acute and chronic forms.[5] Chronic HE (CHE; portal-systemic encephalopathy) is generally a consequence of alcoholic liver cirrhosis and has a high socioeconomic impact. Patients with CHE often demonstrate changes in personality, sleep apnea, altered mood, reduced intellectual capacity, tremor, and irregular muscle tone as well as muscle wasting.[6] HE can also present acutely, due to acute liver failure (ALF) following massive hepatic necrosis or due to viral

Table 1: Summary of the mechanisms and neurological complications of various liver diseases.

Liver disease	Mechanism(s)	Neurological complication(s)
Acute liver failure	Hepatotoxins, cytokines	Cerebral edema and associated increase in intracranial pressure
Chronic liver failure	Hepatotoxins, cirrhosis, viral infection	Neuropsychiatric deficits, seizure, spinal cord injury
Hepatitis A	Inflammatory reaction across blood–brain barrier	Guillain–Barré syndrome (GBS)
Hepatitis B	Blood-borne contact, bodily fluid transfer	GBS, mononeuropathy multiplex associated with polyarteritis nodosa
Hepatitis C	Impaired dopaminergic transmission, parenchymal infiltration	Transverse myelopathy, CNS inflammation, cognitive impairment
Neoplasm	Chemotherapeutic drugs	Brain metastasis, acute mental changes
Non-Wilsonian acquired hepatocerebral degeneration	Manganese	Basal ganglia dysfunction, atypical involuntary movements
Hepatic myelopathy	CNS nutrient deficiencies and hepatotoxins via portocaval shunt	Alzheimer type II astrocyte proliferation, axonal degeneration, demyelination
Nonalcoholic fatty liver disease	Unknown	Cognitive changes, brain volume reduction
Autoimmune liver disease	Unknown	Cognitive impairment, atypical intracortical inhibition

(CNS: Central nervous system)

hepatitis, acetaminophen (Tylenol) toxicity, or exposure to various liver toxins (e.g., acetaminophen, potential drugs of abuse including cocaine, amphetamines, hallucinogens, heroin, antidepressants, anabolic steroids, and anesthetics).[7] Cerebral edema occurs in up to 80% of patients with ALF and represents the most frequent cause of death in these patients due to increased intracranial pressure and cerebral herniation.[8] The only effective treatment presently available is an emergency liver transplantation.[9] The current epidemic of hepatitis A, B, C, D, and E heightens the importance of this growing clinical problem.

Acute Hepatic Encephalopathy

Acute hepatic encephalopathy [(AHE) or fulminant hepatic failure (FHF) or type A HE] generally occurs following massive liver necrosis due to viral hepatitis (i.e., all forms of hepatitis), hepatic neoplasms, vascular causes, or exposure to acetaminophen and other hepatotoxins such as cocaine, amphetamines, hallucinogens, heroin, antidepressants, and anabolic steroids.[10] Acute HE is a life-threatening condition and has an extremely poor prognosis (80-90% mortality) and presents with the abrupt onset of delirium, seizures, and coma.[11]

Neurological Complications

Brain edema (a net increase in total brain water content) is the major neurological complication in AHE.[12] Cerebral edema and associated increase in intracranial pressure leading to brain herniation are the characteristic features of AHE, occurring in up to 80% of patients with AHE and represents the most frequent cause of death in these patients (70% mortality).[13] While the basis for the edema is poorly understood, a preponderance of experimental data favors a cytotoxic mechanism, i.e., an intracellular accumulation of fluid due to the inability of brain cells to adequately regulate their intracellular volume.[14] The only cells in the brain that undergo such swelling are the astrocytes.[15] Astrocyte swelling is seen in humans[16] and in experimental animals with HE[15] as well as in hyperammonemic animals.[17] Magnetic resonance imaging (MRI) also indicates that the brain edema in AHE is cytotoxic. Diffusion-weighted MRI measures the relative motion of water protons across cell membranes [expressed as the apparent diffusion coefficient (ADC)] and is thus capable of distinguishing intracellular from extracellular accumulation of water.[8] A recent diffusion-weighted imaging study found an ADC reduction in patients with ALF, indicating a reduction in the size of the extracellular space, consistent with an intracellular accumulation of water. A recent report also described a reduction in ADC values in a rat model of ALF (galactosamine). We also found a similar ADC reduction in the thioacetamide (TAA) rat model of ALF.[18] The onset of encephalopathy can be rapid and pronounced with the manifestation of asterixis, hepatic coma, delirium, decerebrate posturing, autonomic dysreflexia, and seizures.[12]

Chronic Hepatic Encephalopathy (Type C Hepatic Encephalopathy)

Chronic hepatic encephalopathy is a neuropsychiatric disorder that commonly occurs in the setting of alcoholic cirrhosis and is associated with changes in personality, altered mood, decline in the intellectual capacity, and abnormal muscle tone.[19] The neurological features include signs and symptoms of pyramidal and extrapyramidal dysfunction, brisk tendon reflexes, and flapping tremor. CHE should be distinguished from FHF and episodic unconsciousness ("meat intoxication") in portosystemic shunt encephalopathy. Preliminary results of a prospective evaluation in patients with chronic liver failure revealed a significant correlation between the neuropsychiatric features and globus pallidus hyperintensity on MRI scans.[20]

Neurological Complications

As noted above, CHE (portal-systemic encephalopathy) is generally a consequence of alcoholic liver cirrhosis and viral infection (hepatitis) and represents a high socioeconomic burden. Cognitive indicators in patients with HE range from minor impairments, which are not evident under standard clinical examination protocols, to more apparent findings, with impairments in attention and processing rate.[21] CHE patients progressing to severe HE (acute or chronic HE) may advance to hepatic coma.[21]

Advanced CHE patients can present with a wide range of neurological symptoms including delirium, difficulty thinking, amnesia, personality changes, poor concentration, loss of fine hand movements, poor judgment, as well as permanent neurological conditions, such as seizure and spinal cord injury. In severe cases, patients may also exhibit anxiety, confusion, lethargy, seizures, tremors, and bradykinesia.[22] Some or most of these findings were also observed in animal models of CHE.[23]

HEPATITIS

Several viruses are associated with both AHE and CHE including hepatitis A, B, and C. In addition, AHE often presents with varicella zoster virus, cytomegalovirus, herpes simplex virus, and Epstein–Barr virus.[24]

Hepatitis A

Hepatitis A virus (HAV) infection occurs worldwide, with an estimated 1.4 million cases occurring each year.[25] Hepatitis A can occur intermittently or in a widespread form due to contaminated food or water. HAV is typically transmitted via the orofecal route (either through close personal contact or ingestion of contaminated food or water).[26]

In adults, acute HAV is usually a self-contained infection; ALF manifests in <1% of patients. HAV has an incubation period averaging 28 days, with a range of 15–50 days.[27] Symptomatic illness transpires in >70% of adults with HAV, commencing with the sudden onset of abdominal pain, fever, malaise, nausea, and vomiting.[28] Dark urine, indicative of conjugated bilirubinuria, materializes within a few days to a week of infection. Intrahepatic cholestasis may also be observed.

These are then succeeded by jaundice and pruritus. Jaundice typically peaks within 2 weeks from infection, coinciding with the withdrawal of the original signs and symptoms.[29]

Neurological Complications

Nervous system complications of HAV viral infection appear to be very rare. A variety of neurological syndromes including Guillain–Barré syndrome (GBS) have been reported in patients with serologically confirmed hepatitis A.[30] Unrecognized clinical presentation of hepatitis A with unilateral peripheral acute sensory loss in the prodromal phase of the illness has also been reported. Although rare, GBS is known to occur as a complication in viral hepatitis A cases (as sole peripheral neuropathy).[31] Other neurologic syndromes have also been reported in patients with serologically defined viral hepatitis A and B (see further hepatitis B section) including mononeuritis, auditory neuritis, and seizures.[32] Acute motor and sensory axonal neuropathy (AMSAN) is a specific type of GBS characterized by severe acute onset of distal weakness and affects the sensory nerves and roots. Acute motor axonal neuropathy (AMAN) differs in that it often presents with decreased muscle action potentials and lacking a demyelinating process.[30] Clinical presentations have shown that AMAN and AMSAN can be preceded by *Campylobacter jejuni* enteritis and associated symptoms.[33] However, in recent studies, there was evidence that the AMSAN subtype of GBS was seen following acute HAV infection using clinical evidence and HAV virus–immunoglobulin M (IgM) antibodies in the serum and cerebrospinal fluid (CSF).[30] The exact pathogenesis by which the virus causes the disease is not clear. The involvement of the central nervous system (CNS) in the pathophysiology of the viral disease could be due to direct invasion of the CNS by the virus, as evidenced by the presence of HAV antibodies in the CSF. Therefore, it seems most plausible that transport of antibodies occurs across a disrupted blood–nerve barrier during an inflammatory reaction of nerve roots.[32]

In AMAN and AMSAN, the mechanistic features differ from the pathology of acute inflammatory demyelinating polyradiculoneuropathy (AIDP) such that macrophages invade the periaxonal space, leaving the myelin sheath intact. It has been hypothesized that AMAN and AMSAN are factors in a single type of antibody-mediated immune attack on the axon, but the correlation between AMAN and AMSAN is still unknown.[30,34]

The AMAN cases differ from the AMSAN pattern of GBS via more rapid onset of weakness, in addition to sparing of the dorsal nerve roots; however, the pathologies appear to be similar.[35]

Hepatitis B

Hepatitis B virus (HBV) is a viral infection that affects the liver, capable of causing both chronic and acute disease forms. The infection is transmitted via blood-borne contact or bodily fluid transfer. It is estimated that there are around 257 million HBV carriers in the world, of whom around 900,000 die annually from HBV-related liver disease. The implementation of 95% effective vaccination programs in many countries has resulted in a significant decrease in the incidence of new HBV cases.[36] Nevertheless, HBV infection remains an undeniable cause of decreased quality of life and substantial morbidity and mortality.

Neurological Complications

Tsukada et al. has shown that demyelinating neuropathy is associated with HBV infection. Research studies have shown patients with GBS-type of polyneuropathy and patients with chronic relapsing polyneuropathy associated with HBV infection, and they were examined in search of the pathogenetic factors involved. It was demonstrated that hepatitis B surface antigen (HBsAg) immune complexes were significantly increased in both the sera and the CSF of the patients with GBS. The serum levels of immune complexes were also closely related to the clinical status of the patients. Also, HBsAg-positive labeling of immunofluorescence was found around the endoneural small blood vessels and in the endoneurium. Electron-dense deposits, suggestive of immune complexes composed of HBV, were demonstrated in the endoneurium of the patient with chronic relapsing polyneuropathy. These results suggest that HBsAg immune complexes may be of importance in the etiology of GBS or chronic relapsing polyneuropathy associated with HBV infection.[38]

Lee et al. has extensively described mononeuropathy multiplex (MM) and its relation to HBV infection as "A painful asymmetric sensory and motor peripheral neuropathy involving isolated damage to at least two separate nerve areas. It is a syndrome of diverse causes including diabetes mellitus, demyelinating, infectious, or neoplastic etiology. In association with chronic active hepatitis B, MM associated with polyarteritis nodosa (PAN) is relatively common. Research studies have shown manifestation with multifocal sensorimotor mononeuropathy accompanied by chronic active hepatitis B including vasculitic neuropathies such as PAN. Polyarteritis nodosa is a necrotizing vasculitis of medium-sized arteries; its most prominent clinical manifestations include variable signs such as MM, weight loss, livedo reticularis, hypertension, abnormal renal blood tests, myalgia and arthritis, testicular pain, HBV infection, evidence of vasculitis on abdominal angiography, and abnormal nerve biopsy. Furthermore, HBV infection has been reported in around 30% of patients with PAN, although PAN is a rare complication of hepatitis B."[37]

Chronic hepatitis B is not only a recognized risk factor for the development of an immune-mediated neuropathy, but also a common infection, with it being estimated that there are >300 million affected individuals worldwide.[38]

Hepatitis C

During the chronic stage of hepatitis C virus (HCV) infection, a relatively stable viral load is maintained. However, in cases of coinfection with viruses such as human immunodeficiency virus (HIV), HCV RNA (ribonucleic acid) levels can increase after HIV seroconversion and remain higher than in HCV-only patient populations.[39] The HCV viremia level is inversely correlated with lower CD4 counts in most studies and may temporarily increase with the initiation of antiretroviral therapy or heavy alcohol use.[40]

End-stage HCV occurs when the HCV causes severe liver damage and can no longer function properly. The liver deteriorates over many years, often advancing from inflammation to cirrhosis. Patients are frequently asymptomatic and have only mild symptoms for many years before progressing to cirrhosis.[41]

Common symptoms seen in HCV patients include fatigue and sleep disturbances, along with other indicators such as abdominal pain, anorexia, arthralgia, diarrhea, nausea, and weight loss. Neuropsychiatric conditions (e.g., anxiety and depression) are also common (see further in text).[42]

Neurological Complications

Hepatitis C virus infection has been linked to numerous neurological disorders ranging from encephalomyelitis, leukoencephalitis, and meningeal inflammation to neurodegeneration via spastic quadriparesis and sphincter impairment.[43] The presence of viral genomic material in the brain postmortem signifies a neurological disease correlation. HCV-related transverse myelitis with associated autonomic neuronal dysfunction has also been reported.[44]

Severe demyelination coupled with parenchymal infiltration has been linked to HCV infection via spinal cord biopsy. Disease onset is marked by acute partial transverse and acute transverse myelitis, or spastic paraplegia-associated sensory deficits. Multisegmental spinal involvement and recurrence are common. A patient positive for anti-HCV antibodies but lacking typical HCV symptoms suggests an immune-mediated response leading to neurological complications.[45]

Severe encephalomyelitis has also been linked with chronic HCV infection.[46] MRI reports indicate the presence of CNS damage in the cerebellar and cerebral white matter. Clinical indicators including consciousness, dysfunctional psychomotor, hemianopsia, hemiparesis, urinary retention, and other neurological defects are implicated. Relevant findings have suggested that the risk of HCV infection increases in patients with acute disseminated encephalomyelitis.[47]

Approximately half of HCV-infected patients report cognitive impairment, fatigue, and neuropsychiatric symptoms. During HCV onset, patients commonly present with complications including malaise, attention deficits, and mild amnesia. HCV is a causative agent of various CNS complications ranging from autoimmune disorders to cerebrovascular events.[45] Acute cerebrovascular events including lacunar syndromes and transient ischemic attacks have been reported in HCV patients.[48]

The occurrence of occlusive vasculopathy and vasculitis are well-known progressions.[49] Intracranial stenosis can result from isolated CNS vasculitis.

Multiple case reports have revealed that the CNS ischemic alterations may be correlated with an antiphospholipid-associated syndrome or they might be linked to antineutrophil cytoplasmic antibodies.[50] A promising study has shown HCV-metabolic syndrome association, hypothesizing that HCV infection is a predisposing factor for enhanced carotid wall thickness and atherosclerosis. Thus, the finding suggests that HCV plays a major role in cerebrovascular mortality, particularly in patients with high HCV RNA levels.[46]

Encephalopathic syndromes clinically characterized by altered consciousness, cognitive impairment, dysarthria, and dysphagia are linked with the diffuse association of white matter in HCV patients with circulating anticardiolipin antibodies and/or cryoglobulins.[51] Such patients may present with small lesions in the periventricular white matter and subcortical structures. Alterations in the severe and diffuse infra- and supratentorial white matter, capable of causing vasculitis, have been reported in patients diagnosed with corresponding systemic vasculitis.[45] A recent study documented CNS vasculitis-induced ischemic injury in a patient concurrently suffering from mixed cryoglobulins, peripheral neuropathy, and relapsing multi-infarct encephalopathy.[52] Neuropathological examination of the patient revealed multiple ischemic lesions (diameter: 0.5–3.0 mm) in the white matter of the cerebral hemispheres and cerebellum, accompanied with parenchymal infiltration and lymphocyte aggregates surrounding small vessels. Another recent study has shown the prevalence of vasculitis-induced ischemic changes in a chronic HCV patient with mixed cryoglobulins and sensory neuropathy.[53]

Cognitive decline, functionally characterized by diminished attention, spatial, and visual constructive capabilities, has also been associated with an increased prevalence of periventricular white matter high-intensity signals (WMHIS) on T2-weighted MRI.[53] These patients suggest a relationship between cryoglobulinemia level and the resulting number of impaired cognitive functions; however, no relationship was noted with systemic manifestations of cryoglobulinemia including peripheral neuropathy.[45]

Variations in the WMHIS have shown that vascular disease may trigger the chronic hypoperfusion of white matter and modifications of the blood-brain barrier.[54]

The spectrum of CNS conditions seen in patients with HCV is not confined to the foregoing vasculitic and vasculopathic manifestations, but may also cause inflammatory disorders including acute encephalitis, encephalomyelitis, and meningoradiculitis.[45]

MRI and neuropathological studies have shown patients diagnosed with leukoencephalitis in concordance with the HCV genome[55] or progressive encephalomyelitis with rigidity.[43] Another study has documented a patient suffering from an acute disseminated encephalomyelitis, an autoimmune postinfectious CNS disease developed post HCV infection, supporting the implication of cellular immune-mediated mechanisms in CNS complications of HCV infection.[56]

A recent study consisting of 53 HCV-positive patients with neuropsychiatric conditions showed an increase in choline and myoinositol concentrations in the basal ganglia and white matter, as well as an increase in creatinine, N-acetyl-aspartate (NAA), and N-acetyl-aspartyl-glutamate concentrations in the basal ganglia. These discoveries are consistent with observed HCV-induced chronic inflammation.[57] A study conducted in 2001 showed an increased ratio of choline/creatine (Cho/Cr) in the basal ganglia and the frontal white matter of HCV-infected patients via nuclear magnetic resonance spectroscopy.[58] Additional studies have found a lower NAA/Cr ratio in the frontal gray matter of HCV patients without any change in the Cho/Cr ratio.[59] Both studies suggest the presence of an increased cell membrane turnover and decreased neuronal function.[45] Administration of ondansetron, a competitive antagonist of serotonin receptors (5-HT3), has ameliorated fatigue in HCV-infected patients. A randomized study of 36 HCV-infected patients has also shown improved depression and fatigue scores with ondansetron.[60] These findings have highlighted the importance of serotoninergic pathway dysfunction, which causes fatigue, reduced serotonin synthesis, and reduced serum tryptophan levels.[61,62] Moreover, the results of 15 HCV-infected patients reporting neuropsychiatric symptoms carried out via various neuropsychological tests such as positron emission tomography showed significant declines in striatal and midbrain dopamine transporter availability and decreased metabolism in the limbic, parietal, frontal, and temporal cortices. These findings support the significant role of impaired dopaminergic transmission in causing cognitive impairment in HCV.[59]

Hepatitis C virus infection has also been associated with myopathy and, in a number of cases, inflammatory and noninflammatory myopathies have been reported. The clinical indicators of HCV-linked myopathies range from progressive weakness to relapsing forms, a slight increase in muscle enzymes, and moderate weakness. Pathological features of noninflammatory myopathies include immune-mediated necrotizing myopathy[63] and vacuolar alterations[64] with slow or progressive proximal weakness, and selective type II fiber atrophy in relapsing myopathy. A study by Cortelli et al. has shown oxidative mitochondrial damage in a patient with severe ptosis, diplopia, generalized weakness, and respiratory complications as well as ultrastructural abnormalities of mitochondrial shape and cristae.[65] Additional studies have implicated the ability of HCV to promote tumor necrosis factor-mediated cell death in myocytes.[66]

Functional imaging studies have also identified metabolic changes in the CNS during the progression of HCV infection. Coinfection with HCV is also a potential risk factor for HIV-associated neurocognitive disorder.[67]

Neoplasm

Predominantly solid liver lesions may contain cystic components, as noted in hemangiomas or tumors that have necrotic areas. Conversely, cystic liver lesions may have solid regions, specifically in the malignancy setting. There are many known causes of benign and malignant solid liver lesions.[68]

Common benign hepatic lesions include hepatic hemangioma, hepatocellular adenoma, focal nodular hyperplasia, idiopathic noncirrhotic portal hypertension, and regenerative nodules. Inflammatory pseudotumor is a rare benign solid liver tumor comprised of proliferating fibrous tissue infiltrated by inflammatory cells. The etiology is unknown; however, this lesion frequently occurs in association with a systemic chronic disease.[69]

Common malignant liver lesions include hepatocellular carcinoma, cholangiocarcinoma, and metastatic disease.

The majority of HCCs occur in patients with chronic liver disease or cirrhosis. Thus, older patients with long-standing liver disease are more likely to develop HCC. Large prospective studies, such as that by Colombo et al., have noted a mean presentation age between 50 and 60 years.[70] In certain parts of sub-Saharan Africa, however, the mean presentation age of HCC is decreasing, with the mean presentation age being around 33 years.[71]

Neurological Complications

Neurological complications in liver cancer have not been fully explicated. Between 1995 and 2006, the Yonsei University Health System treated 6,919 patients with HCC. About 62 cases had a brain metastasis diagnosis. And 54 years was the median age at the time of diagnosis.

The median progression period from HCC to brain metastasis diagnosis was just over 18 months. Five patients presented with brain involvement initially. Brain metastasis was associated with intracranial hemorrhage in 54.8% of cases. The most common symptoms exhibited were altered mental status, cephalgia, and motor weakness. The prognosis of HCC patients with brain metastases is extremely poor. However, several subgroups manifested the most favorable survival criteria, with single brain metastasis and proper liver function. For these patients, treatment may significantly improve survival time.[72]

Brain metastases have wide-ranging clinical features and should be suspected in any cancer patient exhibiting behavioral abnormalities or neurological symptoms. In most patients, a steadily expanding neoplasm and its resulting edema cause symptoms.

Although less common, embolization by tumor cells, intratumoral hemorrhage, and obstructive hydrocephalus can cause symptoms.[73]

Acute mental changes are the most common CNS complication due to multiple cancer treatments. AHE commonly occurs after agents such as high-dose cytarabine or methotrexate permeate the blood–brain barrier. Encephalopathy ranges in severity from somnolence and inattentiveness to stupor. Drug withdrawal usually ameliorates the encephalopathy but may require an antidote for full reversal. An example is the reversal of encephalopathy due to administration of ifosfamide via methylene blue.[74]

Chemotherapeutic drugs including L-asparaginase,[75] 5-azacytidine,[76] and cisplatin[77] have been implicated in causing liver injury alongside their antioncogenic effects. This is an important issue since both neoplasm and drug-induced liver injury together can exacerbate existing liver injury, thereby causing CNS dysfunction.

While brain metastasis has been reported in hepatocellular carcinoma cases, it is unclear whether hepatocellular carcinoma alone has any effect on the brain without inducing brain metastasis. This aspect needs to be explored.

Non-Wilsonian Acquired Hepatocerebral Degeneration

The term "acquired hepatocerebral degeneration (AHCD)" is used to mark a division from the heritable Wilson disease. The umbrella term describes a variety of neuropsychiatric abnormalities associated with chronic liver failure, which are clinically distinct from episodes of acute HE.[78] Most documented complications involve basal ganglia dysfunction and include atypical involuntary movements, such as choreoathetosis, dementia, dysarthria, dystonia, tremor, rigidity, pyramidal tract signs, myoclonus, and uncommon ataxia.[79] The presence of neurological symptoms is not linked to the cause of liver failure but seems to correlate with the extent of portosystemic shunting, the number of HE episodes, and blood ammonia levels.[80]

Multiple parenchymal and cholestatic liver diseases are implicated in the onset in AHCD. Most patients with AHCD have signs of portosystemic shunting irrespective of abnormal liver function. There is no defined treatment of AHCD, but recent case reports have emphasized the use of trientine, branched-chain amino acid therapy, and liver transplantation for the treatment of movement disorders. Levodopa may be beneficial in the treatment of AHCD-related parkinsonism.[81] Conventional therapy for HE has not proven effective for AHCD patients. There are sparse and conflicting reports regarding the clinical outcomes of AHCD after liver transplantation.[82,83]

Neurological Complications and Mechanisms

The characteristic presentation of AHCD is that of an extrapyramidal neurological disorder, with balance instabilities and irregular movements. Early symptoms are often characterized by a tremor of the outstretched arms, twitches of the face and limbs, or an unsteady gait. Months or years later, the patient may present with ataxia, dysarthria, and choreoathetosis.[82,84] Mental function may also be affected, occasionally in the form of dementia. Less frequent complications include rigidity, grasp reflexes, nystagmus, intention myoclonus, and hepatic myelopathy (HM). Before presenting with the above symptoms, individuals with AHCD commonly experience several episodes of HE.[85]

Recent evidence has implicated manganese in the pathogenesis of AHCD. Excess consumed manganese is rapidly cleared by the liver before entering the systemic circulation. In patients suffering from both cirrhosis and portosystemic shunting, manganese bypasses the liver and aggregates in the internal globus pallidum, while serum manganese levels may increase or remain stagnant. MRI abnormalities primarily show a signal hyperintensity on T1-weighted images in the internal pallidum. This can also be seen in other cerebral structures including the caudate nucleus, internal capsule, mesencephalon, putamen, and cerebellum and is thought to result from local manganese accumulation.[81]

Neuropathological features are notably similar to those seen in Wilson disease including neurodegeneration and polymicrocavitation in the deep layers of the parietal, occipital, and frontal cortices, the adjacent white matter, the basal ganglia, and the cerebellum, as well as the presence of numerous Alzheimer type 2 astrocytes in cortex and subcortical gray matter, periodic acid–Schiff-positive intranuclear inclusions, and Opalski cells. However, the advanced age of patients, absence of Kayser–Fleischer rings, and normal copper metabolism allow Wilson disease to be excluded.[82]

HEPATIC MYELOPATHY

Hepatic myelopathy is an insidious onset pure motor bilateral progressive and irreversible spastic paraparesis without sensory or bowel or bladder involvement in patients with liver disease in which the neurological dysfunction cannot be attributed to another condition. A progressive spastic paraparesis in patients with liver failure was first described by Leigh and Card in 1949,[86] followed by a comprehensive review of HM by other authors observing HM as a rare complication of cirrhosis, particularly in patients with portosystemic shunts.[86] Pant et al. first described HM surrounding two cases of spastic paraparesis in patients with liver cirrhosis, one with a spontaneous portocaval shunt and the other with a portocaval anastomosis.[88] The archetypal clinical presentation of HM is that of a patient with pre-existing chronic liver disease, developing progressive pure motor spastic paraparesis with minimal sensory deficit and negligible bowel and bladder involvement. The majority of patients report prior episodes of HE and the development of myelopathy often follows the creation of surgical shunts.[89] Prompt and accurate diagnosis of HM is vital due to the ability of patients with early stages of the disease to recover following liver transplantation.[90] Neuropathological findings show demyelination in the lateral corticospinal tracts, with variable degrees of axonal loss.[87] Motor-evoked potential studies may be useful for the early diagnosis of HM, even in patients with preclinical stages of the disease.[91]

Neurological Complications and Mechanisms

The pathogenesis of HM is not fully described. It is widely held that portocaval shunts, or less commonly splenorenal shunts, play a critical role even in the absence of hepatocellular dysfunction.[92] It has been proposed that alteration of the hepatic metabolism leads to deficiencies of CNS essential nutrients, and nitrogenous waste products such as ammonia, mercaptans, and fatty acids bypassing the liver via the portocaval shunt play a contributory role.[91,84] These products cause damage to the axon cylinder, neuronal cell bodies, and myelin.

Moreover, there is a disparity between the tissue reaction in the corticospinal tract and sparing of other spinal cord pathways, where axonal degeneration and demyelination, cytoplasmic astrocytosis, and round-cell infiltration occur, and the reaction in the brain and brainstem, where significant proliferation of Alzheimer type II astrocytes is observed. These distinct sensitivities suggest two pathogenic mechanisms, one responsible for the lesions observed in the brain and brainstem and the other for those seen in the spinal cord. Alternatively, a single factor may be responsible for the generation of both lesions.[93]

Hepatic myelopathy has been shown to be unceasingly progressive, unresponsive to ammonia-lowering therapy and liver transplantation excluding rare reports of recovery.[90] A liver transplant could fully reverse the effects of HM in early-stage patients; however, it has little documented effect in patients with advanced disease.[94]

Nonalcoholic Fatty Liver Disease

Nonalcoholic fatty liver disease is an encompassing term referring to the occurrence of hepatic steatosis in the absence of other causes for secondary hepatic fat accumulation (e.g., substantial alcohol consumption).[95] Clinical histories of NAFLD point toward a natural progression in some individuals to end-stage liver disease.

Nonalcoholic fatty liver disease may progress to hepatocellular carcinoma and cirrhosis and is suspected to be an important trigger of cryptogenic cirrhosis.[96] Obesity is associated with a clinical spectrum of liver abnormalities collectively known as NAFLD, with both diseases sharing increased risk for type 2 diabetes mellitus. NAFLD is divided into two subcategories defined by histologic mechanisms:[97] nonalcoholic steatohepatitis (NASH) and nonalcoholic fatty liver (NAFL).[98]

Nonalcoholic fatty liver disease is seen worldwide and affects all ethnicities and both sexes through distinct manifestations. In the United States, studies utilizing aminotransferase levels report a prevalence of NAFLD of 11%, with most biopsy-based studies reporting a prevalence of NASH of 3–5%.[99] Internationally, NAFLD has a suspected prevalence between 6 and 35% of the world population. In the United States, the prevalence of NAFLD has been increasing over time.[98]

The majority of patients with NAFLD are asymptomatic, although patients with NASH may describe fatigue, general right upper abdominal pain, and malaise.[100] Patients with NAFLD may have an enlarged liver upon physical examination due to fatty infiltration. Hepatomegaly is the presenting sign of NAFLD in some patients. Patients who have developed cirrhosis may have signs of chronic liver disease such as ascites.[101] NAFLD is a precursor of type 2 diabetes (T2D).[102]

Neurological Complications

There exist some forms of liver disease that are not well studied for their involvement in neurological conditions, such as NAFLD. However, patients with NAFLD may eventually develop cirrhosis. Cirrhosis develops when simple steatosis progresses to steatohepatitis and then fibrosis. Among patients with cryptogenic cirrhosis, up to 70% have risk factors for NAFLD.[4] While the risk of disease progression among patients with NAFLD has been evaluated in multiple studies, the results have been variable, and the risk of developing advanced fibrosis among patients with NAFLD is unclear. Patients who develop complications of cirrhosis, such as variceal hemorrhage, ascites, spontaneous bacterial peritonitis, hepatocellular carcinoma, hepatorenal syndrome, or hepatopulmonary syndrome, are considered to have decompensated cirrhosis and have a worse prognosis than those with compensated cirrhosis.[103]

As noted above, NAFLD is associated with metabolic syndrome, incident diabetes, carotid atherosclerosis, and endothelial dysfunction, conditions that, in turn, are strongly linked with brain damage and cognitive impairment.[104] While it is not known whether NAFLD is associated with structural brain measures in humans, a recent study reported no statistically significant associations between NAFLD and hippocampal or white matter hyperintensity volumes or covert brain infarcts.[105] Cognitive function in aged individuals[106] and cognitive changes[107] and brain volume reduction in patients with NAFLD have been identified.[105] Further, NAFLD was shown to induce signs of Alzheimer's disease (AD) in wild-type mice and accelerate pathological signs of AD in an AD model,[108] locomotor activity and stereotypic behavior,[109] insulin resistance, and metabolic disorders with development of brain damage and dysfunction.[110]

While the role of NAFLD in brain dysfunction has been strongly implicated more recently, the mechanism by which NAFLD contributes to the defect in neuronal function is unknown.

Autoimmune Liver Disease

The three main types of autoimmune liver disease (AILD) are autoimmune hepatitis (AIH), primary biliary cirrhosis (PBC), and primary sclerosing cholangitis (PSC). All three are well-defined diseases with diagnosis based on a collection of clinical, serologic, and liver pathology results.[111] AIH is a relapsing idiopathic hepatitis, affecting more women than men across all age groups and ethnicities.[112] PBC is a chronic cholestatic condition predominantly affecting middle-aged females (female : male ratio of 9 : 1) and is distinguished via biochemical cholestasis and granulomatous cholangitis.[113] PSC, also a chronic cholestatic liver disease, is characterized by fibrosing inflammatory damage to the extrahepatic and intrahepatic bile ducts.[114] Although the nature of these diseases is considered autoimmune, the etiology and potential environmental causes of each remain ambiguous.[111]

Neurological Complications and Mechanisms

The etiology of AIH remains unspecified, but evidence indicates a combination of genetic susceptibility and environmental factors, culminating in immune tolerance deficiency leading to T-cell-mediated eradication of hepatocytes.[115] Local gene regulatory networks involving regulatory T-cells are implicated in liver pathogenesis; however, animal models reveal that AIH may result from impaired central tolerance. This has been established by the onset of AIH in mice deficient in medullary thymic epithelial cells.[116]

Primary biliary cirrhosis is associated with malaise, cognitive impairment, and sleeping difficulties. These symptoms allude to the existence of underlying CNS dysfunction. Fatigue develops during exercise due to muscular mechanisms (i.e., peripheral fatigue) and decreased neurotransmitter activation of the motor unit (central fatigue).[117] Patients with PBV have impaired central activation and atypical intracortical inhibition (ICI), suggesting CNS aberrations beyond voluntary control. Both transplanted and nontransplanted patients show similar abnormalities, raising questions concerning the processes underpinning these changes and the longevity of neurological dysfunction in PBC.[118]

While the role of AILD in brain dysfunction has been strongly correlated, the course by which AILD influences the defect in neuronal function is unknown.

CONCLUSION

Neurological complications in liver disease, such as HE, represent an irreversible impairment of neuropsychiatric function which occurs in many conditions including acute and chronic liver failure, viral hepatitis, neoplasm, AILD, non-Wilsonian AHCD as well as in HM.[3,119] In acute and chronic HE, ammonia and cytokines are implicated in the mechanisms of neurological complications, while excess ammonia is implicated in the pathogenesis of non-Wilsonian AHCD as well as in HM. However, the role of liver failure on CNS dysfunction due to drugs of abuse is currently unknown. Additionally, whether agents known to induce CNS dysfunction in acute or chronic HE due to drug toxicity (e.g., elevated blood and brain ammonia and cytokines due to acetaminophen poisoning) also occur in potential drug abuse should be examined.

Certain liver diseases do not demonstrate neurological complications. These include hepatitis D, NAFLD, congestive hepatopathy, etc. The reason for such discrepancies is unknown. However, it is possible that the severity of the disease varies between these liver disorders or the pathogenic factors that are implicated in neurological complications in certain forms of liver disease (e.g., ALF, HCV) may not occur in these liver disorders. Therefore, a careful and exhaustive investigation is needed to identify whether neurological complications occur in these conditions and potential risk factors involved in such processes.

ACKNOWLEDGMENTS

We would like to thank the American Association for the Study of Liver Diseases (AASLD). We also thank Dr Daniel Pelaez, Research Assistant Professor, Department of Ophthalmology, Bascom Palmer Eye Institute, University of Miami Miller School of Medicine, Miami FL, USA, for his helpful comments and suggestions.

CONFLICT OF INTEREST

The authors declare that they have no conflict of interest.

REFERENCES

1. Bhatia SN, Underhill GH, Zaret KS, Fox IJ. Cell and tissue engineering for liver disease. Science Translational Medicine. 2014;6(245):245sr2.
2. Foundation AL. (2016) The progression of liver disease. [online] Available from https://liverfoundation.org/for-patients/about-the-liver/the-progression-of-liverdisease/. [Last accessed February, 2020].
3. Nusrat S, Khan MS, Fazili J, Madhoun MF. Cirrhosis and its complications: Evidence-based treatment. World J Gastroenterol. 2014;20(18):5442-60.

4. Caldwell SH, Crespo DM. The spectrum expanded: Cryptogenic cirrhosis and the natural history of non-alcoholic fatty liver disease. J Hepatol. 2004;40(4):578-84.
5. Jayakumar AR, Rama Rao KV, Norenberg MD. Neuroinflammation in hepatic encephalopathy: Mechanistic aspects. J Clin Exp Hepatol. 2015;5(Suppl 1):S21-8.
6. Butterworth RF. Hepatic encephalopathy. Alcohol Res Health. 2003;27(3):240-6.
7. Hughes RD, Wendon J, Gimson AE. Acute liver failure. Gut. 1991;(Suppl):S86-91.
8. Jayakumar AR, Ruiz-Cordero R, Tong XY, Norenberg MD. Brain edema in acute liver failure: role of neurosteroids. Arch Biochem Biophys. 2013;536(2):171-5.
9. Shokoohi H, Pourmand A, Teng J, Lucas J. Acute liver failure and emergency consideration for liver transplant. Am J Emerg Med. 2017;35(11):1779-81.
10. Wang DW, Yin YM, Yao YM. Advances in the management of acute liver failure. World J Gastroenterol. 2013;19(41):7069-77.
11. Lee WM, Squires RH, Nyberg SL, Doo E, Hoofnagle JH. Acute liver failure: summary of a workshop. Hepatology. 2008;47(4):1401-15.
12. Scott TR, Kronsten VT, Hughes RD, Shawcross DL. Pathophysiology of cerebral oedema in acute liver failure. World J Gastroenterol. 2013;19(48):9240-55.
13. Shaker MC, William D. (2014) Hepatic encephalopathy. [online] Available from http://www.clevelandclinicmeded.com/medicalpubs/diseasemanagement/hepatology/hepatic-encephalopathy/. [Last accessed February, 2020].
14. Michinaga S, Koyama Y. Pathogenesis of brain edema and investigation into antiedema drugs. Int J Mol Sci. 2015;16(5):9949-75.
15. Wetherington J, Serrano G, Dingledine R. Astrocytes in the epileptic brain. Neuron. 2008;58(2):168-78.
16. Bullock R, Maxwell WL, Graham DI, Teasdale GM, Adams JH. Glial swelling following human cerebral contusion: an ultrastructural study. J Neurol Neurosurg Psychiatry. 1991;54(5):427-34.
17. Haack N, Dublin P, Rose CR. Dysbalance of astrocyte calcium under hyperammonemic conditions. PLoS One. 2014;9(8):e105832.
18. Rama Rao KV, Verkman AS, Curtis KM, Norenberg MD. Aquaporin-4 deletion in mice reduces encephalopathy and brain edema in experimental acute liver failure. Neurobiol Dis. 2014;63:222-8.
19. Jones EA, Weissenborn K. Neurology and the liver. J Neurol Neurosurg Psychiatry. 1997;63(3):279-93.
20. Krieger S, Jauss M, Jansen O, Theilmann L, Geissler M, Krieger D. Neuropsychiatric profile and hyperintense globus pallidus on T1-weighted magnetic resonance images in liver cirrhosis. Gastroenterology. 1996;111(1):147-55.
21. National Organization for Rare Disorders. (2011) Hepatic encephalopathy. Available from https://rarediseases.org/rare-diseases/hepatic-encephalopathy/#references [Last accessed February 2020].
22. Rani P. Clerkship-II, Department of Gastroenterology. India: Care College of Pharmacy; 2017.
23. Bajaj JS, Wade JB, Sanyal AJ. Spectrum of neurocognitive impairment in cirrhosis: implications for the assessment of hepatic encephalopathy. Hepatology. 2009;50(6):2014-21.

24. Goldberg E, Chopra S. Acute liver failure in adults: Etiology, clinical manifestations, and diagnosis. UpToDate; 2017.
25. World Health Organization. (2012) Hepatitis A Vaccine Information Sheet. [online] Available from www.who.int › tools › Hep_A_Vaccine_rates_information_sheet [Last accessed February, 2020].
26. Fiore AE. Hepatitis A transmitted by food. Clin Infect Dis. 2004;38(5):705-15.
27. Lemon SM. Type A viral hepatitis: New developments in an old disease. N Engl J Med. 1985;313(17):1059-67.
28. Lednar WM, Lemon SM, Kirkpatrick JW, Redfield RR, Fields ML, Kelley PW. Frequency of illness associated with epidemic hepatitis A virus infections in adults. Am J Epidemiol. 1985;122(2):226-33.
29. Lai M, Chopra S. Hepatitis A virus infection in adults: Epidemiology, clinical manifestations, and diagnosis. UpToDate;2016.
30. Jo YS, Han SD, Choi JY, Kim IH, Kim YD, Na SJ. A case of acute motor and sensory axonal neuropathy following hepatitis A infection. J Korean Med Sci. 2013;28(12):1839-41.
31. Islam S, McDonald JA. Sensory neuropathy in the prodromal phase of hepatitis A and review of the literature. J Gastroenterol Hepatol. 2000;15(7):809-11.
32. Tabor E. Guillain-Barré syndrome and other neurologic syndromes in hepatitis A, B, and non-A, non-B. J Med Virol. 1987;21(3):207-16.
33. Yildirim S, Adviye R, Gül HL, Türk Börü Ü. Acute motor axonal neuropathy (AMAN) with motor conduction blocks in childhood: case report. Iran J Child Neurol. 2016;10(1):65-9.
34. Griffin JW, Li CY, Ho TW, Tian M, Gao CY, Xue P, et al. Pathology of the motor- sensory axonal Guillain-Barré syndrome. Ann Neurol. 1996;39(1):17-28.
35. Dimachkie MM, Barohn RJ. Guillain-Barré syndrome and variants. Neurol Clin. 2013;31(2):491-510.
36. World Health Organization. (2018) Hepatitis B. [online] Available from www.who.int› hepatitis [Last accessed February, 2020].
37. Nam TS, Lee SH, Park MS, Choi KH, Kim JT, Choi SM, et al. Mononeuropathy multiplex in a patient with chronic active hepatitis B. J Clin Neurol. 2010;6(3):156-8.
38. Tsukada N, Koh CS, Inoue A, Yanagisawa N. Demyelinating neuropathy associated with hepatitis B virus infection. Detection of immune complexes composed of hepatitis B virus surface antigen. J Neurol Sci. 1987;77(2-3):203-16.
39. Maier I, Wu GY. Hepatitis C and HIV co-infection: a review. World J Gastroenterol. 2002;8(4):577-9.
40. Singhatiraj E, Suri J, Goulston C. HIV co-infections with hepatitis B and C. J AIDS Clin Res. 2012;3:1-12.
41. Picco M. Hepatitis C: What happens in end-stage liver disease? Mayo Foundation for Medical Education and Research (MFMER), 2018.
42. Chopra S. (2018) Clinical manifestations and natural history of chronic hepatitis C virus infection. [online] Available from https://www.uptodate.com/contents/clinical-manifestations-and-natural-history-of-chronic-hepatitis-c-virus-infection [Last accessed February, 2020]

43. Bolay H, Söylemezoğlu F, Nurlu G, Tuncer S, Varli K. PCR detected hepatitis C virus genome in the brain of a case with progressive encephalomyelitis with rigidity. Clin Neurol Neurosurg. 1996;98(4):305-8.
44. Aktipi KM, Ravaglia S, Ceroni M, Nemni R, Debiaggi M, Bastianello S, et al. Severe recurrent myelitis in patients with hepatitis C virus infection. Neurology. 2007;68(6):468-9.
45. Mathew S, Faheem M, Ibrahim SM, Iqbal W, Rauff B, Fatima K, et al. Hepatitis C virus and neurological damage. World J Hepatol. 2016;8(12):545-56.
46. Sim JE, Lee JB, Cho YN, Suh SH, Kim JK, Lee KY. A case of acute disseminated encephalomyelitis associated with hepatitis C virus infection. Yonsei Med J. 2012;53(4):856-8.
47. Adinolfi LE, Nevola R, Lus G, Restivo L, Guerrera B, Romano C, et al. Chronic hepatitis C virus infection and neurological and psychiatric disorders: an overview. World J Gastroenterol. 2015;21(8):2269-80.
48. Origgi L, Vanoli M, Carbone A, Grasso M, Scorza R. Central nervous system involvement in patients with HCV-related cryoglobulinemia. Am J Med Sci. 1998;315(3):208-10.
49. Arena MG, Ferlazzo E, Bonanno D, Quattrocchi P, Ferlazzo B. Cerebral vasculitis in a patient with HCV-related type II mixed cryoglobulinemia. J Investig Allergol Clin Immunol. 2003;13(2):135-6.
50. Malnick SD, Abend Y, Evron E, Sthoeger ZM. HCV hepatitis associated with anticardiolipin antibody and a cerebrovascular accident. Response to interferon therapy. J Clin Gastroenterol. 1997;24(1):40-2.
51. Monaco S, Ferrari S, Gajofatto A, Zanusso G, Mariotto S. HCV-related nervous system disorders. Clin Dev Immunol. 2012;2012:236148.
52. Serena M, Biscaro R, Moretto G, Recchia E. Peripheral and central nervous system involvement in essential mixed cryoglobulinemia: a case report. Clin Neuropathol. 1991;10(4):177-80.
53. Buccoliero R, Gambelli S, Sicurelli F, Malandrini A, Palmeri S, De Santis M, et al. Leukoencephalopathy as a rare complication of hepatitis C infection. Neurol Sci. 2006;27(5):360-3.
54. Casato M, Saadoun D, Marchetti A, Limal N, Picq C, Pantano P, et al. Central nervous system involvement in hepatitis C virus cryoglobulinemia vasculitis: a multicenter case-control study using magnetic resonance imaging and neuropsychological tests. J Rheumatol. 2005;32(3):484-8.
55. Seifert F, Struffert T, Hildebrandt M, Blümcke I, Brück W, Staykov D, et al. In vivo detection of hepatitis C virus (HCV) RNA in the brain in a case of encephalitis: evidence for HCV neuroinvasion. Eur J Neurol. 2008;15(3):214-8.
56. Sacconi S, Salviati L, Merelli E. Acute disseminated encephalomyelitis associated with hepatitis C virus infection. Arch Neurol. 2001;58(10):1679-81.
57. Bokemeyer M, Ding XQ, Goldbecker A, Raab P, Heeren M, Arvanitis D, et al. Evidence for neuroinflammation and neuroprotection in HCV infection-associated encephalopathy. Gut. 2011;60(3):370-7.
58. Forton DM, Allsop JM, Main J, Foster GR, Thomas HC, Taylor-Robinson SD. Evidence for a cerebral effect of the hepatitis C virus. Lancet. 2001;358(9275):38-9.

59. Heeren M, Weissenborn K, Arvanitis D, Bokemeyer M, Goldbecker A, Tountopoulou A, et al. Cerebral glucose utilisation in hepatitis C virus infection-associated encephalopathy. J Cereb Blood Flow Metab. 2011;31(11):2199-208.
60. Piche T, Vanbiervliet G, Cherikh F, Antoun Z, Huet PM, Gelsi E, et al. Effect of ondansetron, a 5-HT3 receptor antagonist, on fatigue in chronic hepatitis C: A randomised, double blind, placebo-controlled study. Gut. 2005;54(8):1169-73.
61. Cozzi A, Zignego AL, Carpendo R, Biagiotti T, Aldinucci A, Monti M, et al. Low serum tryptophan levels, reduced macrophage IDO activity and high frequency of psychopathology in HCV patients. J Viral Hepat. 2006;13(6):402-8.
62. Jones EM, Gray-Keller M, Art JJ, Fettiplace R. The functional role of alternative splicing of Ca^{2+} activated K^+ channels in auditory hair cells. Ann NY Acad Sci. 1999;868:379-85.
63. Satoh J, Eguchi Y, Narukiyo T, Mizuta T, Kobayashi O, Kawai M, et al. Necrotizing myopathy in a patient with chronic hepatitis C virus infection: A case report and a review of the literature. Intern Med. 2000;39(2):176-81.
64. Zoccolella S, Serlenga L, Amati A, Lavolpe V, Minerva N, Agremorz M, et al. A case of vacuolar myopathy during the course of chronic hepatitis C. Funct Neurol. 2006;21(3):167-9.
65. Cortelli P, Mandrioli J, Zeviani M, Lodi R, Prata C, Pecorari M, et al. Mitochondrial complex III deficiency in a case of HCV related noninflammatory myopathy. J Neurol. 2007;254(10):1450-2.
66. Zhu N, Khoshnan A, Schneider R, Matsumoto M, Dennert G, Ware C, et al. Hepatitis C virus core protein binds to the cytoplasmic domain of tumor necrosis factor (TNF) receptor 1 and enhances TNF-induced apoptosis. J Virol. 1998;72(5):3691-7.
67. Yarlott L, Heald E, Forton D. Hepatitis C virus infection, and neurological and psychiatric disorders: A review. J Adv Res. 2017;8(2):139-48.
68. Schwartz JM, Kruskal JB. (2018) Solid liver lesions: Differential diagnosis and evaluation. [online] Available from https://www.uptodate.com/contents/solid-liver-lesions-differential-diagnosisand-evaluation [Last accessed February, 2020]
69. Bonder A, Afdhal N. Evaluation of liver lesions. Clin Liver Dis. 2012; 16(2):271-83.
70. Colombo M, de Franchis R, Del Ninno E, Sangiovanni A, De Fazio C, Tommasini M, et al. Hepatocellular carcinoma in Italian patients with cirrhosis. N Engl J Med. 1991;325(10):675-80.
71. KimBK, RevillPA, AhnSH. HBV genotypes: Relevance to natural history, pathogenesis and treatment of chronic hepatitis B. Antivir Ther. 2011;16(8):1169-86.
72. Choi HJ, Cho BC, Sohn JH, Shin SJ, Kim SH, Kim JH, et al. Brain metastases from hepatocellular carcinoma: prognostic factors and outcome: Brain metastasis from HCC. J Neurooncol. 2009;91(3):307-13.
73. Brain Mets–aboutcancer.com. (1998) Clinical manifestations and diagnosis of brain metastases. [online] Available from http://www.aboutcancer.com/brain_met_utd_1207.htm [Last accessed February, 2020].
74. Stone JB, DeAngelis LM. Cancer-treatment-induced neurotoxicity: Focus on newer treatments. Nat Rev Clin Oncol. 2016;13(2):92-105.
75. Health NI. Asparaginase. In: Services USDoHH (Ed). Bethesda, MD: US National Library of Medicine; 2017.

76. Bellet RE, Mastrangelo MJ, Engstrom PF, Custer RP. Hepatotoxicity of 5-azacytidine (NSC-102816): A clinical and pathologic study. Neoplasma. 1973;20(3):303-9.
77. Cersosimo RJ. Hepatotoxicity associated with cisplatin chemotherapy. Ann Pharmacother. 1993;27(4):438-41.
78. Finlayson MH, Superville B. Distribution of cerebral lesions in acquired hepatocerebral degeneration. Brain. 1981;104(Pt 1):79-95.
79. Jog MS, Lang AE. Chronic acquired hepatocerebral degeneration: case reports and new insights. Mov Disord. 1995;10(6):714-22.
80. Burkhard PR, Delavelle J, Du Pasquier R, Spahr L. Chronic parkinsonism associated with cirrhosis: a distinct subset of acquired hepatocerebral degeneration. Arch Neurol. 2003;60(4):521-8.
81. Meissner W, Tison F. Acquired hepatocerebral degeneration. Handb Clin Neurol. 2011;100:193-7.
82. Victor M, Adams RD, Cole M. The acquired (non-Wilsonian) type of chronic hepatocerebral degeneration. Medicine (Baltimore). 1965;44(5):345-96.
83. Stracciari A, Guarino M, Pazzaglia P, Marchesini G, Pisi P. Acquired hepatocerebral degeneration: full recovery after liver transplantation. J Neurol Neurosurg Psychiatry. 2001;70(1):136-7.
84. Lewis M, Howdle PD. The neurology of liver failure. QJM. 2003;96(9):623-33.
85. Servin-Abad L, Tzakis A, Schiff ER, Regev A. Acquired hepatocerebral degeneration in a patient with HCV cirrhosis: complete resolution with subsequent recurrence after liver transplantation. Liver Transpl. 2006;12(7):1161-5.
86. Leigh AD, Card WI. Hepato lenticular degeneration: A case associated with posterolateral column degeneration. J Neuropathol Exp Neurol. 1949;8(3):338-46.
87. Zieve L, Mendelson DF, Goepfert M. Shunt encephalomyelopathy. II. Occurrence of permanent myelopathy. Ann Intern Med. 1960;53:53-63.
88. Pant SS, Bhargava AN, Singh MM, Dhanda PC. Myelopathy in hepatic cirrhosis. Br Med J. 1963;1(5337):1064-5.
89. Mendoza G, Marti-Fàbregas J, Kulisevsky J, Escartín A. Hepatic myelopathy: A rare complication of portacaval shunt. Eur Neurol. 1994;34(4):209-12.
90. Weissenborn K, Tietge UJ, Bokemeyer M, Mohammadi B, Bode U, Manns MP, et al. Liver transplantation improves hepatic myelopathy: evidence by three cases. Gastroenterology. 2003;124(2):346-51.
91. Premkumar M, Bagchi A, Kapoor N, Gupta A, Maurya G, Vatsya S, et al. Hepatic myelopathy in a patient with decompensated alcoholic cirrhosis and portal colopathy. Case Reports Hepatol. 2012;2012:735906.
92. Bain VG, Bailey RJ, Jhamandas JH. Postshunt myelopathy. J Clin Gastroenterol. 1991;13(5):562-4.
93. Lefer LG, Vogel FS. Encephalomyelopathy with hepatic cirrhosis following portosystemic venous shunts. Arch Pathol. 1972;93(2):91-7.
94. Kori P, Sahu R, Jaiswal A, Shukla R. Hepatic myelopathy: An unusual neurological complication of chronic liver disease presenting as quadriparesis. BMJ Case Rep. 2013;2013. pii: bcr2013009078.
95. Friedman SL, Neuschwander-Tetri BA, Rinella M, Sanyal AJ. Mechanisms of NAFLD development and therapeutic strategies. Nat Med. 2018;24(7):908-22.

96. Calzadilla Bertot L, Adams LA. The natural course of non-alcoholic fatty liver disease. Int J Mol Sci. 2016;17(5).
97. Byrne CD, Targher G. NAFLD: A multisystem disease. J Hepatol. 2015;62(1 Suppl):S47-64.
98. Born TA. (2013) Nonalcoholic Fatty Liver Disease (NAFLD), Why We Need To Be Responsive: Born Naturopathic Associates, Inc. [online] Available from: http://www.bornnaturopathic.com/blog/health-articles/nonalcoholic-fatty-liver- disease-nafldneed-responsive/ [Last accessed February, 2020].
99. Perumpail BJ, Khan MA, Yoo ER, Cholankeril G, Kim D, Ahmed A. Clinical epidemiology and disease burden of nonalcoholic fatty liver disease. World J Gastroenterol. 2017;23(47):8263-76.
100. Powell EE, Cooksley WG, Hanson R, Searle J, Halliday JW, Powell LW. The natural history of nonalcoholic steatohepatitis: A follow-up study of forty-two patients for up to 21 years. Hepatology. 1990;11(1):74-80.
101. Stengel JZ, Harrison SA. Nonalcoholic steatohepatitis: Clinical presentation, diagnosis, and treatment. Gastroenterol Hepatol (N Y). 2006;2(6):440-9.
102. Lonardo A, Bellentani S, Ratziu V, Loria P. Insulin resistance in nonalcoholic steatohepatitis: necessary but not sufficient—death of a dogma from analysis of therapeutic studies? Expert Rev Gastroenterol Hepatol. 2011;5(2):279-89.
103. Runyon BA. Hepatorenal syndrome. UpToDate; 2009.
104. Filipovic B, Markovic O, Duric V, Filipovic B. Cognitive changes and brain volume reduction in patients with nonalcoholic fatty liver disease. Can J Gastroenterol Hepatol. 2018;2018:9638797.
105. Weinstein G, Zelber-Sagi S, Preis SR, Beiser AS, DeCarli C, Speliotes EK, et al. Association of nonalcoholic fatty liver disease with lower brain volume in healthy middle-aged adults in the Framingham study. JAMA Neurol. 2018;75(1):97-104.
106. Brodersen C, Koen E, Ponte A, Sanchez S, Segal E, Chiapella A, et al. Cognitive function in patients with alcoholic and nonalcoholic chronic liver disease. J Neuropsychiatry Clin Neurosci. 2014;26(3):241-8.
107. Seo SW, Gottesman RF, Clark JM, Hernaez R, Chang Y, Kim C, et al. Nonalcoholic fatty liver disease is associated with cognitive function in adults. Neurology. 2016;86(12):1136-42.
108. Kim DG, Krenz A, Toussaint LE, Maurer KJ, Robinson SA, Yan A, et al. Non- alcoholic fatty liver disease induces signs of Alzheimer's disease (AD) in wild- type mice and accelerates pathological signs of AD in an AD model. J Neuroinflammation. 2016;13:1.
109. Erbas O, Akseki HS, Solmaz V, Aktug H, Taskiran D. Fatty liver-induced changes in stereotypic behavior in rats and effects of glucagon-like peptide-1 analog on stereotypy. Kaohsiung J Med Sci. 2014;30(9):447-52.
110. Ghareeb DA, Hafez HS, Hussien HM, Kabapy NF. Non-alcoholic fatty liver induces insulin resistance and metabolic disorders with development of brain damage and dysfunction. Metab Brain Dis. 2011;26(4):253-67.
111. Washington MK. Autoimmune liver disease: overlap and outliers. Mod Pathol. 2007;20(Suppl 1):S15-30.
112. Decock S, McGee P, Hirschfield GM. Autoimmune liver disease for the non- specialist. BMJ. 2009;339:b3305.

113. Hohenester S, Oude-Elferink RP, Beuers U. Primary biliary cirrhosis. Semin Immunopathol. 2009;31(3):283-307.
114. Williamson KD, Chapman RW. Primary sclerosing cholangitis. Dig Dis. 2014;32(4):438-45.
115. Corrigan M, Hirschfield GM, Oo YH, Adams DH. Autoimmune hepatitis: An approach to disease understanding and management. Br Med Bull. 2015;114(1):181-91.
116. Bonito AJ, Aloman C, Fiel MI, Danzl NM, Cha S, Weinstein EG, et al. Medullary thymic epithelial cell depletion leads to autoimmune hepatitis. J Clin Invest. 2013;123(8):3510-24.
117. Zajac A, Chalimoniuk M, Maszczyk A, Golas A, Lngfort J. Central and peripheral fatigue during resistance exercise: a critical review. J Hum Kinet. 2015;49:159-69.
118. McDonald C, Newton J, Lai HM, Baker SN, Jones DE. Central nervous system dysfunction in primary biliary cirrhosis and its relationship to symptoms. J Hepatol. 2010;53(6):1095-100.
119. Ferenci P. Hepatic encephalopathy. Gastroenterol Rep (Oxf). 2017;5(2):138-47.

CHAPTER

14

The Impact of COVID-19 on Gastroenterology

Her Hsin Tsai

INTRODUCTION

At the time of writing this review, the coronavirus disease 2019 (COVID-19) pandemic is raging across the world with hardly any nation escaping the infection. This infection has preoccupied governments, health establishments and care-workers that are battling to contain it. This disease is caused by the novel coronavirus, now designated severe acute respiratory syndrome coronavirus 2 (SARS-CoV-2). It is primarily an upper respiratory infection. However, it does impact on all specialties in medicine. Needless to say, COVID-19 has had a major impact of on gastroenterology and the effect may linger long after the pandemic is over. The impact on gastroenterology is multi-faceted. Firstly, there is the effect of virus SARS-CoV-2 on the gastrointestinal (GI) tract itself. Secondly, there is the effect naturally of a highly infectious agent on the ongoing care of GI and liver patients. This virus has a particularly deleterious effect on immunocompromised or immunosuppressed individuals. Also, particularly at endoscopy where close contact with the patient and potential contamination with bodily fluids, there is a risk of nosocomial transmission. Finally, there is the effect of the redirection of healthcare priorities to fighting COVID-19 and by the deprivation and reduction of gastroenterology services to chronic GI patients and thus causing a negative impact on many of these important gastroenterology services.[1]

THE STRUCTURE OF SARS-COV-2

SARS-CoV-2 is the strain of coronavirus that causes COVID-19, largely a respiratory illness. SARS-CoV-2 is a positive-sense single-stranded RNA virus. It is a highly contagious agent in humans, and the World Health Organization (WHO) has designated the ongoing pandemic of COVID-19 a Public Health Emergency of International Concern.

SARS-CoV-2 is classed as a strain of severe acute respiratory syndrome-related coronavirus (SARSr-CoV).[2] It is believed to have zoonotic origins and has close genetic similarity to bat coronaviruses, suggesting it emerged from a bat-borne virus reservoir.

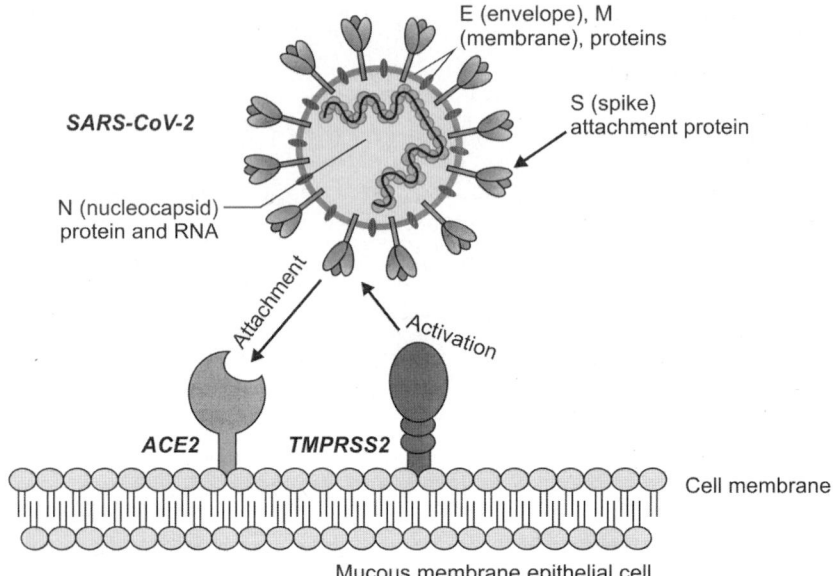

Fig. 1: The attachment of SARS-CoV-2 to host cell.
(ACE2: angiotensin-converting enzyme 2; TMPSS2: transmembrane protease, serine 2)

Each SARS-CoV-2 virion is 50–200 nanometer in size and has four structural proteins, known as the S (spike), E (envelope), M (membrane), and N (nucleocapsid) proteins; the N protein holds the RNA genome, and the S, E, and M proteins together create the viral envelope **(Fig. 1)**. The spike protein is the protein responsible for allowing the virus to attach to and fuse with the membrane of a host cell.

Protein modeling experiments on the spike protein of the virus had suggested that SARS-CoV-2 has significant affinity for the receptor angiotensin-converting enzyme 2 (ACE2) on human cells and can use them as a mechanism of cell entry. Studies have shown that SARS-CoV-2 has a higher affinity to human ACE2 than the original SARS virus strain.[3]

Initial spike protein priming by transmembrane protease, serine 2 (TMPRSS2) is essential for entry of SARS-CoV-2.[4] After a SARS-CoV-2 virion attaches to a target cell, the cell's protease TMPRSS2 cuts open the spike protein of the virus, exposing a fusion peptide. After fusion, an endosome forms around the virion, separating it from the rest of the host cell. Thus the virion escapes lysis by the endosome. The virion then releases RNA into the cell and forces the cell to produce and disseminate copies of the virus, which infect more cells.

EPIDEMIOLOGY

The outbreak was first identified in Wuhan, China, in December 2019. The WHO declared the outbreak a Public Health Emergency of International

Concern on January 30, 2020 and a pandemic on March 11. As of June 9th 2020, more than 7 million cases of COVID-19 have been reported in more than 188 countries and territories, resulting in more than 402,000 deaths with more than 3.2 million people having recovered. However, it is likely that considerable more infections were subclinical or remain undiagnosed.[5]

The virus is primarily spread between people during close contact, most often via small droplets produced by coughing, sneezing, and talking. These droplets would stick to surfaces rather than traveling through air over long distances. Less commonly, people may become infected by touching a contaminated surface and then touching their face. It is most contagious during the first 3 days after the onset of symptoms, although spread is possible before symptoms appear, and from people who do not show symptoms.[6]

THE EFFECT OF SARS-COV-2 ON THE GASTROINTESTINAL TRACT

As the virus enters cells via the ACE2 receptor, there was interest in elucidating which mucosal cells exhibit this receptor. ACE2 is an enzyme attached to the cell membranes of cells in the lungs, arteries, heart, kidney, and intestines. ACE2 is highly expressed in GI mucosal cells from the esophagus to the colon. Early reports of postmortem on patients who had COVID-19 showed virus affecting esophageal tissue.[7] The virus could thus be shown to infect GI mucosal cells and replicate and shed virions into the lumen of the GI tract. Thus it is not surprising that SARS-CoV-2 has been detected in fecal samples of 48% of patients who had diarrheal symptoms. Even patients without GI symptoms of diarrhea may also shed the virus in the stool. Furthermore, virus has been detected in fecal samples of completely asymptomatic patients. Thus the virus may spread while patients were presymptomatic or asymptomatic.[8] More worryingly, this shedding of viruses might last for more than a month.[9] As a result, feces, sputum, even vomitus of potentially infected patients must be considered highly infectious.

Initial reports suggest that GI symptoms are common. The most common symptom is loss of appetite which was found in up to 50% of confirmed infections. This is not surprising as it is often the case in any pyrexial illness as a result of raised inflammatory state and pyrogens. Additionally, those with illness severe enough to be admitted are generally notably anorexic. As well was anorexia, nausea and vomiting is may occur, but this is notably more of a feature in children rather than adults. Diarrhea is variously reported to be present in up to 48% of hospitalized patients but the largest study now published of 7,736 patients with COVID-19, diarrhea was found in only 3.8% of patients.[10] It is hard to explain the differences in reporting, and although the large study was based on retrospective data, it was of a considerably larger population of infected individuals. We have to assume this symptom is not common and perhaps transient. There appears to be similar prevalence of diarrhea in both with mild or severe disease. There are other confounding factors in particular the use of drugs which may cause diarrhea in these patients. This is particularly apposite as antibiotics and antiviral agents are widely used.

Liver function (liver enzyme tests) are abnormal in a significant number of patients. Elevated levels of AST were observed in 112 (18.2%) of 615 patients with nonsevere disease and 56 (39.4%) of 142 patients with severe disease. Elevated levels of ALT were observed in 120 (19.8%) of patients with nonsevere disease and 38 (28.1%) of 135 patients with severe disease.[10] However, in this study it was commented that this could also be due to administered drugs used rather than the infection itself.[10] In another study, 62% of patients requiring ICU treatment were found to have liver injury.[11] Direct virus infection of the liver causing liver damage is possible. As the virus can gain access to the portal blood flow through its binding and infection of small intestinal mucosa. However, to date, postmortem liver studies have failed to show any virus inclusion bodies in the hepatocytes.[12] There are preliminary reports that ACE2 have been detected on bile duct epithelial cells which suggest that it could potentially be infected by SARS-CoV-2 virus.[12]

There have been reports of pancreatic injury associated with COVID-19 infections. In this study, 17% had evidence of pancreatic injury, as manifested by elevated amylase or lipase in routine laboratory studies. The patients did not appear to exhibit clinical pancreatitis. This may again be secondary to respiratory embarrassment or drugs. There is no evidence of direct viral infection of the pancreas.[13]

EFFECT OF COVID-19 ON GASTROINTESTINAL ENDOSCOPY

In infected individuals, virus is shed into the GI tract. This could be virus from nasopharyngeal infected secretions, swallowed by the individual which may survive the gastric acidity and digestive enzymes particularly if there is rapid transit diarrhea present. Also as previously mentioned, the GI tract expresses the receptor ACE2 on the mucosal cells, thus making them vulnerable to infection by the SARS-CoV-2 virus. The proportion of patients in whom stool samples tested positive was between 36% and 53% of all confirmed cases. It has been reported that there is a high accuracy of nucleic acid detection in stool samples. There appears to be no relation between positive rate of the fecal test and the severity of the disease activity or digestive symptoms.[14]

This leads to an obvious concern to the gastroenterologist of its effect on endoscopic procedures. The virus appears to be shed in the feces for up to a month even after the patient becomes symptom free. This may be the case for an unknown number of asymptomatic patients as well. Hence known patients with COVID-19 should be considered as high risk when procedures such as colonoscopy and flexible sigmoidoscopy are carried out. Thus extra precaution, personal protection equipment and scrupulous handwashing should be mandated and disinfection of surfaces in endoscopy rooms, computer mouse and keyboards and all possibly contaminated surfaces is required. This may also apply to all patients as there are an unknown number of asymptomatic patients who may shed the virus in the stool. As a consequence, there will be an increased workload and decreased turnover of endoscopic procedures during this pandemic.[1]

EFFECT OF COVID-19 ON PATIENTS WITH PRE-EXISTING GASTROINTESTINAL DISEASES

Patients with pre-existing GI condition may be at higher risk if infected with COVID-19. This is particularly of concern in patients who are immunosuppressed. The group of major concern are the patients with inflammatory bowel diseases who are on powerful immunosuppressants such as azathioprine and infliximab. Those patients on combination treatments would potentially be at increased risk. Thus national GI organizations have issued warnings and counseled extra-vigilance.[15] The key is to protect them from the infection. This may mean advise to stay at home as much as possible and wearing of masks, social distancing, and scrupulous hygiene. Avoidance of hospitals is desirable and may involve transitioning to e-clinics or telephone clinics.

In the large study reported by Guan et al.,[10] severe cases were more likely to have hepatitis B infection (2.4% vs. 0.6%) than nonsevere cases. This suggests that hepatitis B coinfection may be related to poorer outcome of COVID-19. There is limited data about other underlying chronic liver conditions such as nonalcoholic fatty liver disease, alcohol-related liver disease, and autoimmune hepatitis, and their effect on prognosis of COVID-19.[16] However, those with severe or end-stage liver conditions are likely to be vulnerable to an adverse outcome of the SARS-CoV-2 infection. Patients who have undergone liver transplants would be expected to be vulnerable too as they are immunosuppressed. These patients would need to be likewise protected.

Patients with COVID-19 and cancer were observed to have a higher risk of severe events. Thus several strategies have been proposed, such as intentional postponing of adjuvant chemotherapy or elective surgery on a patient-by-patient basis, stronger personal protection provisions, and more extensive testing.[17] The advice is for all cancer patients and not specifically for GI cancers.

EFFECT OF COVID-19 ON DELIVERY OF GASTROINTESTINAL SERVICES

The final area of concern and perhaps least addressed is the effect of the diversion of healthcare resources to the fight against COVID-19. Other more elective medical services are put on hold and may even have funding pulled. This includes important mortality affecting areas such as cancer diagnosis and screening. Bowel cancer screening may be put on hold, particularly that by flexible sigmoidoscopy. The FIT test version may still be possible but here, there is fear of samples contaminated with SARS-CoV-2 and fear by the postal or delivery services. Bowel cancer screening has well proven survival benefits which may sadly be relegated in importance in the light of the burden that COVID-19 has placed on national health resources.[18] Detection of early stage colorectal cancer has proven benefits with increased survival rates and postponement of detection even by a few months or so may adversely affect it. Additionally, there may be a worryingly number who have mild GI symptoms whose diagnostic procedure may be greatly delayed by the pandemic.[19]

Other GI services that will be affected will be the chronic GI conditions such as inflammatory bowel disease and chronic liver conditions. The suspension of face-to-face clinic consultations during the lockdown is understandable. Some may find that their biologic infusion schedules may be disrupted or postponed. As a consequence, patients with chronic GI diseases such as inflammatory bowel diseases may have to suffer in silence while their management remains suboptimum. Innovative solutions such as mobile apps and E-clinics may be the way forward.

The impact of COVID-19 worldwide on gastroenterology is extensive and its effects may be felt last long after the pandemic is over.

REFERENCES

1. Tsai HH. COVID-19 and the gastroenterologist. Gastro Hep.2020;2:90-1.
2. Gorbalenya AE, Baker SC, Baric RS, de Groot RJ, Drosten C, Gulyaeva AA, et al. The species severe acute respiratory syndrome-related coronavirus: classifying 2019-nCoV and naming it SARS-CoV-2. Nat Microbio. 2020;5(4):536-44.
3. Wrapp D, Wang N, Corbett KS, Goldsmith JA, Hsieh CL, Abiona O, et al. Cryo-EM structure of the 2019-nCoV spike in the prefusion conformation. Science. 2020;367(6483):1260-3.
4. Hoffman M, Kliene-Weber H, Krüger N, Herrler T, Erichsen S, Schiergens TS, et al. SARS-CoV-2 cell entry depends on ACE2 and TMPRSS2 and is blocked by a clinically proven protease inhibitor. Cell. 2020;181(2):271-80.e8.
5. COVID-19 Dashboard by the Center for Systems Science and Engineering (CSSE) at Johns Hopkins University (JHU). ArcGIS. Maryland: Johns Hopkins University; 2020.
6. Centers for Disease Control and Prevention (CDC). "How COVID-19 Spreads". [online] Available from https://www.cdc.gov/widgets/micrositeCollectionViewerMed/index.html [Last Accessed June, 2020].
7. Zhang H, Kang Z, Gong H, Xu D, Wang J, Liet Z, et al. The digestive system is a potential route of 2019-nCov infection: a bioinformatics analysis based on single-cell transcriptomes. BioRxiv. 927806.
8. Cheung KS, Hung IF, Chan PP, Lung KC, Tso E, Liu R, et al. Gastrointestinal manifestations of SARS-CoV-2 infection and virus load in fecal samples from the Hong Kong cohort and systematic review and meta-analysis. Gastroenterology. 2020;S0016-5085(20):30448-0.

9. Tian Y, Rong L, Nian W, He Y. Review article: gastrointestinal features in COVID-19 and the possibility of faecal transmission. Aliment Pharmacol Ther. 2020;51(9):843-51.
10. Guan W, Ni Z, Hu Y, Liang W, Ou C, He J,et al. Clinical Characteristics of Coronavirus Disease 2019 in China. N Engl J Med. 2020;382:1708-20.
11. Huang C, Wang Y, Li X, Ren L, Zhao J, Hu Y, et al. Clinical features of patients infected with 2019 novel coronavirus in Wuhan, China. Lancet. 2020;395:497-506.
12. Zhang C, Shi L, Wang FS. Liver injury in COVID-19: management and challenges. Lancet Gastroenterol Hepatol. 2020;5(5):428-30.
13. Wang F, Wang H, Fan J, Zhang Y, Wang H, Zhao Q. Pancreatic injury patterns in patients with COVID-19 pneumonia. Gastroenterology. 2020;S0016-5085(20): 30409-1.
14. Zhang J, Wang S, Xue Y. Fecal specimen diagnosis 2019 novel coronavirus-infected pneumonia. J Med Virol. 2020.
15. British Society of Gastroenterology. BSG expanded consensus advice for the management of IBD during the COVID-19 pandemic. [online] Available from https://www.bsg.org.uk/covid-19-advice/bsg-advice-for-management-of-inflammatory-bowel-diseases-during-the-covid-19-pandemic/ [Last Accessed June, 2020].
16. Mao R, Liang J, Shen J, Ghosh S, Zhu L, Yang H, et al. Implications of COVID-19 for patients with pre-existing digestive diseases. Lancet Gastroenterol Hepatol. 2020;5(5):425-7.
17. Liang W, Guan W, Chen R, Wang W, Li J, Xu K, et al. Cancer patients in SARS-CoV-2 infection: a nationwide analysis in China. Lancet Oncol. 2020
18. Del Vecchio Blanco G, Calabrese E, Biancone L, Monteleone G, Paoluzi OA. The impact of COVID-19 pandemic in the colorectal cancer prevention. Int J Colorectal Dis. 2020;1-4.
19. Mayor S. COVID-19: impact on cancer workforce and delivery of care. Lancet Oncol. 2020;S1470-2045(20):30240-0.

Index

Page numbers followed by *b* refer to box, *f* refer to figure, *fc* refer to flowchart, and *t* refer to table.

A

Acetaminophen 240
Acquired hepatocerebral degeneration 248
Acute closed-angle glaucoma 169
Acute hepatitis C 226
    infection 226
    treatment of 229
Acute respiratory distress syndrome 10, 261
Acute severe colitis 20
    management of 20
Adalimumab 1, 9, 41
Adaptive arms 70
Adenoma 177
    carcinoma sequence 167
    colonic 163*f*
    detection 171, 173, 174
    hepatocellular 247
Adhesion molecules 67
Adrenocorticosteroids 60
Akkermansia muciniphila 90
Alanine
    aminotransferase 198
    transaminase 227
Alcohol 238
    consumption, substantial 250
Allergic reactions 65
Alzheimer's disease 251
American College of Gastroenterology 132
American Gastroenterology Association 39
American Society of Gastrointestinal Endoscopy 37
Amiselimod 14
Ammonia 250
Amnesia, mild 245
Amoxicillin 108, 112, 113, 119, 120*t*, 121, 122*t*, 123-125, 127, 128

Amphetamines 240
Anabolic steroids 240
Anaerobic luminal bacteria 89
Anal canal 25
Anastomosis 24
Ancylostoma caninum 57
Anemia 4
Angiotensin receptor blockers 31
Angiotensin-converting enzyme inhibitors 31
Anorexia 229, 244
Anti-adhesion agents 7
Antibiotics 20
    side effects 134
Anti-cytotoxic T-lymphocyte-associated protein 4 32
Antidepressants 240
Anti-infliximab antibody 6
Anti-interleukin inhibitors 9
Antimitochondrial antibodies 34
Antineutrophil cytoplasmic antibodies 245
Antinuclear antibodies 34
Anti-programmed cell death
    ligand 1 32
    protein 1 32
Antiretroviral medications 235
Antithyroid antibodie 34
Anti-TNFα therapy 41
Antiviral therapy 233
Apoptotic cells 73*f*
Arthralgia 244
Artificial intelligence 151, 152, 153*f*, 158, 159, 177
    application of 155
    studies of 160*t*
    terminology 152
    use of 177
Artificial neural networks 152, 153, 154*f*
Ascaris 57

Ascitic tap 52
Aspartate aminotransferase 200, 229
Aspirin 32, 207
Asthma 50
Astrocyte swelling 240
Autoimmune diseases 31
Autoimmune disorders 31, 245
Autoimmune liver disease 239, 252
  types of 252
Autonomic neuronal dysfunction 244
Azathioprine 1, 5, 5f, 6, 41, 61
  metabolism 5f

B

B lymphocytes 225
Bacterial biofilm 97
Bacterial infectious diseases 107
Bacteroides
  fragilis 90
  thetaiotaomicron 90
  vulgatus 90
Bariatric surgery 199
Barrett's esophagus 159
Barrett's mucosa 159
Basidiobolomycosis 57
Bat-borne virus 261
Beclomethasone dipropionate 39
Beta-blockers 31, 32
Bifidobacterium
  animalis 40
  breve 90
  longum 90
  strains 126
Bile acid 86
  absorption, abnormal 30
  malabsorption 39, 40
Bile duct cannulation 188
Biological therapy, effect of 22
Biopsy 57t, 121, 126
  colonic 21, 42
  mucosal 52
Bismuth
  based regimen 123
  levofloxacin-amoxicillin treatment 124
  quadruple therapy 115
  salicylate 39
Bleeding 21
  severe colonic 21

Blood
  eosinophilia 74
  investigations 34
    and stool sampling 34
  vessels, superficial 173
Blue laser imaging 173
Body mass index 198
Bone marrow 65
Bowel cancer 265, 266
Brain 58
  ammonia 253
  cells 240
  edema 240
  herniation 240
Budesonide 39, 40, 61
Buscopan 169
  use of 178

C

Calcinosis 31
Campylobacter 33
  jejuni 242
Canagliflozin 203
Cancer 10, 199
  cells 76
Capillaria 57
Carbohydrates 59, 197
Carcinogenesis 96
Carcinoma
  colonic 21
  mucinous 96
Cecal intubation rate 167
Celiac disease, screening for 39
Cells
  preservation of 95
  sensitive, structure of 154
  types of 13
Cenicriviroc 205-207
Central nervous system 8, 239, 242
Cerebral edema 240
Cerebrospinal fluid 242
Chemokines 67
Chemotherapeutic drugs 248
Cholangiocarcinoma 247
Cholangiography, percutaneous transhepatic 185
Cholangiopancreatography, endoscopic retrograde 184
Cholangitis, primary sclerosing 21

Cholestatic liver
   diseases 248
   function 184
Cholesterol 198, 205
Cholestyramine 39, 40
Chromoendoscopy 171, 178
   conventional 171
   dye-based 171
   virtual 171
Chronic hepatitis
   C 223, 227, 228
      infection 227
      treatment of 230
   prevention of 196
Churg-Strauss syndrome 58
Cirrhosis 201, 229, 232
   compensated 232
   primary biliary 252
Clarithromycin 108, 109, 112-114, 120t, 121, 123, 125, 127
   resistance 109, 125
Closed-angle glaucoma 169
Clostridium difficile 30, 33
Coagulation, abnormal 184
Cocaine 240
Coeliac disease 30
Colectomy 21, 23
   risk of 20
   subtotal 23
Colitis
   collagenous 29, 32, 36
   eosinophilic 49, 54f
Colon 24, 87f
   cancer 10
   removal of 24
Colonic mucosal patterns, visualization of 171
Colonocytes 88
   exfoliated 91
Colonoscopes, standard 176
Colonoscopy 167, 172
   cap-assisted 174, 174f
   high-definition 170
   risks of 35
   technology 170
   water-assisted 170
   wide-angle 176
Colorectal cancer 71, 74, 77f, 86, 95, 167
   risk of 21

Colorectal carcinoma
   cell 75
   prevention of 167
Colorectal mucus 73f, 92, 95f, 97f
Colorectal neoplasia 161
Comorbid disease, exacerbation of 186
Concomitant therapy 113
Confocal laser endomicroscopy 36
Consciousness 244
Conventional therapy 248
Convolutional neural networks 152, 153
Coriobacteriaceae 30
Coronavirus 261
   disease 261
   strain of 261
Corticosteroids 60
Cotton's consensus 185
COVID-19 on
   delivery of gastrointestinal services, effect of 265
   gastroenterology, impact of 261
   gastrointestinal endoscopy, effect of 264
   patients with pre-existing gastrointestinal diseases, effect of 265
Crohn's disease 11, 30, 71, 92
Cryoglobulinemia 245
Cryoglobulins 245
Cryptitis 37
Cytokines 10, 12, 67, 72, 253
   proinflammatory 61
   receptors 11
Cytomegalovirus 241
Cytotoxic cationic proteins 65
Cytotoxic T-cells 74

D

Damage-associated molecular patterns 75, 77
Dapagliflozin 204
Deep learning 154f, 155f
Deep mucosal biopsies 52
Degranulation 77
Delirium 240
Dendritic cells 74
Desulfovibrio desulfuricans 90
Detoxification 238
Device-assisted colonoscopy 174

Diabetes mellitus
   treatment of 200
   type 1 31
   type 2 197, 202, 251
Diarrhea 57, 58, 244, 263
   bloody 1
   chronic nonbloody watery 33
   functional 33
   treatment of 30
   watery nonbloody 29
Digestive symptoms 264
Diminutive adenomas, diagnosis of 178
Dipeptidyl peptidase-4 inhibitors 202
Diplopia 246
Direct-acting antivirals 228
   development of 196
   different classes of 230*fc*
Disease flare, indicator of 3
Double-wire technique 189
Duodenal involvement 54*f*
Dysbiosis 92
Dysmotility 50
Dyspepsia 131
   functional 131
Dysphagia 49, 50
Dysplasia 21, 22
   high-grade 21, 22
   low-grade 21, 22
Dysreflexia, autonomic 240
Dysregulations, transcriptomic 93

E

Early gastric cancer 131
   detection of 159
Eczema 50
Elafibranor 205
Elbasvir 234
Electrolyte solutions 190
Electronic chromoendoscop 35
Elemental diet 59
Encephalomyelitis 244
Encephalopathic syndromes 245
Encephalopathy
   acute hepatic 240
   chronic hepatic 241
   hepatic 227, 238, 239, 241
   multi-infarct 245
   portal-systemic 239, 241
Endocuff 175, 175*f*
Endorings 175

Endoscopic bile duct balloon dilatation 189
Endoscopic mucosal resolution 15
Endoscopic ultrasound 188
Endoscopy 52, 109
   lower gastrointestinal 161
   stack 164
   white-light 172
English Bowel Cancer Screening Programme 169
Enteritis 49
Enterocytes 88
Enteroendocrine cells 88
Enzyme 88
   activity 5
   immunoassay 226
Eosin stain staining 55
Eosinophilic gastroenteritis 49, 59
   classification 49
   clinical
      assessment 50
      course 58
      features 50
   diagnosis 55
   differential diagnosis 55
   epidemiology 50
   natural history 58
   pathogenesis 50
   small bowel involvement of 55*f*
Eosinophilic gastrointestinal diseases 59, 62
   researcher 58
Eosinophilic gastrointestinal disorders 49, 50
Eosinophilopoiesis 66*f*
Eosinophils 55, 60, 65-67, 70-72, 73*f*, 74, 94, 97
   constitute 65, 70
   cut-off levels of 57*t*
   functions of 68
   human 65
   maturation 65
   migration of 67
   secretory functions of 67
Epithelial barriers 65
Epithelial cell 68
   colonic 88
Epithelial surface 91
Epithelium 72
   intestinal 91

Epstein-Barr virus 241
Erythema 35
Erythrocytes 73*f*
Escherichia coli 40, 97
Esomeprazole 32, 121
Esophageal cancer, diagnosis of 159
Esophageal disease 49
Esophageal dysmotility 31
Esophageal tissue 263
Esophagitis, eosinophilic 49
Esophagogastroduodenoscopy 36
Esophagus 49
Estimated glomerular filtration rate 234
Etrasimod 14
 efficacy of 14
Etrolizumab 9
European Association for Study of Liver 207
European Helicobacter and Microbiota Study Group 109
European Microscopic Colitis Group 40
Exogenous hormone therapy 30
Extracellular DNA trap formation 77, 97
Eyes 51

F

Fatigue 229
 central 252
 peripheral 252
Fatty acids 250
Fatty liver disease, nonalcoholic 196, 206, 207, 215, 216, 238, 239, 250, 251, 265
Fecal immunochemical test 176
Fecal transplant 42
Fetal scalp monitors 233
Fever 4
 low-grade 229
Fibrosis 229, 238
 advanced 215*f*
 regression 198
Flexible spectral imaging color enhancement 173
Fluoroquinolones 127
 quadruple therapy 123
Focal liver lesion detection 157
Focal nodular hyperplasia 247
Food allergies 50
Fuji intelligent chromoendoscopy 35
Fujifilm endoscopes 173
Full-spectrum endoscopy 177
Fusobacterium nucleatum 97

G

Galactosamine 240
Gamma
 activated sequence 11
 activation factor 11
 glutamyl transferase 203
Gastric
 antral mass 58
 cancer
  endoscopic detection of 160*t*
  infiltrative 57
 epithelium 123
 hydrochloric acid 86
 malignancy 164
  diagnosis of 159
 obstruction 51
Gastritis, eosinophilic 49, 53*f*
Gastroenterology 151
Gastrointestinal
 bleeding 58, 238
 conditions, group of 49
 diseases 33
 endoscopy 159
 mucus structure 87*f*
 physicians 151
 physiology 98
 radiology 155
 symptoms 263
 tract 86
Generic biosimilars 2
G-eye colonoscopy 177
Glucagon-like peptide-1 200, 207
 receptor agonists 202
Goblet cell 88, 89, 97
 adjacent 89
 depletion 96
 development 69
 mucus-producing 97
Granulocyte
 leukocytes 65
 macrophage colony-stimulating factor 66
Grasp reflexes 249
Grazoprevir 234
Guanidine monophosphate synthetase 5
Guanosine monophosphate synthetase 5

Guillain-Barré syndrome 242
Gut bacteria 88
Gut immune system, maintenance of 70
Gut inflammation, mediators of 1
Gut microbiota 94
Gut mucus 86, 89-90, 98

H

H2 receptor antagonist 32
Hallucinogens 240
Healthy liver 238
Heart 58
    disease 199
    failure, worsening 204
Helicobacter pylori 106, 108, 111, 116, 134
    antibiotic resistance 127
    clarithromycin resistance 127
    cure rate 107
    eradication 108, 124, 126, 128-131, 132*t*, 133
        failure 123, 127
        regimens 115, 117, 129
        therapy 108, 126, 131, 134
        treatment 116, 126
    gastritis 107
    growth of 124
    infection 106-110, 112, 113, 119, 120*t*, 122-125, 127, 133, 134
        after treatment 133
        cure of 130
        eradication of 122*t*
        risks of 129
        treatment of 106*b*, 106*t*, 107, 123, 125, 133
    isolates 113
    regimens 110
    related disease 131
    resistance of 123
    strains 114
    therapy 107, 129, 130
    treatment 110, 111, 129, 131, 132
        failure 134
        testing after 132
Hemangioma, hepatic 247
Hemianopsia 244
Hemiparesis 244
Hemodialysis 226

Hemorrhage 10
Hepatic coma 240
Hepatic failure, fulminant 240
Hepatic fat accumulation 197
Hepatic tissue 238
Hepatitis 238, 240, 241
    A 239, 241, 242
        virus 241
    autoimmune 252, 265
    B 239, 243
        chronic 244
        complications of 243
        surface antigen 243
        virus 243
    C 227, 234, 239, 244
        diagnosis 227
        during pregnancy, treatment of 232
        epidemiology 223
        management of 223
        pathogenesis 224
        therapeutics 231
        treatment 229, 233, 234
        viremia 227
        virus infection 196, 223, 224*f*, 225, 225*f*, 226*fc*, 227, 229, 230, 234, 244, 246
    virus infection 223
Hepatobiliary-pancreatic disorders 184
Hepatocellular carcinoma 196, 226
    development of 204
Hepatopathy, congestive 238
Hepatorenal syndrome 227
Heroin 240
Herpes simplex virus 241
Homeostasis, immunological 238
Hormonal balance 238
Host cell exfoliation 91
Human immunodeficiency virus 234, 244
Human intestinal tract 65
Human leukocyte antigen 30
Hybrid therapy 115
Hydration, intravenous 190
Hypereosinophilic syndrome 57
Hyperplastic polyps 167, 177
    types of 167
Hypertension 198

Index

I

Idiopathic noncirrhotic portal 247
Ileal pouch 24
    anal anastomosis 22, 24
    formation 24
    procedures 23
Ileostomy 23, 24
    defunctioning 23, 24
    permanent 22, 25
Immune
    cells 97
        transepithelial migration of 74
    checkpoint inhibitor 31, 32, 36
    complexes 243
    system, activation of 29
Immunomodulators 41
Infertility, risk of 24
Inflammatory bowel disease 6, 19, 31, 57, 71, 86, 92, 266
    prevalence of 1
    surgery for 23
Inflammatory bowel disorder 29
Inflammatory cells 37, 247
    abundance of 95f
Inflammatory conditions, treatment of 12
Infliximab 1, 15, 41
    monotherapy 6
    plus azathioprine 6
    serum 6
Innate arms 70
Inner mucus layer 87, 94
Insulin 198
    glucose-dependent 200
Interferon 11
    regulatory factor 11
    sensitivity determining region 225
    stimulated response element 11
Intestinal microbiome, role of 206
Intestinal mucosal barrier, functionality of 68
Intestinal protective barrier, component of 88
Intestine, small 87f
Intracellular accumulation 240
Intracellular tight junctions 88
Ipragliflozin 203
    group 204
Irritable bowel syndrome 2

J

Jak-stat pathway 11f
Jaundice 184, 242
John Cunningham virus 8

K

Kidney 58
    disease 234

L

Lactobacillus
    acidophilus 40
    johnsonii 90
    plantarum 90
    reuteri 90
    rhamnosus 90
    strains 126
Lamina propria 30, 37, 67-70, 75, 89
    cellularity 35
    intestinal 88
Langerhans cell histiocytosis 58
Lansoprazole 32, 121
Laparoscopy 52
Leaving scar tissue 238
Leukoencephalitis 244
Leukoencephalopathy, progressive multifocal 8
Levofloxacin 122t, 123
    bismuth quadruple 124
    resistant strains 123
    therapy 122
Linitis plastica 52, 57
Lipolytic digestive enzymes 86
Lipoprotein, low-density 205
Liraglutide 200, 207
Liver
    biopsy 198, 203
    cancer, primary 223
    cirrhosis, alcoholic 239, 265
    conditions, chronic 266
    disease 202, 228, 238, 239, 239t, 249, 253
        end-stage 201, 238
        neurological complications in 238
        stage of 238
    enzyme tests 264
    failure 238
        acute 239
        chronic 239, 253

fibrosis 228
   stages 205
  function 264
   abnormal 248
  lesions 156
   diffuse 158
  toxins 240
  transplantation 238
Low-birth weight infants 232
Lungs 58
Lymph glands 51
Lymph nodes 13
Lymphocytes 8, 30
  intraepithelial 37
Lymphocytic colitis 29, 32, 36
Lymphoid cells 68
  innate 70
Lymphoid organs 13
Lymphoid tissue
  gut-associated 69
  mucosa-associated 131
Lymphoma 131

M

Maastricht consensus report 132
Machine learning 152, 153, 154f, 155f
Macrophages 73f, 74, 94, 97
Major colorectal diseases 65, 70
Malaise 245
Malignant cells, exfoliated 97
Malignant diseases, treatment of 157
Malignant lesions, chemotherapy of 157
Mature eosinophils
  functional characteristics of 65
  migration of 66f
  structural characteristics of 65
Mayo score 2
Medical management, failure of 21
Menopausal hormone therapy 30
Mepolizumab 62
Mercaptans 250
Mercaptopurine 1, 5
Mesalamine 39, 40
Metabolic syndrome 196, 200
Metalloproteinase 30, 88
Metastatic disease 247
Metformin 200, 207
Methotrexate 41
Methylmercaptopurine 5

Methylthioinosine monophosphate 5
Metronidazole 110, 111, 114, 116, 123, 125-128
Microbiome 90
  manipulation 206
Microscopic colitis 29, 30, 33, 34t, 36t, 42
  antibiotics 40
  clinical features 33
  development of 32t
  diagnosis 34
  disease activity index 38, 38t
  environmental factors 31
  epidemiology 29
  lifestyle modification 38
  management 38
  medications 39
  pathophysiology 29
  prescribed medications 31
  probiotics 40
  risk factors 33
  surgery 42
Migration 91
Modern health delivery system 158
Mononeuropathy multiplex 243
Motor axonal neuropathy, acute 242
Mucosa 52, 95, 171, 173
  colonic 29
Mucosal Addressin-cell adhesion
    molecule 8
Multidisciplinary team 19
  part of 19, 158
Multidrug-resistant transporter genes 118
Multifactorial disease 74
Multi-light technology 173
Multiorgan failure 238
Myelopathy, hepatic 239, 249, 250
Myoclonus 248, 249
Myopathies
  inflammatory 246
  noninflammatory 246

N

N-acetyl-aspartate 246
N-acetyl-aspartyl-glutamate
    concentrations 246
Narrow-band imaging 160-162, 163f, 172
Natalizumab 8
Nausea 229, 244

Neoplasm 238, 239, 247, 253
Neoplastic lesions 159
Neurotoxicity, risk of 40
Neutrophils 67, 73f, 94, 95f, 97
    derived etosis 97
    extracellular traps 76
Nitroglycerine, transdermal 190
Nitroimidazole 112, 113, 123
Nonbismuth quadruple sequential and concomitant regimens 123
Non-nucleoside inhibitor 230
Nonsteroidal anti-inflammatory drugs 31, 32, 34, 190
Non-Wilsonian acquired hepatocerebral degeneration 239, 248
Nucleoside inhibitor 230
Nucleotide inhibitor 230
Nystagmus 249

O

Obesity, complications of 216
Obeticholic acid 205, 207
Oddi dysfunction, sphincter of 184
Oddi pressure 190
Olympus medical systems 176
Omalizumab 62
Omeprazole 32, 118, 121, 125
Optimized 5-ASA therapies 4
Optimized immunosuppressive therapies 4
Optimizing anti-TNF treatments 5
Optimizing conventional therapies 2
Oral contraceptive pill 30
Organ failure 186
Orlistat 200
Ozanimod 14

P

Pain, abdominal 57, 58, 229, 244
Painful red eye 169
Pancreatic duct 188
    stenting 189
Pancreatic inflammation 186
Pancreatitis Across Nations Clinical Research and Education Alliance 186
Pancreatogram, endoscopic 184
Paneth cells 88

Panproctocolectomy 23
Pantoprazole 32, 121
Parasitic infestations 51, 57
Parvimonas micra 97
Pediatric obesity 215
Pelvic
    dissection 24
    sepsis 25
Penicillin allergy 125
Pentoxifylline 41
Peptic ulcer 130
Peptostreptococcus stomatis 97
Peroxisome proliferator-activated receptor 201, 207
Pioglitazone 201
Polyarteritis nodosa 58, 243
Polymerase chain reaction 228
Polyneuropathy, chronic relapsing 243
Polypeptide, glucose-dependent insulinotropic 202
Polyps
    adenomatous 167
    colonic 162t
    detection of 161, 167, 174
Portal hypertension, presence of 228
Positive predictive value 159, 160
Positron emission tomography 158
Post-endoscopic retrograde cholangiopancreatography pancreatitis 184, 185
Pouch
    function 24
    procedure 23
    vaginal fistula 24
Precut sphincterotomies 189
Proctectomy, completion 23, 25
Proctocolectomy 23, 25
Prophylactic pancreatic stent 189
Prostate cancer 10
Protein
    nonstructural 225, 230
    tyrosine kinase family 11
Proteolytic granzyme 76
Proton-pump inhibitor 31, 32, 107, 120t, 230
    combination of 122t
    dose of 117
Proximal colon retroflexion 169
Pruritus 242
Pseudotumor, inflammatory 247

Psychomotor, dysfunctional 244
Ptosis, severe 246
Pylorus, thickened 53f
Pyramidal tract signs 248

Q

Quadruple regimen 125
Quinolone 117, 127

R

Rabeprazole 121
Rapid cell death 67
Rapid mucus renewal 88
Raynaud's phenomenon 31
Rectal cancer 10
Rectal malignancy, risk of 23
Rectal stump
    dehiscence, risk of 23
    management of 23
Rectal tumors, low 24
Rectum 24, 25
    removal of 24
Red blood cells 37
Reflux 50
Renal papillary cancer 10
Reslizumab 62
Retroflexion 169
Rheumatoid
    arthritis 31
    factor 34
Rhinitis 50
Ribonucleic acid 223, 226, 244
Rifabutin 119
    therapy 119, 124
Rosiglitazone 201
Ruminococcus
    gnavus 90
    torques 90

S

Saccharomyces boulardii 126
Sanger sequencing 228
SARS-CoV-2
    on gastrointestinal tract, effect of 263
    structure of 261
    to host cell, attachment of 262f
Saturated fats 198
Scar tissue 238
Sclerodactyly 31
Seizures 240
Selective serotonin reuptake inhibitors 31, 32, 34
Selonsertib 205, 207
Sensory axonal neuropathy 242
Sentinel cells 89
Serotonin-norepinephrine reuptake inhibitors 34
Sertraline 32
Serum fasting glucose 203
Sessile serrated polyps 167
Sigmoid eosinophilic colitis,
    colonoscopic appearance of 54f
Sjogren's syndrome 31
Skin 51
    cancers, nonmelanoma 10
Small bowel obstruction 24
Sodium
    cromoglycate 61
    glucose cotransporter 203
Somatostatin 190
Spectrum bias 152
Sphincteroplasty 189
    pancreatic 189
Sphincters 24
Sphingosine 1-phosphate 12, 13
    receptor modulators 12, 13f
Sphingosine kinase 13
Sphingosine lyase 13
Standard six-food elimination diet 59
Standard triple therapy, efficacy of 120t
Statins 31, 204, 207
Steatohepatitis 251
    nonalcoholic 196, 207, 251
Steroids 20, 25, 39, 42
    dependency 21
    long-term 21
Stiff nonpliable mucosa 35
Stoma
    management of 19
    permanent 24
Stomach 87f, 159
    marked antral thickening of 53f
Stone diseases, surgery for 184
Stool urgency 33
Strongyloides 51, 57